Essentials of
Writing
Biomedical
Research Papers

Essentials of Writing Biomedical Research Papers

Mimi Zeiger, M.A.

LECTURER IN SCIENTIFIC WRITING
CARDIOVASCULAR RESEARCH INSTITUTE
UNIVERSITY OF CALIFORNIA, SAN FRANCISCO

McGRAW-HILL, INC.
Health Professions Division
New York   St. Louis   San Francisco   Colorado Springs   Auckland
Bogotá   Caracas   Hamburg   Lisbon   London   Madrid   Mexico
Milan   Montreal   New Delhi   Paris   San Juan   São Paulo
Singapore   Sydney   Tokyo   Toronto

ESSENTIALS OF WRITING BIOMEDICAL RESEARCH PAPERS

1 2 3 4 5 6 7 8 9 0 MAL MAL 9 8 7 6 5 4 3 2 1 0

This book was set in Century Schoolbook by Harper Graphics. The editors were William Day and Lester A. Sheinis. The production supervisor was Annette Mayeski. The cover was designed by José Fonfrias. The text was designed by Rita Naughton. Project supervision was by Spectrum Publisher Services, Inc.
Malloy Lithographers, Inc., was printer and binder.

ISBN 0-07-072833-X

Library of Congress Cataloging-in-Publication Data

Zeiger, Mimi.
    Essentials of writing biomedical research papers / Mimi Zeiger.
        p.   cm.
    Includes bibliographical references.
    Includes index.
    ISBN 0-07-072833-X
    1. Medical writing—handbooks, manuals, etc.   2. Technical
writing—Handbooks, manuals, etc.   I. Title.
    [DNLM: 1. Writing. WZ 345 Z46e]
    R119.Z45   1991
    808'.06661—dc20
    DLC
    for Library of Congress   90-13222
                                                                             CIP

Contents

Section II THE TEXT OF THE BIOMEDICAL RESEARCH PAPER 91

Chapter 4 THE INTRODUCTION 93

Chapter 5 MATERIALS AND METHODS 113

Chapter 6 RESULTS 141

CONTENTS **vii**

Chapter 7 **DISCUSSION** **165**

Functions   165
Content   165
Organization   171
Length   188
Details   188
Summary of Guidelines for Discussions   **191**
Example of a Clearly Organized Discussion   193
Exercise 7.1   Overall Story in a Complex Discussion   198
Exercise 7.2   Content and Organization in a Discussion   202

Section III **SUPPORTING INFORMATION**   **207**

Chapter 8 **FIGURES AND TABLES**   **209**

Figures   209
Tables   224
Telling a Story   237
Summary of Guidelines for Figures and Tables   **240**
Exercise 8.1   Design of Figures and Tables and Their Relation to the Text   245
Exercise 8.2   Table Design and Relation to the Text   246

Chapter 9 **REFERENCES**   **247**

Purposes   247
Selecting References   247
Accuracy   248
Incorporating References Into the Text   249
Systems for Citing References   251
Summary of Guidelines for References   **253**
Exercise 9.1   Accuracy of References   254

Section IV **THE OVERVIEW**   **255**

Chapter 10 **THE ABSTRACT**   **257**

Function   257
Abstracts of Results Papers   257
Abstracts of Methods Papers   271
Indexing Terms   273
Abstracts for Meetings   274
Summary of Guidelines for Abstracts   **278**
Exercise 10.1   The Content of Abstracts   281
Exercise 10.2   Length of Abstracts   283

Chapter 11 **THE TITLE**   **284**

Functions   284
Content of Titles for Results Papers   284
Content of Titles for Methods Papers   287

Preface

Essentials of Writing Biomedical Research Papers grew out of a course in scientific writing given to postdoctoral fellows in cardiovascular research. The course was started by Julius H. Comroe, Jr., M.D., the founder and first director of the Cardiovascular Research Institute at the University of California, San Francisco. Since 1978, when I began teaching this course, I have been assessing writing problems in drafts of research papers and discovering which principles of writing authors need to consider to make their writing clear. In addition, I have been adapting drafts of papers by young authors into examples and exercises that illustrate these writing principles. The result of these efforts is this book.

A special feature of this book is its emphasis on structure and storytelling. The book explains how to construct both individual paragraphs and each section of a research paper so that each paragraph, each section, and finally the paper as a whole tell a clear story.

Other special features of this book are numerous specific principles of clear biomedical writing (summarized as checklists at the end of each chapter), numerous examples of unclear writing followed by clearer revisions, and numerous exercises coupled with one or more revisions. The examples and exercises are taken mainly from drafts and also from some published biomedical research papers. The revisions are models that students can imitate in their own papers.

Several instructors have used this book successfully in courses on biomedical writing given to graduate students, postdoctoral fellows, and junior faculty all over the world. Because the students have limited time available, the course is usually brief and intensive, running about 24 hours for 4, 6, or 12 weeks or about 35 hours for one week.

In preparing this book over the past several years, I have received help from many people. First, I am indebted to Dr. Comroe. The syllabus for his writing course gave me a solid jumping-off point, and his dedicated teaching was inspirational. Second, I am indebted to the numerous postdoctoral fellows who worked on their papers with me to the point of near-perfection necessary for use as teaching examples. Without their willingness to pursue perfection and their generosity in allowing me to publish their original and revised drafts as examples and exercises, this book would not have been possible. Similarly, I am indebted to the authors of published papers, and to their publishers, who have graciously allowed me to use parts of their papers as examples and exercises. These papers provided some of the most useful and stimulating examples and exercises in this book. In addition, I am grateful to the many participants in the writing classes whose insightful revisions have enriched this book. I am also grateful to the many scientists who prevented me from making gruesome errors in science. No doubt some errors remain, but I hope readers will be able to see past scientific problems to understand the writing principles being illustrated. Finally, I especially want to thank seven people: Bobbi Angell, an illustrator affiliated with the New York Botanical Garden, who made the hand-drawn figures in this book, and Paul Sagan, an editor in the Cardiovascular Research Institute, University of California, San Francisco, who prepared the computer-drawn figures, for their fine work and cheerful spirit throughout many revisions; David F. Teitel, M.D., Associate Professor of Pediatrics, University of California, San Francisco, Harold Schultz, Ph.D., Associate Professor of Physiology, University of Nebraska Medical Center, Omaha, and Thomas Pisarri, Ph.D., Assistant Research Physiologist, Cardiovascular Research Institute, University of California, San Francisco, who kindly and efficiently helped me write and rewrite revisions for a few challenging exercises; and Stanton A. Glantz, Ph.D., Professor of Medicine, University of California, San Francisco, and Bryan K. Slinker, D.V.M., Ph.D., Assistant Professor of Medicine and of Physiology and Biophysics, University of Vermont, who tirelessly and graciously advised me on scientific and statistical questions throughout the development of this book. They are the special sort of consultant that every English instructor working in science needs—knowledgeable, sensible, and generous.

THE GOAL: CLEAR WRITING

THE PURPOSE OF THIS BOOK

Most readers agree that much of the biomedical literature is badly written (Woodford, 1967). The problem with most biomedical research papers is that they lose the forest for the trees. The extreme example is a paper that gives overwhelming details about what others have found ("review of the literature"); exhaustive lists of variables measured (generally written as an alphabet soup of abbreviations); a blizzard of data in the form of means, standard errors, and P values; and a meandering "discussion" of the data. No story is told; no message emerges. But science is not data. Data are the raw material of science. It is what you do with data that is science—the interpretation you make, the story you tell.

The purpose of this book is to show you how to marshal the details of a biomedical research paper into a comprehensible story that has a clear message. To achieve this purpose, the book presents numerous specific principles of clear writing and illustrates each principle with examples of murky writing followed by revisions showing how the ideas can be written more clearly. The numerous specific principles and the examples followed by revisions are two special features of this book. Another special feature is the exercises in each chapter, coupled with one or more revisions at the end of the book. The exercises provide opportunities both to recognize appropriate and inappropriate application of the writing principles (reading exercises) and to put the principles into practice (writing exercises). The revisions of examples and of the writing exercises can be used as models for your own writing.

The reason for doing exercises is that application of the principles of writing requires judgment. There are few if any "rights" and "wrongs" in writing. Rather there are better and worse choices. The point, then, is to develop your judgment so that you can make better choices. To help develop your judgment in making these choices, you can compare your critiques of the reading exercises and your revised versions of the writing exercises with those given in the revisions at the end of this book. These revisions have been synthesized from a number of drafts and comments by students over several years. Bear in mind, however, that there is no such thing as a perfect paper. In fact, you may disagree with some choices made in the revisions. That is OK. The process of revision is endless. The revisions of the exercises in this book are therefore intended only as improvements, not as ultimate perfection.

Most examples and exercises in this book are taken from pre-publication drafts written by junior researchers who were in post-doctoral training positions in cardiovascular research. These examples are not intended to show the ultimate level of excellent writing but rather a reasonable level of clarity achievable by young researchers early in their careers. People interested in writing may want to try to make their writing lively as well as clear. In fact, that is the ultimate goal. But the goal of this book is only clarity.

REASONS FOR WRITING CLEARLY

Many if not most scientists love to work in the laboratory but hate to write papers. But writing is at least as important as doing experiments, and writing clearly is important not only to your readers but also to yourself.

Write Clearly to Ensure That Your Readers Understand Your Message

Think of yourself as a reader for a moment. What kind of papers do you like to read? Short, meaty, and clear most likely. Well, then, write short, meaty, clear papers yourself. Short, meaty, clear papers are the most likely to be understood. The truth of this proposition will come home to you as you read examples of biomedical writing in this book and discover how easy it is to get the wrong message. If you can make mistakes, so can your readers.

Who are these readers? Certainly they include scientists who do research in your field. But this is just the core of the audience. The complete spectrum of potential readers ranges from graduate students to Nobel laureates and includes many readers whose native language is not English. Furthermore, many of your readers may not be in your field. Eventually all scientists begin to read outside their fields: you can dig your trench only so deep; sooner or later you start finding links with other specialties. These links often lead to exciting scientific discoveries. So it is important that scientists from outside your field can read your paper. Finally, and perhaps most importantly, most readers are only half awake when they are reading your paper, perhaps late at night or on a bus or plane somewhere. Because of this wide range of backgrounds of potential readers and because of their semiconscious state while they are reading, the burden of clarity rests on you, the author. The reader's job is to follow the author's thinking and to agree or disagree; it is not to decode and reconstruct the paper. Thus, if you want your readers to get your message, you will have to make it abundantly clear to them.

The standard of clarity that we will use goes back to Quintilian, a Roman rhetorician who lived in the first century A.D.: *clear writing is writing that is incapable of being misunderstood.* Note that this is a much tougher standard than saying that clear writing is writing that can be understood.

Write Clearly to Clarify Your Own Thinking

Holding to this tough standard of clear writing has a second benefit: it will help you clarify your own thinking (Woodford, 1967). Many people have the idea that they know what they want to say and all they need to do is write it down. But this is rarely the case. Rather, writing helps you discover what you mean. As you write, you often find that the direction of your thoughts changes, and you may end up with an answer to a slightly different question from the one you asked at the beginning of your research. This evolution of thought is a great advantage of writing. Another advantage is that faulty reasoning is exposed, because as you read what you have written, you will find lapses in logic and inconsistencies that will stimulate you to rethink what it is that you really mean.

Thus, there are two good reasons why it is desirable to write clearly: first, to be sure that you yourself know what you mean, and second, to be sure that you get your message across to your readers.

THE SCOPE OF THIS BOOK

This book deals with the type of publication that forms the major portion of a research scientist's bibliography—journal articles that report results of original research. It also includes some comments on methods papers (papers that report new or improved methods, apparatus, or materials). It does not deal with other types of papers, such as theoretical papers, case reports, and review articles. Although the examples come primarily from one area of biomedical research, many of the writing principles apply to papers in other areas of science as well.

THE APPROACH TAKEN IN THIS BOOK

The approach taken in this book is to explain and illustrate what a clearly written biomedical research paper is. The process of getting a paper written is touched on only lightly. The idea behind this approach is that if you know what you are aiming at, you will have a better chance of reaching it. Thus, this book does not deal with what you do first and what you do second but rather with what the end product should look like if it is to be clear.

Specifically, this book deals with the choice of words and the arrangement of words into larger and larger structures that tell a story. The emphasis on structure and storytelling is the fourth special feature of this book.

The first section of this book is devoted to the building blocks of writing (word choice, sentence structure, and paragraph structure). The second, third, and fourth sections examine the structure of individual parts of a biomedical research paper in turn: first the text (Introduction, Materials and Methods, Results, Discussion); then supporting information (figures, tables, and references); and finally the overview (abstract, title, and the big picture, which assesses the structure of the paper as a whole, to ensure that all the parts work together to tell a story and send a single, clear message).

This book is developmental. The later chapters build on writing principles presented in the earlier chapters. In particular, the chapters on the parts of the research paper (Chaps. 4–7) and the chapter on the big picture (Chap. 12) build on principles of paragraph structure. Thus, the book starts with the smallest unit of writing (words) and works up to the largest unit (the entire paper).

A lot of writing principles are included in this book. A summary of the principles for each topic is included at the end of each chapter, and an overview of the main principles is given below.

AN OVERVIEW OF THE MAIN PRINCIPLES OF WRITING PRESENTED IN THIS BOOK

Since the problem with most biomedical research papers is that they lose the forest for the trees, the solution is to build a structure into the paper so that the forest is clear. Each of the four parts of the text of a biomedical research paper has its own structure.

Introduction

The Introduction follows a standard structure: the funnel. A funnel starts broadly and then narrows. Thus, in a biomedical research paper, the Introduction funnels from something known, to something unknown, to the question the paper is asking. The Introduction may end with the question or may go on to state the experimental approach to answering the question. An example of an Introduction that has a funnel shape is given in Example 1 below.

Example 1   Introduction

A *Known*
B *Unknown*
C *Question*

D *Experimental approach*

AIt is known that several general anesthetics, including *barbiturates, depress* the bronchomotor response to *vagus* nerve stimulation (1, 7, 9). **B**However, the *site* of this *depression* has not been determined. **C**To determine which *site* in the *vagal* motor pathway to the bronchioles is most sensitive to *depression by barbiturates*, **D**we did experiments in isolated rings of ferret trachea in which we stimulated this pathway at four different sites before and after exposure to barbiturates.

An important detail to notice in this Introduction is that the key terms in the question (italicized) repeat words in the statements of what is known and unknown. Repeating key terms is important because the repetition makes it obvious that the question follows inevitably from what is known and unknown. It is important that the question follows inevitably and is stated clearly because the rest of the paper depends on the question. Specifically, Methods tells what you did to answer the question, Results tells what you found that answers the question, and the Discussion states and explains the answer to the question. To avoid losing the forest for the trees in a biomedical research paper, the trick is to use the question as the touchstone for selecting and organizing ideas in each section of the paper.

Materials and Methods

The structure of the Materials and Methods section is essentially chronological. You start by describing what you did first to answer your question and end by describing what you did last. In addition, because Materials and Methods is usually a long section, it is divided into subsections according to the type of information. For example, in a study that makes an intervention and then measures some variables, one possible structure is as follows:

Preparation
Protocol
Methods of Measurement
Analysis of Data

In the Methods section, the most important subsection for presenting the forest is often the protocol. The protocol gives the overview of what you did to answer the question and thus is the framework against which the details of methods make sense.

Three components need to be pulled together in the protocol:

- The independent variable (the variable you manipulated)
- The dependent variable (the variable you measured)
- All controls

An example of a protocol that has all three components is given in Example 2. (This example is from a different paper than Example 1.)

Example 2 Protocol

E Independent variable
F Dependent variable +
baseline
G Detail
H Sham control

ETo stimulate pulmonary C-fiber endings, in each of the 9 dogs we injected capsaicin (10–20 µg/kg) into the right atrium. **F**At 10-s intervals for 60 s before (baseline) and 60 s after each injection, we measured secretions from tracheal submucosal glands. **G**Injections were separated by resting periods of about 30 min. **H**As a control, in the same 9 dogs we measured secretion in response to injection of vehicle (0.5–1.0 ml) into the right atrium.

Results

In the Results section, the overall structure is either chronological, to correspond with the structure of Methods (for example, when two or more series of experiments were done), or in the order of most to least importance to the question (for example, when chronological order would make the important results difficult to find). (Similarly, some parts of the Methods section can be organized from most to least important; for example, for a long, complicated calculation, state the final calculation first and then go back and explain the earlier calculations.)

In addition, within each paragraph of the Results section, organize the ideas from most to least important. Thus, state an important result in the first sentence, and state less important results and supporting details in later sentences, as in Example 3.

Example 3 Results

I Important result

J, K Less important results

IIncubation of rings of fetal lamb ductus arteriosus in arachidonic acid increased production of prostaglandin E_2 to 3.5 times above baseline (Fig. 1). **J**This increase was blocked when the rings were incubated in arachidonic acid in the presence of indomethacin. **K**In the control series of experiments, prostaglandin E_2 production measured at the same 90-min intervals did not change.

In this paragraph, note that the control results (J, K), which are least important, are last. Also note that a "ballpark value" (3.5 times) is given instead of the exact data, which are presented in a figure. Finally, note that in the first sentence, the method appears as the subject of the sentence ("Incubation of rings of fetal lamb ductus arteriosus in arachidonic acid") and the result is in the verb and completer ("increased production of prostaglandin E_2 to 3.5 times above baseline"). Thus, the method is subordinated and the first sentence, the most prominent sentence in the paragraph, states the result, which is the most important statement in the paragraph.

Discussion

For the Discussion section there is no prescribed structure. However, there are some general guidelines. The first and most important guideline is to state the answer to the question at the beginning of the Discussion. The reason for stating the answer at the beginning is that the answer is the most important statement in the paper, so it should appear in the most prominent position: first. Immediately after stating the answer, give supporting evidence. An example of the first paragraph of a Discussion in which the first sentence states the answer to the question and the rest of the paragraph gives supporting evidence is given in Example 4.

Example 4 Beginning of a Discussion

L Answer

M, N Support for improvement

1 *L*In this study, we have shown that <u>a 42-day course of dexamethasone leads to sustained improvement in pulmonary function and improves neurodevelopmental outcome in very low birth weight infants who are at high risk of developing bronchopulmonary dysplasia.</u> *M*Evidence of improved pulmonary function is that after a 42-day course of dexamethasone given to our preterm infants who were ventilator and oxygen dependent at 2 weeks of age, the durations of positive pressure ventilation, of supplemental oxygen, and of hospitalization were less than those in control infants, who received saline placebo. *N*Evidence of improved neurodevelopmental outcome is that the infants who received the 42-day course of dexamethasone had a lower incidence of neurologic handicap and significantly higher scores on the Bayley Scales of Infant Development than did infants in the control group.

After stating and supporting the answer, organize the remaining topics from most to least important, beginning with the topic most closely related to the answer. Indicate the organization by using topic sentences to state the point of each paragraph. The reader should be able to read the first sentence of every paragraph in the Discussion section and see the structure of the Discussion, as in Example 5, which continues the Discussion begun in Example 4.

Example 5 Middle of a Discussion

2, 3 Serious complications

2 Importantly, we did not observe any of the serious complications of dexamethasone administration suggested by previous, uncontrolled trials (14, 15, 17). (etc.)

3 However, some infants may have had adrenocortical suppression, since mean serum cortisol levels were significantly lower in infants who received the 42-day course of dexamethasone than in control infants. (etc.)

4 Support for 42-day therapy

4 We have also found that the duration of dexamethasone therapy is important. (etc.)

5, 6 Other complications

5 Two points regarding the clinical courses of infants in our study are worth noting. First, the only two infants who developed pneumothoraces during the study period were receiving dexamethasone. (etc.)

6 Second, retinopathy was found in a very high number of infants in all three groups. (etc.)

The middle of this Discussion moves from most to least important topics. After the answer to the question is stated at the beginning of the Discussion (that the therapy is beneficial, see Example 4), the middle of the Discussion goes on first to comment on serious complications, which, if present, would undermine the therapy, then to explain why a long treatment (42 days) is needed, and finally to explain points not asked in the question that are interesting but less important (other complications).

This organization is clear from reading the topic sentences. Note that the first sentence of paragraph 5 is the topic sentence for both paragraph 5 and paragraph 6; the second sentence of paragraph 5 is the topic sentence for paragraph 5 alone.

The Discussion cannot just stop. It must clearly come to an end. Two standard ways of ending are to restate the answers and to state applications or implications of the answers, or you can do both. For the Discussion in Examples 4 and 5, the author restated the answers and also the point about complications, thus pulling the message of the paper together (Example 6).

Example 6 Ending of a Discussion

O Answers

P Complications

7   ^{O}In summary, we have shown that dexamethasone therapy for 42 days leads to sustained improvement in pulmonary function and improves neurodevelopmental outcome in very low birth weight infants who are ventilator and oxygen dependent at 2 weeks of age and therefore are at high risk of developing bronchopulmonary dysplasia. ^{P}Although dexamethasone use may be associated with adrenocortical suppression, it is not associated with an increased incidence of major complications, including infection, hypertension, and growth failure.

This ending reinforces the message of the paper and feels conclusive.

Note that the answer in the final paragraph in the Discussion is virtually identical to the answer in the first paragraph. This exact repetition of answers is important. If the answers were different, we would not know which one to believe.

Finally, it is important that the answer answers the question asked. The question focuses the entire paper for the reader. If the answer does not answer the question asked, the reader will be confused, as in Example 7.

Example 7 Question and Answer Mismatch

Question: We asked whether liquid leaks directly from edematous lung.
Answer: We conclude that liquid leaks across the visceral pleura.

In this example, the answer actually does answer the question, but that is not obvious because the key terms are different. To make clear that the answer answers the question asked, and thus to make the message of the paper clear, use the same key terms in the question and answer, as in the revision of Example 7.

Revision

Question: We asked whether lung edema leaks into the pleural space.
Answer: We conclude that lung edema leaks into the pleural space.

The rest of this book explains in greater detail how to follow these guidelines so that you will be able to write a biomedical research paper in which both the trees and the forest are clear.

USING THIS BOOK

Whether you are using this book by yourself or in a class, read each chapter carefully and be sure that you understand all of the principles. Most importantly, take the time to write each exercise carefully. It is not enough to read through an exercise quickly and think briefly about what you would do to revise it. The way you will learn is by struggling with the exercises, trying to apply the relevant writing principles. When you compare your revisions with the ones at the end of the book, you may find that you did the same thing as done in the revisions, or you may have done something very different. Your revisions may be better. But even if you missed the point, the struggle will have been valuable. The important thing is to grapple with words on paper, because the only way to learn to write is by writing. So do not peek at the revisions; give yourself the opportunity to make your own mistakes and achieve your own successes and thus to develop judgment in applying the principles of writing.

Some of the exercises are rather difficult. Try to spend the time needed to understand these exercises, and try not to get stuck in the scientific details. Also, the examples and exercises come almost exclusively from cardiovascular research, an area that may be unfamiliar to some readers. Again, try to think about the writing, not the science. For some readers it may actually be easier to understand writing problems in a field outside their own.

When you start applying the writing principles in this book to your own writing (using the summaries at the ends of the chapters as checklists), you will find that no paper can follow all of the principles exactly. Every paper has its own story to tell and its own organizational challenges—some detail that does not fit anywhere, some topic that interrupts the story line. This is why writing a biomedical research paper is difficult. There is no absolute formula. Every paper is different. You will need judgment and creativity to apply the principles in this book to your own writing, and these skills take time to develop. Sometimes you may be stumped. If possible, consult an experienced teacher of scientific writing or an experienced author's editor, or consult a colleague who writes clearly. Otherwise, if a writing principle is confusing to you or you cannot make it work, ignore it. It is more important that the science is accurate than that the writing is "perfect." As you gain experience in writing, you should be able to bend the rules as necessary to make your paper say what you want to say. The goal is not to follow all the rules but to have a clearly written paper.

THE BUILDING BLOCKS OF WRITING

Writing uses words. There are two things you can do with words—choose them and arrange them. The first chapter of this book deals with choosing words. Most of the rest of the book deals with arranging words. The arranging is in increasingly larger units of thought—sentences, paragraphs, sections of a biomedical research paper, and the research paper as a whole.

Words, sentences, and paragraphs are the building blocks of writing. In later chapters of this book, the principles of word choice, sentence structure, and paragraph structure will be expanded to apply to the sections of a biomedical research paper and to the research paper as a whole.

CHAPTER 1

WORD CHOICE

The choice of words to use in biomedical research papers is governed by a few basic principles. The first exercise in this chapter is designed to help you discover these principles by evaluating words in sentences. The principles are stated and discussed in detail in the revisions at the end of this book. These principles are the most important concepts in this chapter.

The second exercise addresses a different issue—distinguishing between words whose meanings are similar but not exactly the same. One reason that distinguishing between words is difficult in English is that English is a particularly rich language, incorporating some half a million words and having an abundance of synonyms and near synonyms. Another reason that distinctions are difficult is that English, like all other languages, is constantly changing. Fortunately, the meanings of most words remain essentially the same over the centuries. Lungs are still lungs and to increase is still to increase (but see Exercise 1.2). However, over time, the meanings of some words change to serve the needs of the people who speak the language. One way that words change is by taking on extra meanings. Some words even come to mean their opposite. For example, "scan" means both "to glance at quickly" (as in "to scan a list of titles") and "to scrutinize closely." Furthermore, in the last 15 or 20 years, "scan" has taken on a new meaning in medicine: "to examine the human body for the presence or localization of radioactive material." In addition, "scan," which was only a verb before, is now also a noun, meaning a picture of the distribution of radioactive material in some part of the body. Thus, at any given moment, some words in the language are in flux. Exercise 1.2 focuses on several sets of words that biomedical researchers tend to confuse. Twenty years from now, different words might be included in this exercise.

In the remaining pages of this chapter, the words in Exercise 1.2, and also several other words, are defined and examples of their use are given.

In all the examples and exercises in this chapter, we will be looking at words in context, not in isolation. The reason is that words are not "good" or "bad" individually; rather, words must be viewed in the context of a given sentence and, as we will see, in a given paragraph and, indeed, in the paper as a whole.

There is no final authority on the use of words in English. The standard used in scholarly writing (including biomedical research papers) is the practice of educated writers. For specific guidance on the meanings and existence of individual words, Americans use unabridged dictionaries such as *Webster's Third New International Dictionary of the English Language Unabridged* (Webster's Third). For specific guidance on current usage of words, see the usage notes in *The American Heritage Dictionary of the English Language.*

■ *EXERCISE 1.1: PRINCIPLES OF WORD CHOICE*

The words underlined in the examples in this exercise illustrate problems in word choice frequently found in biomedical research papers.

1. *Improve the word choice in Examples 1-26. (It is OK to use a dictionary.) If you are not sure of how to improve the word choice, guess.*

2. *In each of the six groups of examples, the underlined words all violate one principle of word choice. Identify the principle of word choice that is being violated by each group of words. Write the principle on the line after the Roman numeral. Note: This exercise can be done in conjunction with reading* The Elements of Style *by Strunk and White (see Literature Cited).*

3. *Write a list of guidelines for the use of abbreviations in biomedical research papers.*

I. _____

1. Renal blood flow was <u>drastically compromised</u> when the aorta was obstructed.

2. The short-circuit current remained increased for <u>several</u> hours.

3. The <u>change</u> in short-circuit current produced by 10^{-5} M major basic protein was 85% of the maximal response to isoproterenol. A higher concentration of major basic protein would therefore probably have produced only a minimal further increase in the short-circuit current.

4. The cells were <u>exposed</u> to lipoprotein-deficient serum for 48 h.

5. <u>Animals</u> were studied in utero 4–9 weeks later.

6. In isolated, perfused dog lungs, infusion of serotonin <u>was associated with</u> an increase in microvascular pressure.

7. We found a linear increase in the percentage of early loss of microspheres <u>with</u> a doubling of coronary arterial pressure.

8. <u>With</u> inhalation of amyl nitrate, compliance decreased.

9. Maximal coronary vasodilatation <u>with</u> carbochromen had other effects.

10. The salicylates are rapidly absorbed <u>with</u> a peak plasma salicylate concentration within 2 h.

11. The osmotic pressure of plasma was subtracted from the osmotic pressure of plasma <u>with</u> heparin.

II. _____

12. Blood samples were drawn from the 5 <u>female</u> and 3 <u>male children</u> at ½, 1, 2, 3, and 4 h <u>following</u> the <u>initiation</u> of dialysis.

13. All heat-stable materials <u>utilized</u> in the isolation and processing of solutions to be injected into mice were sterilized <u>prior to</u> use.

14. These ganglia contained 1-40 neuronal <u>perikarya</u>.

15. The Doppler signal displayed continuous, low-frequency blood flow that was directed <u>hepatopetally</u>.

III. _____

16. After 4 h <u>of hemodialysis</u>, we abruptly ended the hemodialysis procedure.

17. Oxygen uptake in response to drugs <u>was examined and found to</u> vary considerably.

18. Maximal coronary blood flow further decreased endocardial diameter and increased wall thickness during systole. Both <u>the decrease in systolic endocardial diameter and the increase in systolic wall thickness</u> were greater when the pericardium was closed.

IV. A. _____

19. We <u>vortexed</u> the tubes.

20. We <u>endorphinized</u> the dogs.

21. We studied the effect of clonidine on the hindleg reflexes of the <u>spinalized</u> rat.

22. We <u>hemorrhaged</u> the dogs.

23. Sufficient dialyzed protein was added to 200 ml of properly <u>pH'd</u> gold.

IV. B. _____

24. After <u>cutdowns</u> of a femoral artery and vein, we removed the left fourth to eighth ribs.

25. Scintillation fluid was added to the <u>hot</u> samples.

26. The trachea was intubated and the lamb was <u>placed on</u> a Harvard ventilator.

IV. C._____

27.   [A]This study measured the responses of forearm blood flow (<u>FBF</u>) and forearm vascular resistance (<u>FVR</u>) after isometric handgrip exercise (<u>IHE</u>) and related them to plasma norepinephrine (<u>NE</u>) and epinephrine (<u>E</u>) in 12 normotensives (<u>N</u>) and 14 primary hypertensives (<u>PH</u>). [B]<u>IHE</u> was performed at 30% of maximum voluntary contraction using a calibrated dynamometer. [C]Systolic blood pressure (<u>SBP</u>), diastolic blood pressure (<u>DBP</u>), heart rate (<u>HR</u>), <u>FBF</u>, <u>FVR</u>, <u>NE</u>, and <u>E</u> were measured in the resting arm before and after <u>IHE</u>. [D]Pre-exercise <u>SBP</u> and <u>DBP</u> were higher in <u>PH</u> than in <u>N</u>. [E]<u>FVR</u> was similar in <u>PH</u> and <u>N</u>. [F]<u>NE</u> was higher in <u>PH</u> compared to other matched normotensives. [G]After <u>IHE</u>, <u>SBP</u> and <u>DBP</u> were increased 18% and 19%, respectively, in <u>PH</u> and 16% and 25% in <u>N</u>. [H]<u>HR</u>, <u>NE</u> and <u>E</u> were increased in <u>PH</u> and <u>N</u>. [I]Group differences were not significant. [J]Pre and post <u>IHE</u> <u>FBF</u> was similar in both groups. [K]<u>FVR</u> increased in both groups. [L]The findings indicate that skin and muscle arteriolar resistance at rest and during stress in <u>PH</u> with enhanced sympathetic tone are not different from <u>N</u>, and suggest that other hemodynamic abnormalities, perhaps increased cardiac output and splanchnic resistance, mediate the excessive neural tone and raise blood pressure.

Guidelines for Using Abbreviations in Biomedical Research Papers:

■ *EXERCISE 1.2: WORDS CARELESSLY INTERCHANGED*

Underline the word in each set of words within parentheses that makes the best sense in the sentence. It is OK to look words up in a dictionary. After you finish this exercise, check your answers by reading the definitions that appear on the next several pages.

1. This response was blocked by phentolamine but was not (affected, effected) by propranolol.

2. The digoxin (amount, concentration, content, level) was increased from 0.5 to 2.5 ng/ml.

3. This procedure permits early identification of a (clotted, clogged) catheter.

4. Drug therapy (included, consisted of) 0.25 mg of digoxin per day, 750 mg of procainimide every 4 h, and 40 mg of propranolol 4 times a day. No other drugs were used.

5. Preganglionic stimulation (enhances, increases) norepinephrine release from terminals within the superior cervical ganglion.

6. Increased knowledge of cardiac muscle function has greatly (enhanced, improved) our ability to detect and quantify disorders of myocardial contraction.

7. Treatment with methylprednisolone after the lesion is established significantly (enhances, speeds) recovery.

8. At frequent (intervals, periods) we measured pH, P_{O_2}, and P_{CO_2} in arterial blood, and during each (interval, period) of study we measured pulmonary blood flow two or three times.

9. We studied the responses of the following (parameters, variables): heart rate, cardiac output, oxygen consumption, and systemic vascular resistance.

10. We used three anesthetic (regimes, regimens, regiments).

11. Seventy-five percent nitrous oxide (represents, is) a subanesthetic concentration in the dog.

12. Ultracentrifugally isolated lipoproteins consist of a mixture of particles of (varying, various) sizes and functional characteristics.

WORDS CARELESSLY INTERCHANGED

Careful writers distinguish between words that more casual writers carelessly interchange, such as the following sets of words.

D E F I N I T I O N	**E X A M P L E**
ABILITY, CAPACITY	
Ability. The mental or physical power to do something, or the skill in doing it.	Optimal oxygen transport depends on the remarkable *ability* of hemoglobin to combine with oxygen.
Capacity. The full amount that something can hold, contain, or receive.	The oxygen *capacity* of 1 g of hemoglobin is 1.39 ml of oxygen.
ACCURACY, PRECISION, REPRODUCIBILITY	
Accuracy. The degree of conformity of a measurement to the known or true value of the quantity measured.	The *accuracy* of the polygraphic method for estimating the efficiency of oxidative phosphorylation was checked by the conventional manometric technique.
Precision. Broadly, the degree of refinement with which a measurement is made or reported.	The value 3.43 shows greater *precision* than the value 3.4, but it is not necessarily more accurate.
Reproducibility. The degree to which related measurements, made under the same circumstances, can be duplicated.	The *reproducibility* of the method, as analyzed in 18 series of sequential measurements in 12 dogs, was excellent.
AFFECT, EFFECT	
Affect (verb). To act on or influence.	How smoking *affects* the health is still a matter of concern to physicians.
Effect (noun). A resultant condition.	We studied the *effect* of epinephrine on glucose kinetics in dogs.
ALTERNATELY, ALTERNATIVELY	
Alternately. Following by turns: first one, then the other.	The mice were *alternately* fed and deprived of food.
Alternatively. Involving a choice between two or more courses of action or possibilities.	The dog's weight can be controlled by diet or, *alternatively*, by drugs.
AMONG, BETWEEN	
Among. In the midst of. "Among" is used to express the relation of one thing to a group of many surrounding things. It is not used to express the relation of two things.	We found one intact test tube *among* the broken ones.

Between. Expresses the relation of two or more things as individuals.

There were no significant differences *between* the three experimental groups.

AMOUNT, CONCENTRATION, CONTENT, LEVEL

Amount. The total bulk, or quantity, of that which is measured.

The *amount* of DNA isolated from the left ventricle of the rats was 600 µg.

Concentration. The amount of a substance contained in a given amount of another substance; the strength or density of a solution.

The *concentration* of DNA in the left ventricle of the rat is 1.5 µg/mg of tissue. The ventricle weighs 400 mg. Therefore, the ventricular *content* of DNA is 600 µg.

Content. The total amount of a substance in another substance.

Level. [1]Position along a vertical axis; [2]relative position or rank on a scale. [3]"Level" is also used as a general term for amount, concentration, or content.

[1]The chest was opened at the *level* of the fifth rib.
[2]Cardiac output and heart rate did not increase above normoxic *levels*.
[3]Blood sugar *levels* (that is, concentrations) remained stable throughout the experiment.

CAN, MAY

Can. Denotes the power, or ability, to do something.

Homogeneous cell lines of short duration *can* be achieved with cloning techniques.

May. Refers either to possibility or to permission.

This mechanism *may* also be the cause of the ozone effect noted in two other studies.

CLOT, CLOG

Clot. To form into a thick, viscous, or coagulated mass.

The milk was *clotted* by the addition of a coagulant.

Clog. To block up, to obstruct; to become obstructed or choked up.

The valves of the car were *clogged* with carbon.

CONTINUAL, CONTINUOUS

Continual. Intermittent, occurring at repeated intervals.

The experiments were hampered by *continual* infections in the rat colony.

Continuous. Uninterrupted, unbroken continuity.

The machine made a *continuous* hum.

INCIDENCE, PREVALENCE

Incidence. Number of cases developing per unit of population *per unit of time.*

According to data from the American Lung Association, the *incidence* of tuberculosis is 100 cases per 100,000 persons per year.

Prevalence. Number of cases existing per unit of population *at a given time*; more loosely, the degree to which something occurs (how widespread, how common it is).

The *prevalence* of tuberculosis in the Bay Area at the present time is 300 cases per 100,000 persons.

INCLUDE, CONSIST OF

Include. To have as a part or member; to be made up of, at least in part; to contain. "Include" often implies an incomplete listing.

Conditions that increase intra-abdominal pressure also increase the likelihood of significant reflux. These conditions *include* obesity, ascites, and pregnancy.

Consist of. To be made up of, to be composed of.

Pre-prolactin and ovalbumin *consist of* 228 and 385 residues, respectively.

INCREASE, AUGMENT, ENHANCE, IMPROVE, SPEED

Increase. A general word that means to become or to make greater in some respect, such as size, quantity, number, degree, value, or intensity.

Although the insulin concentration *increased*, the insulin/glucose ratio decreased.
Blood pressure *was increased* by intravenous injection of epinephrine.

Augment. A more formal word that generally implies to increase by addition, often to increase something that is already of a considerable size, amount, etc.

Confiscation of the monasteries greatly *augmented* the resources of the crown.

Enhance. An evaluative word that means to add to something already attractive, worthy, or valuable, thus increasing its value.

The neat polished floors were *enhanced* by fine Arabian carpets.

Improve. To advance to a better state or quality; to make better.

The patient's condition did not *improve* after chemotherapy.

Speed. To hasten.

Lying in bed for 10 days *speeds* recovery from a back injury.

INTERVAL, PERIOD

Interval. The time between two specified instants, events, or states.

Period. The time during which events or states occur.

Electrical testing was performed at 5-min *intervals* for a *period* of 30 min after the administration of insulin.

LOCATE, LOCALIZE

Locate. To determine the position of something; to find its location.

We *located* a fetal hindleg and delivered it through a small incision in the uterine wall.

Localize. (With an object) To confine or fix in a particular area or part. (Without an object) To collect or accumulate in or be restricted to a specific or limited area.

Hot applications helped to *localize* the infection.
Iodine tends to *localize* in the thyroid.

MILLIMOLE, MILLIMOLAR, MILLIMOLAL

Millimole (mmol). An *amount, not* a concentration.

Millimolar (mM). A *concentration, not* an amount.

Millimolal. A *concentration, not* an amount.

A 0.5 *millimolar* solution contains 0.5 *millimole* of a solute in 1 liter of solution (*or*, a 0.5 mM solution contains 0.5 mmol/liter of solution.) The final volume is 1 liter.

A 0.5 *millimolal* solution contains 0.5 mmol of a solute in 100 grams of solvent. The final volume may be more or less than 1 liter.

MUCUS, MUCOUS

Mucus. The noun.

Mucous. The adjective.

Mucus is a viscous secretion of the *mucous* membranes.

OPTIMAL, OPTIMUM

Optimal. The adjective; never used as a noun.

Optimum. The noun; often used as an adjective.

An organism will grow best under *optimal* conditions.

The *optimum* is the most favorable set of conditions for the growth or reproduction of an organism.

PARAMETER, VARIABLE, CONSTANT

Constant. A constant is a quantity that is fixed, that is, the same wherever it is found.

Parameter. A parameter is not fixed absolutely, as a constant is. A parameter can change. But a parameter is fixed for a given system. Thus, a parameter is a characteristic, that is, a definer, of a system.

Variable. A variable is a quantity that can change in a given system. Thus, a variable is not a characteristic (definer) of a system.

Note: The mean and standard deviation of a given population are *parameters*. Estimates of the mean and standard deviation (obtained from a random sample from that population) are *statistics*.

Recommendation: Do not use "parameter" unless you are discussing an equation. You probably mean "variable" or one of its numerous synonyms, such as "factor," "characteristic," "condition," "criterion," "index," or "measure." If you mean "perimeter"(!), use "perimeter."

Pi is a *constant*; 2 is a *constant*.

Parameters from saturation experiments (the dissociation constant, K_D, and the receptor concentration, B_{max}) were determined by an analysis of bound ligand as a function of free ligand.

The concentration of a drug in the blood plasma as a function of time after injection is a *variable*.

In a process for which growth rate is proportional to mass—represented, for example, by $dm/dt = km$—there is an exponential relationship between the *variables* mass, m, and time, t; m grows exponentially as t increases (see the equation below). The exact shape of the exponential increase depends on the value of the *parameter* k, which is different for different systems. The value of k determines the exact nature of the exponential relationship for the specific system (see the graph below). If k is large (for example, 1.0), the growth rate is rapid; if k is small (for example, 0.005), the growth rate is slow. The variables mass and time can take on many values in each system. The *parameter k* has a fixed value for each system.

Equation: $m(t) = m_0 e^{kt}$

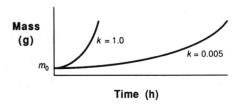

Mass (g)

$k = 1.0$

$k = 0.005$

m_0

Time (h)

PRONE, SUPINE

Prone. Lying or placed so that the face and the belly are downward.

We placed the dog *prone* on the table so that we could examine its back.

Supine. Lying or placed on the back (spine) with the face and the belly up.

We placed the apneic man *supine* and applied rhythmic pressure to his rib cage.

REGIME, REGIMEN, REGIMENT

Regime. A governmental or social system.

Life was better under the old *regime*.

Regimen. A systematic plan.

The exercise *regimen* of a ballet dancer is strenuous.

Regiment. A unit of soldiers consisting of at least two battalions.

The *regiment* was ordered to march.

REPRESENT, BE

Represent. To serve as a sign or symbol of; to take the place of.

Each data point *represents* one measurement of airway resistance.

Be. Equal, constitute.

Alcohol *is* a depressant of the central nervous system.

VARIOUS, VARYING

Various. Distinct, diverse, different.

"We used *various* concentrations" means that you used several different concentrations.

Varying. Changing, fluctuating.

"We used *varying* concentrations" means that the concentrations changed during the experiment.

CHAPTER 2

SENTENCE STRUCTURE

English sentences are clearest, most forceful, and easiest to understand if they are simple and direct. If instead sentences are complicated and indirect, the reader is slowed down and even confused. Five problems that commonly interfere with simplicity and directness in sentences in scientific research papers are

- Not expressing the core of the message in the subject, verb, and completer
- Piling nouns into noun clusters
- Packing too many ideas into one sentence
- Having unclear antecedents of pronouns
- Not putting parallel ideas in parallel form

Having one or two of these problems in one or two sentences in a research paper will not completely undermine the paper's clarity. But sentence after sentence containing these problems creates a definite reading difficulty. And when problems in sentence structure appear in combination with problems in word choice (see Chap. 1) and paragraph structure (see Chap. 3), clarity is seriously compromised.

We will examine these five problems, and also five lesser problems, in this chapter.

EXPRESS THE CORE OF THE MESSAGE IN THE SUBJECT, VERB, AND COMPLETER

A sentence is most likely to be simple and direct if the subject, verb, and completer convey the core of the message. To ensure that they do, make the topic the subject of the sentence and put the action of the sentence in the verb. (The topic is what the sentence is talking about. The action is what the topic is doing or what is being done to it.)

Make the Topic the Subject of the Sentence

Example 2.1   The <u>children</u> with arteriovenous shunts **had** the shunts opened, heparin injected, and the arterial and venous sides of the shunt clamped.

In this sentence, the subject and verb are <u>children</u> **had**. But the topic of this sentence is not children, and the message is not about children having something (as it would be, for example, in the sentence, "The children had diabetes mellitus"). This sentence has three topics—shunts, heparin, and the sides of the shunt—and the message of the sentence is about what happened to them. Therefore, these terms should be the subjects of the sentence.

Revision   In the children who had arteriovenous shunts, the <u>shunts</u> **were opened**, <u>heparin</u> **was injected**, and the arterial and venous <u>sides</u> of the shunt **were clamped**.

In this revision, the topics are the subjects of the sentence, and the subjects and verbs convey the message of the sentence.

Put the Action in the Verb

Verbs express action in English. If the action of a sentence is expressed by the main verb, the sentence is natural and direct and easy to understand. If, instead, the action is expressed in a noun, the sentence is oblique, tangled, and more difficult to understand.

Three common ways of expressing action in a noun instead of in a verb are (1) to put the action in the *subject* of the sentence, (2) to put the action in the *object* of the verb, and (3) to put the action in a *prepositional phrase*.

Action Inappropriately in the Subject

Example 2.2   An <u>increase</u> in heart rate **occurred.**

In this example, the verb (**occurred**) does not express the action of the sentence. Instead, the subject of the sentence (<u>increase</u>) expresses the action. As a result, the grammar does not coordinate with the meaning, and the sentence is complicated and indirect.

To revise a sentence whose action is in the subject, the trick is to

- Omit the subject and the preposition that follows it (here "increase in").
- Replace the vague verb (here "occurred") with the action from the omitted subject (here "increase" becomes "increased").

Revision   Heart rate **increased**.

In the revised sentence, the grammar and the meaning coincide. That is, the subject states the topic (heart rate) and the verb expresses the action (increased). Thus, the sentence is simple and direct.

In addition, the revised sentence has fewer words than the original sentence and hence is more efficient.

Action in the Subject:	An increase in heart rate occurred.	(6 words)
Action in the Verb:	Heart rate increased.	(3 words)

Note also that the verb of the original sentence, **occurred**, is vague and general. It does not contribute to the *meaning* of the sentence (the meaning is in the subject) but simply performs the *function* of a verb. It could be replaced by another general verb, such as "was seen" or "was noted," without appreciably altering the meaning of the sentence.

Finally, if we compare the subjects and verbs of the two sentences, we see that the subject and verb of the revised sentence (heart rate **increased**) express the core of the message, whereas the subject and verb of the original sentence (increase **occurred**) express only part of the core—the action but not the topic. Thus, when the action is in the verb, the sentence is simpler, more direct, and more efficient than when the action is in the subject.

Action Inappropriately in the Object

Example 2.3 The new drug **caused** a *decrease* in heart rate.

Revision The new drug **decreased** *heart rate*.

In this example, the action is expressed by the object (*decrease*), and the true object (heart rate) is sidetracked into a prepositional phrase. Thus, the subject, verb, and object of the original sentence (drug **caused** a *decrease*) express less of the sentence's message than do the subject, verb, and object of the revised sentence (drug **decreased** *heart rate*). Again, when the action is in the verb, the sentence is simpler, more direct, and more efficient than when the action is in the object.

To revise a sentence whose action is in the object, omit the verb (here "caused") and make a new verb from the object (here "a decrease" becomes "decreased").

Action Inappropriately in a Prepositional Phrase

Prepositions are words such as "of," "for," "on," "in," "to," "with."

Example 2.4 *WITH* BILATERAL LEG VESSEL CONGESTION, the compliance of forearm vessels increased significantly.

In this example, the action in the first part of the sentence is expressed in the object of a preposition ("congestion," the object of "with"), and there is no verb. As a result, the sentence is dense and difficult to read. The sentence becomes simpler and clearer when the action is expressed by a verb (and when the vague term "with" (see Exercise 1.1) is replaced by the precise term "when").

Revision WHEN THE VESSELS IN BOTH LEGS **WERE CONGESTED**, the compliance of forearm vessels increased significantly.

Note that in the revision, the fancy term "bilateral" can be omitted.
In the next example, the suppressed verbs are not so obvious as in the first example.

Example 2.5 *WITH* HYPOXIA OF LONGER DURATION OR SEVERER DEGREE, the shortening phase may get progressively briefer.

Revision WHEN HYPOXIA **LASTS** LONGER OR **IS** MORE SEVERE, the shortening phase may get progressively briefer.

This revision illustrates that a crucial factor for clarity in a sentence is expressing action in a verb.
Verbs are the lifeblood of an English sentence. Omitting them (by putting the action in a prepositional phrase) or weakening them (by putting the action

in the subject or object and adding a vague verb) saps the sentence of its lifeblood and makes the sentence dense and difficult to read.

This problem can be viewed numerically: sentences become easier to read as the proportion of verbs to nouns increases. The proportion of verbs to nouns is maximal when all action is expressed by verbs. This is the natural way to write in English. When sentences are written unnaturally, with the action in a noun, the ratio of verbs to nouns decreases, and the sentences become proportionally more difficult.

Action in the		*Verbs: Nouns*
Subject:	An <u>increase</u> in <u>heart rate</u> **occurred**.	1:2
Verb:	<u>Heart rate</u> **increased**.	1:1
Object:	The new <u>drug</u> **caused** a <u>decrease</u> in <u>heart rate</u>.	1:3
Verb:	The new <u>drug</u> **decreased** <u>heart rate</u>.	1:2
Prepositional Phase:	With <u>hypoxia</u> of longer <u>duration</u> or severer <u>degree</u>, the shortening <u>phase</u> **may get** progressively briefer.	1:4
Verb:	When <u>hypoxia</u> **lasts** longer or **is** more severe, the shortening <u>phase</u> **may get** progressively briefer.	3:2

Dramatic reversals in the verb-noun ratio, such as the reversal illustrated in the last pair of sentences above, emphasize the advantage of putting the action in the verb.

To check your writing, ask yourself what action you want each sentence to express, and then make sure that you express this action in a verb.

How to Find Action That Is Not in the Verb

- Look for *weak verbs*, such as "occurred," "showed," "caused," "produced," "was achieved," "was observed," "was noted."
- Look for *nouns made from verbs*. These nouns have special endings:

Ending	*Example*
-tion	prolongation, inhibition, formation, decomposition
-ment	measurement, assessment
-ence	occurrence, existence
-al	removal

- Look for *"increase"* and *"decrease"* used as nouns instead of as verbs. (The verb in the sentence will generally be a weak verb.)

   Example: An <u>increase</u> in heart rate **occurred**.

- Look for *"with"* followed by a noun made from a verb.

   Example: *With* the <u>occurrence</u> of <u>increases</u>, . . .

   (Note that this group of words contains action but no verb.)

After putting the action in a verb, check that the core of the message is in the subject, verb, and completer.

■ *EXERCISE 2.1: EXPRESS THE CORE OF THE MESSAGE IN THE SUBJECT, VERB, AND COMPLETER*

Make the topic the subject in the following sentences.

1. The adults ended dialysis with a plasma acetate concentration almost double that of the children.

2. The patient showed no change in symptoms.

3. The patient was begun on 6 g of aspirin daily and had resolution of his arthritis.

Action Inappropriately in the Subject

Put the action in the verb in each of the following sentences. (Omit the subject and the preposition that follows it; replace the vague verb with the action from the omitted subject.)

4. A progressive decrease in the death rate occurred.

5. Evaporation of ethanol from the mixture takes place rapidly.

6. Removal of potassium perchlorate was achieved by centrifugation of the supernatant liquid at $1400 \times g$ for 10 min.

7. Measurements of blood pH were made with a Radiometer capillary electrode.

8. Prolongation of life for uremic patients has been made possible by improved conservative treatment and hemodialysis.

9. An abrupt increase in minute ventilation and respiratory frequency occurred in all dogs as exercise began.

Action Inappropriately in the Object

Put the action in the verb in each of the following sentences. (Omit the verb. Make a new verb from a noun that expresses action.)

10. We made at least two analyses on each specimen.

11. Infusion of tyramine produced a decrease in cutaneous blood flow.

12. These agents exert their action by inhibition of synthesis of cholesterol by the liver.

13. This net difference in osmolarity causes a flux of water into the cerebrospinal fluid, causing increased pressure.

Action Inappropriately in a Prepositional Phrase

Put the action in the verb in each of the following sentences. (Use a different word instead of "with" and substitute a verb for the noun that contains action.)

14. A capsule of amyl nitrite was crushed and held in front of the nose for 20 s with normal respiration maintained.

15. Calcium is translocated across the membrane along with the formation of a phosphorylated enzyme intermediate. Calcium is then released into the lumen with the simultaneous decomposition of the phosphorylated intermediate enzyme into the unphosphorylated enzyme and ADP plus phosphate.

DO NOT PILE NOUNS INTO NOUN CLUSTERS

Noun Clusters

One noun is commonly used to modify another in English. Examples include "blood flow," "protein metabolism," "lung function," and "ion concentration." But adding another noun (or nouns) onto an already existing noun pair is confusing. (For a detailed treatment of this topic, see Woodford, <u>Scientific Writing for Graduate Students</u>, p. 52.)

Example 2.6   filament length variability

Example 2.7   air spaces phospholipid pool

At first glance, it is not easy to see what these terms mean. The terms are clearer if they are not compacted into clusters.

Untangling Noun Clusters

To untangle a noun cluster, start from the end and work your way to the beginning, supplying the appropriate prepositions, as in the revisions shown here:

Revisions   variability <u>of</u> filament length
phospholipid pool <u>in</u> the air spaces
(*or*: pool <u>of</u> phospholipids <u>in</u> the air spaces)

The prepositions make clear how the nouns are related to each other. Note that the preposition used to translate a cluster into understandable English is not always the same. Here "of" and "in" are used. Also note that the revised versions are all longer than the original versions. This is OK. The goal is clarity, not brevity.

Cautionary Note

Not all sequences of nouns are noun clusters. Some noun pairs and even triplets are so well established that they have become single words. For example, even though "heart rate" looks like two words, it is actually one word. So when untangling noun clusters, treat such terms as single words. Be careful to distinguish between terms that have become single words and those that have not. (Check an unabridged dictionary.)

Adjective Added to a Noun Cluster

The problem is compounded when an adjective is added to a noun cluster.

Example 2.8   *chronic* sheep experiments

Example 2.9:   *peripheral* chemoreceptor stimulation

What is chronic—the sheep or the experiments? What is peripheral—the chemoreceptors or the stimulation? For the answer to be clear, *only one noun* must be placed after the adjective.

Revisions   *chronic* **experiments** <u>in</u> sheep
stimulation <u>of</u> the *peripheral* **chemoreceptors**

Note that "chronic" modifies the last noun in its cluster ("experiments") but "peripheral" modifies the first noun in its cluster ("chemoreceptor"). Since there is no predictable pattern for determining which noun the adjective modifies, the clearest practice is to write the idea the long way, not as a cluster.

Noun Being Modified Missing From the Noun Cluster

Ultimate confusion arises when the noun that the adjective modifies is omitted from the noun cluster altogether.

Example 2.10   To assess for *zero drift*, we checked each catheter in saline at 38°C.

What is zero drift? It sounds like it means "no drift." Actually, it means "drift of the zero point."

Revision   To assess for *drift of the zero point*, we checked each catheter in saline at 38°C.

Recommendation: Treat clusters like abbreviations. Do not use them if you can possibly avoid them. If you are forced to use one, write it the long way the first time you use it; then use the cluster.

■ *EXERCISE 2.2: UNTANGLING NOUN CLUSTERS*

Untangle the noun clusters in the following sentences by adding the appropriate preposition or prepositions, and other words as needed. Start at the end of the cluster and work your way to the beginning.

Noun + Noun

1. Shunt blood clotting occurred after 5 days.

2. The precipitate was further purified by sucrose density gradient centrifugation.

3. Title: "Blood-Brain Barrier CSF pH Regulation"

Adjective + Noun + Noun

In your revision, do not omit the adjective. Put only one noun after the adjective (italicized).

4. The antigen was prepared from *whole* rat liver homogenates.

5. T_4 stimulated choline incorporation into *primary* fetal lung cell cultures.

Adjective + (   ) + Noun

Add the missing noun.

6. Normal and ulcerative colitis serum samples were studied by paper electrophoresis.

7. There was no significant difference between resting lactates and exercising lactates.

DO NOT PACK TOO MANY IDEAS
INTO ONE SENTENCE

Short sentences are easier to understand than long sentences. Therefore do not pack too many ideas into one sentence either by stringing ideas together or by talking about more than one thing at a time.

Do Not String Ideas Together

Example 2.11   *(53 words)*

In one patient who had numerous vegetations, the echocardiogram correctly predicted a large vegetation (15 mm) attached to the right coronary cusp but failed to detect the 4- to 5-mm lesions found at surgery on the remaining two cusps, whereas in another patient, the echocardiogram correctly predicted lesions on all three cusps.

In this example, the first idea ends before "whereas." The second idea belongs in a separate sentence.

Revision

In one patient who had numerous vegetations, the echocardiogram correctly predicted a large vegetation (15 mm) attached to the right coronary cusp but failed to detect the 4- to 5-mm lesions found at surgery on the remaining two cusps. However, in another patient, the echocardiogram correctly predicted lesions on all three cusps.

Talk About One Thing at a Time

A long sentence that strings ideas together is difficult to read. Even more difficult is a sentence that talks about two ideas at once or a sentence in which one idea is nested inside another. In Example 2.12, two ideas are being discussed at once: elution order and extent of separation.

Example 2.12   *(43 words)*

The elution order and extent of separation of these two isoenzymes are *quite different* from those achieved on DEAE-cellulose chromatography of α-chymotryptic-digested S1, *where light chain 1 emerges first, followed by a well-resolved second peak of light chain 3*.

The ideas in Example 2.12 are easier to understand when they are written in separate sentences:

Revision

The elution order of these two isoenzymes, *light chain 3 followed by light chain 1*, is *the reverse* of that achieved by DEAE-cellulose chromatography of α-chymotryptic-digested S1. Similarly, the extent of separation is *reversed, the peak of light chain 1 being much better resolved than the peak of light chain 3*.

Note that putting the ideas in separate sentences also allows precise statement of what the differences in elution order and extent of separation are (italicized).

In the next example, three ideas are presented in one sentence: the purpose of the experiment, how the experiment was done, and a description of the patients. Furthermore, the description of the patients is nested inside the explanation of how the experiment was done.

Example 2.13   *(47 words)*

To study the mechanisms involved in the beneficial effects of hydralazine on ventricular function in patients who have chronic aortic insufficiency, a radionuclide assessment of ventricular function was performed in 15 patients with pure aortic insufficiency, functional capacity I or II, at rest and during supine exercise.

Revision A

To study the mechanisms involved in the beneficial effects of hydralazine on ventricular function in patients who have chronic aortic insufficiency, a radionuclide assessment of ventricular function was performed in 15 patients at rest and during supine exercise. All patients had pure aortic insufficiency and were in functional capacity I or II.

In Revision A, the description of the patients is presented in a separate sentence. However, it might be even better to put all three ideas in separate sentences, as in Revision B.

Revision B

Our aim was to assess the mechanisms involved in the beneficial effects of hydralazine on ventricular function in patients who have chronic aortic insufficiency. For this assessment, we did a radionuclide study of ventricular function in 15 patients at rest and during supine exercise. All patients had pure aortic insufficiency and were in functional capacity I or II.

In Revision B, the purpose is separated from the statement of what was done. In addition, the description of the patients is put in a separate sentence. Thus, each sentence talks about one thing, and the ideas are easier to understand.

In general, to avoid overloaded sentences, keep sentences as short as possible. A numerical guideline you can use is to have a mean sentence length of no more than 22 words per sentence. Note that this is a mean value. If you have two or three long sentences, balance them by writing a short sentence. The short sentence will have a strong impact, as you can see in Revision A above. To make this impact work to your advantage, put an important idea in the short sentence.

In papers that have especially difficult scientific content, short sentences are particularly important. The harder the science, the simpler the writing must be.

■ EXERCISE 2.3: OVERLOADED SENTENCES

In your own writing or in a journal article, find a sentence that has too many ideas packed into it and rewrite it as two or more simpler sentences.

Overloaded Sentence:

Revision:

BE SURE THAT THE ANTECEDENTS OF PRONOUNS ARE CLEAR

An antecedent is the word that a pronoun refers to. In Example 2.14, "methods" is the antecedent of the pronoun "they" and "conditions" is the antecedent of the pronoun "that."

Example 2.14 We used these <u>methods</u> because *they* enabled us to measure loss of microspheres under <u>conditions</u> *that* are normally used to assess blood flow.

If the antecedent of a pronoun is unclear, the reader may have trouble understanding the sentence. The antecedent of a pronoun can be unclear for at least two reasons.

More Than One Antecedent

One reason that the antecedent of a pronoun can be unclear is that the sentence may contain more than one possible antecedent.

Example 2.15 The presence of disulfide <u>bonds</u> in oligopeptides may restrict the formation of ordered <u>structures</u> in sodium dodecyl sulfate solution. Once *they* are reduced, the predicted conformation can be fully induced.

In this example, "they" is ambiguous. It could refer to either "bonds" or "structures," or even "oligopeptides." To make the meaning clear, the possible solutions are to revise the sentence structure or to repeat the noun. Here the simplest solution is to repeat the noun, as in the revision below:

Revision The presence of disulfide <u>bonds</u> in oligopeptides may restrict the formation of ordered <u>structures</u> in sodium dodecyl sulfate solution. Once <u>the bonds</u> are reduced, the predicted conformation can be fully induced.

Example 2.16 <u>Laboratory animals</u> are not susceptible to <u>these diseases</u>, so research on *them* is hampered.

In Example 2.16, the intended antecedent is "diseases." To make the sentence clear, one solution is simply to repeat "these diseases," as in Revision A.

Revision A Laboratory animals are not susceptible to <u>these diseases</u>, so research on <u>these diseases</u> is hampered.

Another solution is to change the sentence structure. The advantage of changing the sentence structure in this case is that the inelegant repetition of "these diseases" can be avoided.

Revision B Research on <u>these diseases</u> is hampered because laboratory animals are not susceptible to *them*.

In Revision B, "them" can refer only to "these diseases" because it is not reasonable for the object ("them") to refer to its own subject ("laboratory animals").

As this example demonstrates, one of the two solutions to an ambiguous sentence that has more than one antecedent will usually work.

No Antecedent

A second reason the antecedent of a pronoun can be unclear is that no antecedent is present. This situation occurs when the word "this" is used alone at or near the beginning of a sentence to refer to a concept implied in the previous sentence.

Example 2.17   Tyson et al. abruptly occluded the venae cavae before analyzing the heart beats. As a result of _this_, the volume of the right heart rapidly decreased.

In this example, the implied concept, and thus the antecedent of "this," is the occlusion procedure. To make the antecedent of "this" immediately clear, the solution is to write "this" followed by a category term implied by the details in the previous sentence. In this example, the detail "abruptly occluded" belongs to the category "procedure" (that is, occluding is a procedure), so a clearer way to write the beginning of the next sentence is "As a result of this procedure. . . ."

Revision A   Tyson et al. abruptly occluded the venae cavae before analyzing the heart beats. As a result of this procedure, the volume of the right heart rapidly decreased.

But even "this procedure" is not optimally clear. For greatest clarity, use the _tightest fitting category_. In this example, the tightest fitting category is not "procedure" but "occlusion," that is, the name of the specific procedure. Note that "occlusion" is simply the noun form of the verb "occluded" in the previous sentence. Using another form of the same word is always the tightest fitting category.

Revision B   Tyson et al. abruptly occluded the venae cavae before analyzing the heart beats. As a result of this occlusion, the volume of the right heart rapidly decreased.

Now that the meaning of "this" is clearly stated, the reader's job is much easier.

In summary, antecedents of pronouns can be unclear (1) if the sentence contains more than one antecedent and (2) if no antecedent is stated. The solutions for the first problem are either to restate the noun or to change the sentence structure. The solution for the second problem is to add the tightest fitting category term after the pronoun.

One other point worth noting is that antecedents of pronouns should be part of the text. Subtitles are not part of the text.

Example 2.18   Hearts.
Those used for this study were taken from 13 litters of newborn hamsters.

Revision   <u>Hearts</u>.
The <u>hearts</u> used for this study were taken from 13 litters of newborn hamsters.

Items in parentheses, including references, are not part of the text.

Example 2.19   In previous studies, fetal sheep responded to asphyxia with immediate femoral vasoconstriction, which was abolished by sciatic nerve section (8). However, despite nerve section, delayed vasoconstriction occurred, and <u>they</u> speculated that it resulted from circulating catecholamines.

Who are "they"?

Revision   In previous studies, fetal sheep responded to asphyxia with immediate femoral vasoconstriction, which was abolished by sciatic nerve section (8). However, despite nerve section, delayed vasoconstriction occurred, and <u>the investigators</u> speculated that it resulted from circulating catecholamines.

The point is that the text should make sense even if all subtitles and all items in parentheses are omitted.

■ *EXERCISE 2.4: CLEAR ANTECEDENTS OF PRONOUNS*

More Than One Antecedent

In the sentence below, the pronoun (underlined) could refer to more than one antecedent. Revise this sentence to make the meaning clear either by restating the noun or by changing the sentence structure.

1. To decrease blood volume by about 10% in a few minutes, blood was pooled in the subjects' legs by placing wide congesting cuffs around the thighs and inflating <u>them</u> to diastolic brachial arterial pressure.

No Antecedent

In the sentences below, the pronoun (underlined) has no stated antecedent. In addition, sentence 3 has more than one possible antecedent. Revise these sentences to make the meaning clear. Use the tightest fitting category.

2. After repeated ultracentrifugation, the apolipoprotein A-I content of high-density lipoproteins was reduced to about 65% of the original serum value, but no A-II was lost. <u>This</u> suggests that the binding environments of these two apolipoproteins in high-density lipoproteins differ.

3. A large bolus of contrast material decreases the relative error by producing a larger change in CT number. <u>This</u> is limited by the relative difficulty of administering a bolus and by the patient's tolerance.

PUT PARALLEL IDEAS IN PARALLEL FORM

Parallel ideas are ideas that are equal in logic and importance. Parallel ideas should be written in parallel form, either as a pair or as a series.

Pairs

The value of writing parallel ideas in parallel form is that the form of the first idea prepares the reader for the form of the next idea. As a result, readers can concentrate all of their attention on the ideas, not on the form.

Example 2.20 A   Cardiac output decreased by 10% but. . . .

This beginning creates an expectation. What do you expect to come next? In general, a contrasting idea. (This is the expectation created by "but.") Specifically, another variable and a contrasting action—no change, an increase, or a decrease by a different percentage. (This is the expectation created by the form of the beginning of the sentence.) Thus, you expect a sentence like one of these:

Example 2.20 B

Contrasts:

Cardiac output decreased by 10% BUT blood pressure was unchanged.
Cardiac output decreased by 10% BUT heart rate increased by 20%.
Cardiac output decreased by 40% BUT blood pressure decreased by only 10%.

| VARIABLE | ACTION | % | VARIABLE | ACTION | % |
| (subject) | (verb) | (completer) | (subject) | (verb) | (completer) |

Note that in all these examples the group of words after "BUT" is in the same form as the group of words before "BUT": subject (name of the variable), verb (how the variable acted), completer (percentage of change), if relevant.

These examples are contrasts, but other kinds of ideas can also be parallel.

Example 2.21

Similar Ideas: We hoped <u>to increase the complete response</u> AND <u>to improve survival</u>.

    Pattern: infinitive + object AND infinitive + object

Example 2.22

Alternatives: In dogs, about 20% of plasma glucose carbon is recycled via tricarbon compounds EITHER <u>in cold</u> OR <u>at neutral ambient temperature</u>.

    Pattern: EITHER prepositional phrase OR prepositional phrase

In this example, note that "in cold" and "at neutral ambient temperature" are in parallel form even though the specific prepositions ("in," "at") are different. All that matters for parallel form is that both items are prepositional phrases.

Example 2.23

Comparisons: <u>Pulmonary blood flow</u> WAS ALWAYS GREATER THAN <u>renal blood flow</u>.

Pattern: *noun WAS GREATER THAN noun*

Example 2.24

Comparisons: Cardiac output WAS HIGHER <u>in the experimental group</u> THAN <u>in the control group</u>.

Pattern: *WAS HIGHER prepositional phrase THAN prepositional phrase*

If parallel ideas are not written in parallel form, the logical relation of the ideas (similarity, alternatives, contrast, comparison) is obscured.

Example 2.25   This lack of response could have been due to damage of a cell surface receptor by the isolation procedure, but it could also be that isolated cells do not respond normally because the cells are isolated.

In this sentence, the groups of words before and after "but" are not parallel, so it is not immediately obvious that the second half of the sentence is giving another possible reason for the lack of response. (Note that "it" does not refer to "this lack of response.")

Revision A   This lack of response could have been due to damage of a cell surface receptor by the isolation procedure, but it could also have been due to the fact that isolated cells do not respond normally because they are isolated.

In this revision, the ideas before and after "but" are in parallel form, and "it" refers appropriately to "this lack of response." However, this sentence can be written more simply, as follows:

Revision B   This lack of response could have been due to damage of a cell surface receptor by the isolation procedure or simply to the fact of isolation, which could alter normal cell responses.

In this revision, the ideas are easier to understand because the repetition of "could have been due to" and one repetition of "isolated" have been omitted. In both revisions, the author's intention of presenting alternative reasons is clear because the ideas are written in parallel form.

Note that certain types of words indicate the need for parallel form. These are *conjunctions*, such as "and," "or," and "but," and *terms that indicate comparisons*, such as "greater than," "less than," and "different from." Whenever you write these conjunctions or terms, check to make sure that the ideas they link are in parallel form.

Three Problems in Writing Comparisons

Three problems arise in writing comparisons: overuse of "compared to," comparison of unlike things ("apples and oranges"), and absolute statements disguised as comparisons.

Overuse of "Compared To"

In comparisons containing a comparative term, such as "higher," "greater," "lower," "less," the accompanying term should be "than," not "compared to."

Example 2.26 We found a <u>higher</u> K_D at 37°C <u>compared to</u> 25°C.

Revision We found a <u>higher</u> K_D at 37°C <u>than at</u> 25°C.

Note the repetition of "at" in the revision for the parallel form.
"Compared to" should not be used with "decreased" or "increased" because the meaning is ambiguous.

Example 2.27 Experimental rabbits had a 28% <u>decrease</u> in alveolar phospholipid <u>as compared to</u> control rabbits during normal ventilation.

Did alveolar phospholipid decrease (A) in both experimental and control rabbits? (B) only in experimental rabbits? (C) in neither group?

A *Decrease in both groups*

Revision A Experimental rabbits had a <u>28% greater decrease</u> in alveolar phospholipid <u>than did</u> control rabbits. . . .

B *Decrease only in experimental rabbits*

Revision B Experimental rabbits had a <u>28% decrease</u> in alveolar phospholipid <u>but control rabbits had no decrease.</u> . . .

C *Decrease in neither group*

Revision C Experimental rabbits had <u>28% less</u> alveolar phospholipid <u>than did</u> control rabbits. . . .

In these revisions, the topic (alveolar phospholipid) is not the subject. The revisions below make the topic the subject.

Revision D Alveolar phospholipid <u>decreased 28% more</u> in experimental rabbits than in control rabbits.

Revision E Alveolar phospholipid <u>decreased by 28%</u> in experimental rabbits <u>but did not decrease</u> in control rabbits.

Revision F Alveolar phospholipid <u>was 28% less</u> in experimental rabbits than in control rabbits.

Because "decrease compared to" has at least three possible interpretations, "compared to" should not be used with "decreased" (or with "increased").

Comparison of Unlike Things

Although everyone is aware that "you cannot compare apples and oranges," such comparisons are common in scientific research papers.

Example 2.28 These <u>results</u> are similar to <u>previous studies</u>.

Revision A These <u>results</u> are similar to <u>the results of</u> previous studies.

Note that a pronoun ("that" or "those") can often be used to avoid repeating the noun:

Revision B   These <u>results</u> are similar to <u>those</u> of previous studies.

Example 2.29   Activation-controlled <u>relaxation</u> in these membrane-deprived cells **resembled** intact <u>myocardium</u> from frogs.

Revision   Activation-controlled <u>relaxation</u> in these membrane-deprived cells **<u>resembled</u> that in** intact myocardium from frogs.

When to Add "That" or "Those" to a Comparison.   To decide whether to add "that" or "those" (or to repeat the noun), determine whether the comparative term is all together in one spot or is split. (In Examples 2.28 and 2.29, the comparative terms, "are similar to" and "resembled," are all together in one spot.) If the comparative term is all together in one spot, "that" or "those" is needed. If the comparative term is split, "that" or "those" is not needed.

Example 2.30

Comparative term together: (add "that" or "those")	Losses at 34 min <u>were greater than</u> **those** at 4 min.
Comparative term split: (do not add "that" or "those")	Losses <u>were greater</u> at 34 min <u>than</u> at 4 min.

Absolute Statements Disguised as Comparisons

Absolute statements should not be written as if they were comparisons.

Example 2.31   This medium contains about 4-5 mM phosphate compared to Schneider's medium.

Actually, this medium contains about 4-5 mM phosphate *regardless* of the concentration of phosphate in Schneider's medium. The concentration is an absolute value and does not depend on any other concentration.

Revision   This medium contains 4–5 mM phosphate; Schneider's medium contains 9–10 mM phosphate.

If you want to compare the two concentrations, write the following sentence: "In this medium, the concentration of phosphate (4–5 mM) is about half that in Schneider's medium (9–10 mM)."

Series

In all the preceding examples, two terms are in parallel form, but more than two terms can be in parallel form, as in the following examples of parallel series.

Example 2.32   We   washed out   the lungs   five times with Solution I,
                          instilled   8–10 ml   of the fluorocarbon-albumin
                                                    emulsion into the trachea,
                   and   incubated   the lungs   in 154 mM NaCl at 37°C for 20
                                                    min.

Pattern: verb   +   object   +   completer

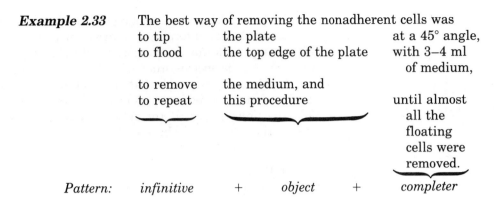

Example 2.33

The best way of removing the nonadherent cells was

to tip	the plate	at a 45° angle,
to flood	the top edge of the plate	with 3–4 ml of medium,
to remove	the medium, and	
to repeat	this procedure	until almost all the floating cells were removed.

Pattern: *infinitive*   +   *object*   +   *completer*

In a series, as in a pair, the form of all the parallel items must be the same. In Examples 2.32 and 2.33, the parallel items are all verbs ("washed," "instilled," " incubated") followed by objects and other completers, and infinitives ("to tip," "to flood," "to remove," "to repeat") followed by objects and other completers.

Two Problems of Parallelism

A frequent problem of parallelism is the confusion between a pair and a series. This confusion results in strange hybrids.

Example 2.34   The D225 modification contains 12.5 mg of cysteine HCl, 50 mg of methionine and has a final volume of 115 ml.

In this example, the first two values (12.5 mg, 50 mg) set up an expectation: we expect a third value after "and." Instead we get a verb ("has"). But "has" is not parallel to "12.5 mg" and "50 mg." Rather, "has" is parallel to "contains," and there is no third value parallel to 12.5 mg and 50 mg. To signal that there are only two values, "and" should be placed between the two values, as in Revision A (not a comma, as in the original version).

Revision A   The D225 modification contains 12.5 mg of cysteine HCl <u>and</u> 50 mg of methionine and has a final volume of 115 ml.

However, having two "ands" joining different levels of parallel items in one sentence is inelegant. To avoid this inelegance, a semicolon can be used in place of the second "and."

Revision B   The D225 modification contains 12.5 mg of cysteine HCl <u>and</u> 50 mg of methionine; <u>its final volume is 115 ml</u>.

Another problem of parallelism is the proper use of paired conjunctions. Paired conjunctions are "both . . . and . .," "either . . . or . . .," "neither . . . nor . . .," and "not only . . . but also. . . ."

Example 2.35   The mechanical response of heart muscles depends <u>on</u> BOTH the absolute osmolal increase AND <u>on</u> the species studied.

Revision: The mechanical response of heart muscles depends BOTH <u>on</u> the absolute osmolal increase AND <u>on</u> the species studied.

For parallel form, the group of words between "both" and "and" must be in exactly the same form as the group of words after "and." In the revision, both groups of words are prepositional phrases ("on the absolute osmolal increase," "on the species studied").

Another way to check that the sentence is in parallel form when paired conjunctions are used is to look just at the relative positions of the conjunctions and the prepositions. If the first conjunction (here "both") comes *after* the preposition ("on") and the second conjunction (here "and") comes *before* the preposition ("on"), that is,

<u>on</u> BOTH x
AND <u>on</u> $y,$

something is wrong. Either both conjunctions must come before both prepositions:

BOTH <u>on</u> x
AND <u>on</u> y

or the preposition must come only before the first conjunction:

<u>on</u> BOTH x
 AND $y.$

An Extra Advantage of Parallelism

In addition to being clear, an extra advantage of parallelism is that it allows you to avoid repetition.

Example 2.36 The young subjects could readily accommodate blood volume changes in other compartments, but the middle-aged subjects could not readily accommodate blood volume changes in other compartments.

Revision The young subjects could readily accommodate blood volume changes in other compartments, but the middle-aged subjects could not.

Example 2.37 Pulse rate **decreased** by 40 beats/min, systolic blood pressure **declined** by 50 mmHg, and cardiac output **fell** by 18%.

In Example 2.37, the authors thought that repeating "decreased" would be boring, so they used different verbs each time. But this variation of "decreased" detracts from the items that actually are different. To avoid boring repetition without succumbing to distracting variation, simply omit the second and third verbs:

Revision Pulse rate **decreased** by 40 beats/min, systolic blood pressure by 50 mmHg, and cardiac output by 18%.

Omitting these verbs works because the parallel form creates the expectation of repetition and thus strongly implies the omitted verbs.

■ *EXERCISE 2.5: PARALLELISM IN SENTENCES*

Correct the faulty parallelism in the following sentences. (Number 3 is tricky.)

Pairs

1. Cardiac output was less in the E. coli group than the Pseudomonas group.

2. Left ventricular function was impaired in the dogs that received endotoxin and the control dogs.

3. Pulsation of the cells or cell masses may be quick and erratic or may occur at fairly regular and leisurely intervals. (*What do you expect after "quick and erratic or"? Make your revision as simple as possible.*)

Series

4. The tubes were spun on a Vortex mixer for 10 s, stored at 4°C for 2 h, and then they were centrifuged at $500 \times g$ for 10 min.

5. Tracheal ganglion cells have been classified on the basis of their spontaneous discharge (12), according to their electrical properties (5), and whether vasoactive intestinal peptide is present or absent (8).

Hybrids

6. Phenylephrine increased the rate of mucus secretion, the output of non-dialyzable ^{35}S and caused a net transepithelial movement of Na towards the mucosa.

7. The fractions were centrifuged, resuspended in a small volume of buffer, and a sample of cells was counted in an electronic cell counter.

Paired Conjunctions

In your revision, do not omit the paired conjunctions, <u>underlined</u>.

8. Even the highest dose of atropine had no effect on <u>either</u> baseline pulse rate <u>or</u> on the vagally stimulated pulse rate.

9. An impulse from the vagus nerve to the muscle has to travel <u>both</u> through ganglia <u>and</u> post-ganglionic pathways.

10. The internal pressure must <u>not only</u> depend on volume <u>but also</u> the rate of filling.

■ *EXERCISE 2.6: PARALLELISM IN COMPARISONS*

Revise sentences 1 and 2 so that they use "than" instead of "compared to."

1. The greater stability in this study compared to the previous study resulted from more accurate marker digitization.

2. Total microsphere losses were greater at 34, 64, and 124 min when compared to 4 min.

Revise sentence 3 to avoid ambiguity.

3. We frequently observed a decrease in mean coronary arterial pressure compared to mean aortic pressure after carbochromen injection.

Revise sentences 4–6 so that they compare comparable things.
(Rule: Add "that" or "those" or repeat the noun when the comparative term is all together in one spot, but not when the comparative term is split.)

4. The loss of apolipoprotein A-I from high-density lipoproteins during ultracentrifugational isolation was greater than during other isolation methods.

5. Losses of apolipoprotein A-I during other isolation methods were smaller in comparison to ultracentrifugation.

6. Like subfragment 1, the protein composition of heavy meromyosin was homogeneous.

AVOID WRITING FLAWS

In addition to the five common writing problems explained above, there are five writing flaws to avoid. These flaws are (1) the subject and verb do not make sense together, (2) the subject and verb do not agree, (3) helping verbs are omitted, (4) modifiers are dangled, and (5) sentences containing information in parentheses do not make sense. When one of these flaws appears, the reader is slowed down and may even need to reread the sentence to figure out the intended meaning.

Be Sure That the Subject and Verb Make Sense Together

Example 2.38   The <u>appearance</u> of nondialyzable ^{35}S in the luminal bath **was measured**.

Can appearance be measured?

Revision A   The <u>amount</u> (OR concentration, rate of appearance, rate of secretion) of nondialyzable ^{35}S in the luminal bath **was measured**.

Revision B   The <u>appearance</u> of nondialyzable ^{35}S in the luminal bath **was noted**.

Be Sure That the Subject and Verb Agree (See Strunk and White, I.9.)

Example 2.39   The <u>esophagus, stomach, and duodenum</u> of each rabbit **was** examined.

Although "rabbit was" sounds right, the subject of the sentence is actually plural—"esophagus, stomach, and duodenum"—so the verb must be plural.

Revision   The <u>esophagus, stomach, and duodenum</u> of each rabbit **were** examined.

Do Not Omit Helping Verbs

Example 2.40   The <u>tissue</u> **was minced** and the <u>samples</u> **incubated**.

"Tissue" is singular, so "was minced" is the correct verb. But "samples" is plural, so carrying over the "was" is not grammatically correct.

Revision   The <u>tissue</u> **was minced** and the <u>samples</u> **were incubated**.

Example 2.41   Contrast medium **was infused** at a steady rate into the injection port, and the <u>flow</u> **calculated** from the observed change in CT number at equilibrium.

"Flow," like "contrast medium," is singular, so carrying over the singular helping verb "was" is grammatically correct. However, the second part of the sentence could be misread, because "calculated" could seem like an adjective ("flow that was calculated"), and the reader could get to the end of the sentence and still be waiting for the verb. To prevent misreading, it is clearest to repeat the helping verb.

Revision   Contrast <u>medium</u> **was infused** at a steady rate into the injection port, and the <u>flow</u> **was calculated** from the observed change in CT number at equilibrium.

Avoid Dangling Modifiers *(See Strunk and White, I.11.)*

Example 2.42   Blood flow was allowed to return to baseline before proceeding with the next occlusion.

In this sentence, blood flow seems to be proceeding with the next occlusion. The reason is that the first part of the sentence is passive, whereas the second part is active. Thus, "proceeding" dangles; that is, it has no noun to modify. The solutions are either to make both parts of the sentence active or to make both parts passive. In the active sentence, "proceeding" modifies "we." In the passive sentence, "proceeding" is omitted.

Revision A   We **allowed** blood flow to return to baseline before **proceed-**
(Active)   **ing** with the next occlusion.

Revision B   Blood flow **was allowed** to return to baseline before the next
(Passive)   occlusion **was begun**.

Example 2.43   In changing from a standing to a recumbent position, the heart expands noticeably in all directions.

In this sentence, "changing" dangles because it modifies an inappropriate noun. Thus, the heart appears to be changing from a standing to a recumbent position. For clarity, put the experimental subject or the experimental animal into the sentence.

Revision   When <u>the subject</u> changes from a standing to a recumbent position, the heart expands noticeably in all directions.

Be Sure That Sentences Containing Information in Parentheses Make Sense

Example 2.44   Pentobarbital (10^{-6} M) had no effect, 10^{-5} M slightly depressed the response, and 5×10^{-5} M almost abolished the response.

If the reader skipped over the information in parentheses, which is a legitimate reading technique, the sentence would not make sense. The point is that a certain *concentration* of pentobarbital did not have an effect, not that *pentobarbital* did not have an effect.

Revision   At 10^{-6} M pentobarbital had no effect, at 10^{-5} M it slightly depressed the response, and at 5×10^{-5} M it almost abolished the response.

Note the use of parallel form for the series of three items in the revision.

SUMMARY OF GUIDELINES FOR WRITING SIMPLE, DIRECT SENTENCES

Express the core of the message in the subject, verb, and completer.
> Make the topic the subject of the sentence.
> Put the action in the verb.

Do not pile nouns into noun clusters.

Do not pack too many ideas into one sentence.
> Do not string ideas together.
> Talk about one thing at a time.
> Aim for a mean sentence length of no more than 22 words per sentence.

Be sure that the antecedents of pronouns are clear.
> For a pronoun that has more than one possible antecedent, either restate the noun instead of using a pronoun or change the sentence structure.
> For a pronoun (usually "this") that has no stated antecedent, add the tightest fitting category term after the pronoun.

Put parallel ideas in parallel form.
> Make contrasts, similarities, alternatives, and comparisons parallel.
> Use "than" for comparisons, not "compared to."
> Do not compare apples and oranges.
>> When the comparative term is all together in one spot, add "that" or "those."
>> When the comparative term is split, do not add "that" or "those."
> Do not write absolute statements as comparisons.
> Do not confuse pairs and series.
> Use parallel form with paired conjunctions.
> Use parallel form to avoid repetition.

Avoid writing flaws.
> Be sure that the subject and verb make sense together.
> Be sure that the subject and verb agree.
> Do not omit helping verbs.
> Avoid dangling modifiers.
> Be sure that sentences containing information in parentheses make sense.

CHAPTER 3

PARAGRAPH STRUCTURE

Even if a paper has perfect word choice and perfect sentence structure, it can be difficult to understand if the paragraphs are not clearly constructed. Each paragraph must be constructed to tell a story. Readers should be able to follow the story of each paragraph whether or not they understand the science.

For a paragraph to tell a clear story,

- The ideas in the paragraph must be organized.
- The continuity, that is, the relationship between ideas, must be clear.

ORGANIZATION

A paragraph should have a topic sentence and logically organized supporting sentences. A *topic sentence* is a sentence that gives an overview of all the other sentences in a paragraph. This overview states either the topic or the point of the paragraph. *Supporting sentences* are sentences that say something specific about the topic or the point stated in the topic sentence. Supporting sentences should be organized in a logical way that best tells the story indicated by the topic or the point stated in the topic sentence.

The strategy of paragraph structure is to create an expectation (in the topic sentence) and then fulfill it (in the supporting sentences). Thus, the ideal position for a topic sentence is at the beginning of the paragraph so that readers will know what the paragraph is about before they read it.

In practice, not every paragraph must have a topic sentence. For example, the first paragraph of a Materials and Methods section in which animal experiments are described is often about the surgical preparation of the animals. This paragraph conventionally begins with a sentence something like this: "Twenty rabbits were anesthetized with. . . . " That is, the paragraph jumps right into the first step instead of using a topic sentence (such as "The rabbits were prepared for the experiments as follows"). Because the convention of beginning the surgical preparation paragraph by describing anesthesia is so strong, no topic sentence is needed. However, in the vast majority of paragraphs, providing a topic sentence is most helpful to the reader. Get in the habit of writing a topic sentence when you write a paragraph.

Examples 3.1–3.3 below all begin with a topic sentence. In addition, each paragraph is organized logically to tell the story of the point made in the topic sentence and thus to fulfill the expectation that the topic sentence creates.

Structure

A Topic sentence
B States first theory

C Explains a detail of B

D States second theory

E Explains a detail of D

F States third theory

Example 3.1

A There are three different theories put forward for the very slow relaxation of catch muscles of molluscs. *B* One theory holds that catch is due to some unusual property of myosin in these muscles that produces a slow rate of detachment (12). *C* In this theory, paramyosin would have no special role beyond that of providing the long scaffolding on which the myosin is positioned as well as the mechanical strength for the large tensions developed. *D* The second theory holds that tension is developed by actin-myosin interaction but is maintained by paramyosin interactions (13, 14). *E* Because the thick filaments are of limited length, interaction would have to occur through fusion of thick filaments (15). *F* A third theory, to which I subscribe, pictures a structural change in the paramyosin core affecting the rate of breaking of myosin-actin links at the filament surface (5, 16).

Example 3.1, which is from an Introduction to a journal article, has a topic sentence and logically organized supporting sentences. The point of the topic sentence is that three theories exist. The supporting sentences briefly describe each theory in turn. This sequence of descriptions fulfills the expectation created by "three different theories" in the topic sentence. The order for the three theories is not random, but proceeds from least to most important. That is, the *pattern of organization* is *enumeration of specifics from least to most important*. Thus, the author first describes the two theories she rejects and then describes the theory she accepts. The reasons for her rejection are implied in the extra sentence about each of the first two theories (sentences C and E). The rest of the paper goes on to explain the third theory at greater length.

Structure

A Topic sentence

B Assessment of distribution
  B₁ First step

  B₂ Second step
C Assessment of size and shape

D Explanation of a detail from C

Example 3.2

A To determine the distribution, size, and shape of ganglion cell bodies in the tracheal neural plexus, we examined individual cell bodies in their entirety at $100\text{–}400\times$ with a compound light microscope. *B₁* For the assessment of distribution, first each ganglion cell body that was stained by the acetylcholinesterase reaction product or that was bordered by acetylcholinesterase-positive ganglion cell bodies was classified according to its location in the tracheal neural plexus; *B₂* then the number of cell bodies in each ganglion was counted. *C* For the assessment of the size and shape of each ganglion cell body, the major (a) and minor (b) axes of the cell body were measured with a calibrated reticle in the eyepiece of the microscope, and, based on these dimensions, the mean caliper diameter, the volume ($\pi ab^2/6$), and the aspect ratio (a/b) were calculated. *D* Mean caliper diameter was calculated by the formula for a prolate ellipsoid of rotation as described by Elias and Hyde (1983).

In Example 3.2, which is from the Methods section of a journal article, the topic of the paragraph is how three variables (distribution, size, and shape) were assessed. The supporting sentences are organized in the same order as the variables are named in the topic sentence. That is, the *pattern of organization* is *enumeration of specifics in the announced order*. However, unlike Example 3.1, in which each theory was described separately, Example 3.2 describes only one variable separately and two variables (size and shape) together, because these two variables were assessed by the same measurements. Thus, the content is not forced into a preconceived structure or organized according to a preconceived principle; rather, the ideas are organized according to the content, that is, according to the way the assessment was actually done.

Note also that only one supporting sentence is needed to explain how distribution was assessed but that two sentences are needed to explain how size and shape were assessed. The second sentence about size and shape (D) explains a detail from the first sentence (C). Thus, the numbers of sentences used for each subtopic in a paragraph do not necessarily have to be the same. The length of an explanation, like the organization, depends on the content.

Structure

A Topic sentence
B, C Supporting evidence

D, E Exception

Example 3.3

A "Pulmonary" nerve endings were relatively insensitive to phenyl diguanide (table 1, fig. 3B). *B* Of 25 "pulmonary" nerve endings tested, only 10 were stimulated when this drug was injected into the right atrium, and in only one of these did firing exceed 2.2 impulses/s. *C* (If the latter ending be excluded, the average peak frequency of the endings stimulated was only 1.7 impulses/s.) *D* The exception, which fired with an average frequency of 17.4 impulses/s at the peak of the response, was encountered in the only dog in which right atrial injection of phenyl diguanide evoked reflex bradycardia within the pulmonary circulation time (latency 2.2 s). *E* Moreover, in this dog arterial pressure fell, whereas in all other dogs it rose, but only after sufficient time had elapsed for the drug to reach the systemic circulation.

In Example 3.3, which is from the Results section of a journal article, the point of the topic sentence is that "pulmonary" nerve endings were relatively insensitive. The supporting sentences are organized according to the type of evidence: first, evidence supporting the point; second, the exception that does not support the point. That is, the *pattern of organization* of this paragraph is *pro-con*. In a pro-con paragraph, the contradictory evidence could come either first or last. There is no single "correct" organization for this type of paragraph. The organization depends on the point you are making and the quality of the evidence you have.

Number and Position of Topic Sentences

So far we have been examining paragraphs that have only one topic sentence. However, a paragraph can have more than one topic sentence. Often a paragraph has two topic sentences—one at the beginning of the paragraph and one at the end. The first topic sentence can state either the topic or the point of the paragraph. The last topic sentence either states or restates the point of the paragraph (see the revision of Example 3.26 below).

Because the positions of prominence in a paragraph are the beginning (most prominent) and the end (second most prominent), the ideal positions for two topic sentences are the beginning and the end. However, it is not always possible to put the topic sentences at the beginning and the end. Sometimes a logical step is needed before the first topic sentence can be stated. And sometimes a supporting sentence is needed after the last topic sentence. As a result, the first topic sentence will be the second sentence in the paragraph, and the last topic sentence will be the second-to-last sentence in the paragraph. This situation is illustrated in Example 3.4.

Structure

A Finding and implication

Example 3.4

A Like Karoum et al. (21), we estimated the half-life of ganglionic dopamine to be considerably less than 1 h, which indicates a very rapid rate of turnover.

B Topic sentence (speculation based on A)

C Finding that supports B

D Finding used to interpret C

E Interpretation of C based on D

F Topic sentence (speculation restated)

G Support for F

B Although measures of total dopamine turnover cannot distinguish between the rates of turnover associated with SIF cells and principal neurons, from our results we suspect that this rapid rate of turnover is accounted for primarily by precursor dopamine in principal neurons. *C* We based this suspicion on our finding that within 1 h after injection of the synthesis inhibitor α-MT, and 40 min after injection of the synthesis inhibitor NSD-1015, the ganglionic dopamine content had dropped by about 60%, leaving some 7 pmol of dopamine that was resistant to further significant depletion for at least 3 h. *D* To interpret these data, we used Koslow's finding that approximately 40% of the dopamine in the rat superior cervical ganglion is stored in SIF cells (26). *E* Applying this figure to our measure of ganglionic dopamine (18 pmol/ganglion) would mean that about 7 pmol of dopamine is contained in SIF cells. *F* Therefore, we speculate that the 7 pmol of dopamine remaining 1 h after synthesis was inhibited represents SIF cell dopamine that is slowly turning over, whereas the 60% that is rapidly depleted represents precursor dopamine in principal neurons that is rapidly turning over. *G* This notion is consistent with reports which have shown that SIF cell catecholamines have a very slow turnover in the rat superior cervical ganglion (32, 41).

In Example 3.4, which is from the Discussion section of a journal article, the first sentence presents a finding and an implication of that finding. The implication is that the rate of dopamine turnover is rapid. The next sentence, which is the topic sentence of the paragraph, moves on from that implication by making a related point—that the rapid rate of turnover is probably accounted for primarily by precursor dopamine in principal neurons. Sentences C–E present the details that support this point. Sentence F is another topic sentence that restates the point more specifically. Sentence G supports sentence F by citing published findings.

It is also possible to view Example 3.4 as having three topic sentences: sentence A states the general topic (rapid rate of turnover); sentence B states the point (that the rapid rate of turnover is probably accounted for primarily by precursor dopamine in principal neurons); and sentence F restates the point more specifically.

Thus, it is not always possible to put the topic sentence in the ideal position. Still, the goal is to put the topic sentence at the beginning of the paragraph (if the paragraph has only one topic sentence) or at the beginning and the end (if the paragraph has two topic sentences), because these are the positions of prominence.

Patterns of Organization for Supporting Sentences

As we have seen in the examples above, one way that a paragraph can be organized is according to a standard pattern. The patterns that we have seen so far are *enumeration of specifics from least to most important* (Example 3.1), *enumeration of specifics according to the announced order* (Example 3.2), and *pro-con* (Example 3.3). We will examine other standard patterns later in this chapter (comparison-contrast and parallel structure) and also in the chapters on the Introduction (funnel), Materials and Methods (chronological order), and Results and Discussion (most to least important). These patterns occur frequently in scientific research papers. However, some paragraphs, particularly those in the Discussion section, are not organized according to a standard pattern but instead are organized according to the logic of the story the author wants to tell, as we saw in Example 3.4 above.

EXERCISE 3.1: PARAGRAPH ORGANIZATION

PART 1

Below are three versions of the same paragraph from a Results section. Which version is clearest? Why? What is wrong with the other two versions? If you do not like any of these versions, write a fourth version that is better.

Version 1

^AChanging the pH of the perfusion fluid from 7.4 to 6.9 or from 7.4 to 7.9 had no influence on either electrical potential difference or oxygen consumption. ^BLactate and pyruvate concentrations, however, decreased at pH 6.9, their ratio remaining unchanged. ^CAt pH 7.9, lactate concentrations increased significantly by one-third, whereas pyruvate concentrations decreased by approximately the same fraction, thus doubling the lactate-pyruvate ratio (Fig. 1).

Version 2

^AChanging the pH of the perfusion fluid from 7.4 to either 6.9 or 7.9 had no influence on either electrical potential difference or oxygen consumption. ^BHowever, it did affect lactate and pyruvate concentrations (Fig. 1). ^CAt pH 6.9, the concentrations were lower than those at pH 7.4, but the ratio remained unchanged. ^DAt pH 7.9, lactate concentrations were one-third higher than those at pH 7.4 and pyruvate concentrations were lower by about the same fraction, thus doubling the lactate-pyruvate ratio.

Version 3

^ADecreasing the pH of the perfusion fluid from 7.4 to 6.9 had no effect on either electrical potential difference or oxygen consumption, but it did decrease lactate and pyruvate concentrations, though without altering their ratio (Fig. 1). ^BIncreasing the pH of the perfusion fluid from 7.4 to 7.9 again had no effect on electrical potential difference or oxygen consumption, but it increased lactate concentrations by one-third and decreased pyruvate concentrations by about the same fraction, thus doubling the lactate-pyruvate ratio (Fig. 1).

Version # _____ is clearest.

Strengths of This Version: *Weaknesses of the Other Versions:*

PART 2

Below is a paragraph from a Results section in which the details in the supporting sentences (B–E) are not organized in the way that most clearly supports the topic sentence (A). The question is, how should the details in B–E be organized to best support the point made in A? To answer this question, we need to see that the paragraph is a comparison and contrast of the effects of two agents during two conditions—air infusion and recovery. A paragraph of comparison and contrast can be organized in any of three ways:

- *Whole by whole (here, all results for air infusion and then all results for recovery)*

- *Part by part (here, results for lymph flow, then results for the lymph-to-plasma protein concentration ratio, and finally, results for lymph protein clearance)*

- *Similarities and differences, or differences and similarities (here, all variables that changed and then all variables that did not change, or vice versa)*

1. *How is the paragraph below organized?*_____

   (To figure out the organization, write the topic of sentences B, C, D, and E in the margin and compare your topics with the three statements above.)

2. *How should this paragraph be organized to best support the point made in the topic sentence, that is, to carry out the organization that the topic sentence*

   implies? _____

3. *Revise the paragraph so that the supporting sentences clearly support the topic sentence. In your revision, (a) do not change the topic sentence; just reorganize the ideas in the supporting sentences; (b) make the logical sequence clear: lung lymph flow decreased; the lymph-to-plasma protein concentration ratio was unchanged; therefore, lymph protein clearance decreased; (c) avoid repetition.*

   (Note: "Lymph dynamics" in sentence A is the category term for lymph flow, lymph-to-plasma protein concentration ratio, and lymph protein clearance.)

*A*Both the alpha adrenergic agonist and the antagonist affected lung lymph dynamics slightly during the air infusion but not during recovery. *B*During the air infusion, the alpha agonist phenylephrine decreased lung lymph flow by 25%, whereas the alpha antagonist phentolamine had the opposite effect (Fig. 2). *C*During recovery, neither agent had a significant effect on lymph flow though lymph flow still tended to decrease after phenylephrine and to increase after phentolamine. *D*Neither agent changed the lymph-to-plasma protein concentration ratio either during the air infusion or during recovery. *E*Therefore, phenylephrine decreased lymph protein clearance during the air infusion and phentolamine increased it, but neither agent had any effect during recovery.

CONTINUITY

Even if a paragraph is well organized—that is, has a topic sentence and logically organized supporting sentences, the story of the paragraph can be difficult to follow if the paragraph does not have continuity. Continuity is the smooth flow of ideas from sentence to sentence (and from paragraph to paragraph). For a paragraph to have continuity, the reader must understand not merely what each sentence says but also *why* the author is writing each sentence, and why at this point in the paragraph. How does the sentence contribute to the story?

For example, in Example 3.1 above, sentence C begins "In this theory." If this introductory link were omitted, we would still understand what the rest of the sentence is saying, but we would no longer know why the author is saying it. That is, we would not see how sentence C relates to sentence B.

An explicit relationship between every pair of sentences is the essence of continuity. The next pages present prerequisites for continuity and several techniques for providing explicit links to create continuity between sentences.

Prerequisites for Continuity

Organized Ideas

Organization (see previous pages) is the basis of continuity. It is difficult, if not impossible, to have a smooth flow of ideas if the ideas are not organized.

No Missing Steps

In addition to the ideas being organized, all key steps in the logic must be presented if a paragraph is to have continuity.

Example 3.5

A As expected, serum glucose decreased to about 800 mg/dl by the sixth hour of insulin infusion. *B* It was elected to stabilize serum glucose at this level to allow for osmotic equilibration. *C* An estimate of net total body glucose per hour was made as follows: . . . .

This paragraph is difficult to follow because sentence C is not linked to sentence B: we do not know why the authors estimated net total body glucose.

Revision

A As expected, serum glucose decreased to about 800 mg/dl by the sixth hour of insulin infusion. *B* To allow for osmotic equilibration, we stabilized serum glucose at this level by adding to the fluid infusion an amount of glucose equivalent to the net loss of total body glucose. *C* We estimated net loss of total body glucose as follows: . . . .

In this revision, the missing step (underlined) that links serum glucose to total body glucose has been provided, thus making the paragraph easy to follow. This addition creates the continuity that was missing from the original version.

Techniques of Continuity

Once all the ideas are organized and all the steps are provided, several techniques can be used to link ideas, thus making the story easy to follow. These techniques include

1. Repeating key terms
2. Keeping a consistent order
3. Keeping a consistent point of view
4. Putting parallel ideas in parallel form
5. Signaling the subtopics of a paragraph
6. Using transitions to indicate relationships between ideas

Repeating Key Terms

Almost everyone remembers being told not to repeat the same word twice in a sentence, a paragraph, or some other unit. This advice is valuable for avoiding repetition of a word within a sentence, as shown in the second revision of example 1 in Exercise 2.4, which avoids repetition of "congesting cuffs." But this advice does not hold for key terms.

Key terms are words or phrases that name important ideas dealt with in a paragraph. Key terms can be either technical terms, such as "contractility" (as in Example 3.6 below), or nontechnical terms, such as "theories" (Example 3.1 above) or "decrease" and "increase" (Example 3.8 below). Repeating key terms from sentence to sentence is the strongest technique for providing continuity. For example, in the revision of Example 3.5, repetition of the key terms "serum glucose" and "net loss of total body glucose" holds the paragraph together. In Example 3.1 above, "theories," which appears in every sentence except E, is the main key term that holds the paragraph together. Other key terms that contribute to continuity in this paragraph are "catch" (sentences A and B), "muscles" (A, B), "myosin" (B, C, D, F), "paramyosin" (C, D, F), and "interaction" (D, E). In Example 3.2 above, the main key terms that link the sentences together are "distribution" (sentences A, B), "size" (A, C), "shape" (A, C), and "ganglion cell bodies/body" (A, B, C). In addition, "mean caliper diameter" links sentences C and D.

Repeat Key Terms Exactly. Repeating key terms from sentence to sentence links ideas unmistakably. Varying key terms is distracting, if not downright confusing.

Example 3.6

Digitalis increases the <u>contractility</u> of the mammalian heart. This change in <u>inotropic state</u> is a result of changes in calcium flux through the muscle cell membrane.

What is "inotropic state"? How does it relate to the previous sentence? The answer is that "contractility" and "inotropic state" mean the same thing. If no difference in meaning is intended, why use two different terms and risk confusing the reader?

Revision

Digitalis <u>increases</u> the <u>contractility</u> of the mammalian heart. This <u>increased contractility</u> is a result of changes in calcium flux through the muscle cell membrane.

In this revision, the continuity is clearer because the key term "contractility" is repeated exactly. In addition, the notion of increasing is repeated, rather than being generalized to "change." Repetition of two key terms makes the continuity even stronger.

Generally, using a synonym instead of repeating the key term does not work. Repeating key terms works like a knee-jerk reaction; no thinking is involved. Even if you do not speak the language, you can see that the word is the same. But using a synonym requires a mental manipulation and thus puts more of a demand on the reader. For example, in Example 3.2 above, changing "ganglion cell body" (sentence A) to "neuronal cell body" in sentence B would confuse some if not all readers, because readers might think that the different terms refer to different things. Thus, for clear continuity, the key term must be repeated exactly. This is not the place for creativity.

Repeat Key Terms Early in the Sentence.   Continuity is clearest if the key term is repeated early in the sentence. If the key term is delayed until the end of the sentence, the continuity is broken and the reader is kept in suspense temporarily, as in Example 3.7, which is a permutation of the revision of Example 3.6:

Example 3.7

Digitalis increased the contractility of the mammalian heart. Changes in the calcium flux through the muscle cell membrane cause this increased contractility.

The more delayed the repetition of the key term, the less obvious the continuity.

But won't this repetition of key terms be boring? To answer this question for yourself, please read the following excerpts from published papers.

Addition of the external resistor (1.37 cm $H_2O/(L/s)$) produced a marked increase in the real part and magnitude of impedance at all frequencies, a slight increase in the imaginary part, a phase curve that increased less rapidly with frequency, and a slight decrease in the resonant frequency. These changes are consistent with a significant increase in the total system resistance and a smaller increase in system inertance.

Did you notice the repetition of "increase" in this paragraph? Did it bother you?

Severe congenital valvar aortic stenosis is usually due to a grossly deformed aortic valve that will probably need complete replacement at some time. Nevertheless, when surgical relief is necessary in young children, a palliative valvotomy is usually preferred to valve replacement for two main reasons. The first is that the aortic valve annulus is often small, so any prosthetic or homograft valve either may be difficult to insert or will be small, and thus will almost certainly need to be changed as the child grows. The second reason is that none of the present artificial valves is likely to last a lifetime, so the longer aortic valve replacement is deferred, the more likely it is that a better valve will be available. Therefore, the simpler palliative operation is favored, especially in small children.

Did the repetition of "valve" in this paragraph bother you?

One way to avoid boring readers by too much repetition is to use a category term plus "this" or "these."

Example 3.8

Maximal coronary blood flow further decreased endocardial diameter and increased wall thickness during systole. <u>Both the decrease in systolic endocardial diameter and the increase in systolic wall thickness</u> were greater when the pericardium was closed.

Revision

Maximal coronary blood flow further decreased endocardial diameter and increased wall thickness during systole. <u>Both of these changes</u> were greater when the pericardium was closed.

Another way to avoid repetition is to condense the information. For example, in the Results section, you do not need to report every increase and every decrease—just the important ones.

When repetition of key terms seems excessive to you, keep in mind that as the writer you are more aware of repetition than the reader is. Most readers do not begin to notice a word until the third time they read it. So you do not have to start worrying about repetition being boring until the fourth time you use a word.

If you can do nothing to avoid repetition that seems boring to you, remember that the goal of scientific writing is clarity. If the choice is between boring readers and confusing them, bore them.

Do Not Use One Term for Two Meanings. Diametrically opposite to the use of different terms for conveying one meaning (or varying key terms) is the use of one term for conveying different meanings.

Example 3.9

. . . reduction of reduced glutathione. . . .

What does this phrase mean? "Reduced glutathione" must mean glutathione that has been deoxidized. Presumably "reduction" does not also mean "deoxidized" but "decreased." It is clearest to write "decrease in reduced glutathione," if that is what you mean.

Summary.   In summary, to link ideas clearly,

- Do not vary key terms. Repeat the key term, or use a category term plus "this" or "these," or condense the information.
- Do not keep the reader in suspense. Repeat the key term early in the sentence.
- Do not use one term to convey two different meanings. Use different terms to convey different meanings.

■ *EXERCISE 3.2: REPEATING KEY TERMS*

In the following paragraph from an Introduction, four key terms from the first two sentences—"blood products," "intracranial hemorrhage" "timing," and "method"—are not repeated in the third sentence, so the relation between the three sentences is not easy to see.

1. *In your revision, make the key terms the same throughout the paragraph.*

2. *In your revision, also try to clarify what "timing" and "method" mean, either by defining these terms or by changing them to other terms.*

*A*Blood products are used frequently in the care of sick preterm infants, but their use may increase the risk of intracranial hemorrhage. *B*Clinicians may be able to decrease the risk of intracranial hemorrhage by optimizing the timing and method of blood product administration. *C*We therefore studied the effects of the rapidity of volume expansion on cerebral blood flow and intracranial pressure in small preterm infants within the first 7 days after birth.

Keeping a Consistent Order

If you list two or more items in a topic sentence and then go on to describe or explain them in supporting sentences, *keep the same order*: if the items in the topic sentence are A, B, C, the supporting sentences should explain first A, then B, and last C. Thus, the reader's expectation is fulfilled. Furthermore, the supporting sentences should include all the items mentioned in the topic sentence and should not add any items *not* mentioned in the topic sentence.

To ensure that the reader knows you are talking about the same things in the supporting sentences as in the topic sentence, *repeat key terms exactly*.

In the supporting sentences, *avoid interrupting the sequence of explanations* with other information.

An example of a paragraph in which consistent order is used is Example 3.2 above. In Example 3.2, the topic sentence (A) mentions distribution, size, and shape of ganglion cell bodies. The next sentence (B) describes distribution, and the sentence after that (C) describes size and shape—the same order as in the topic sentence.

Another example is Example 3.10 below. In this example, the topic sentence lists three items clearly. The supporting sentences explain the three items in the same order as in the topic sentence and use exactly the same key terms. Unfortunately, other information had to be explained between the second and third items (sentences D and E explain the second item; sentence F prepares for the third item). This interruption makes the paragraph difficult to read because fulfillment of our expectation of hearing about the third item is so long delayed.

Example 3.10

^{A}Samples of **inspired, end-tidal**, and **mixed-expired** gases were taken during the 2-h wash-in period. ^{B}**Inspired** gas samples were collected proximal to the non-rebreathing valve. ^{C}**End-tidal** gas samples were collected through a catheter, the tip of which was placed near the tracheal end of the endotracheal tube. ^{D}The endotracheal tube was connected to the non-rebreathing valve with flexible <u>Teflon</u>® tubing whose internal volume was approximately <u>100 ml</u>. ^{E}<u>Teflon</u>® was used to avoid the absorption and release of anesthetic that occur with plastics such as polyethylene, and the added <u>100 ml</u> of dead space was used to prevent contamination of end-tidal samples with inspired gas. ^{F}Expired gases were conducted via a flexible Teflon® tube to an aluminum mixing chamber. ^{G}**Mixed-expired** gas samples were collected distal to the aluminum mixing chamber. ^{H}All gas samples were collected in 50-ml glass syringes that were stored upright (to produce a slight positive pressure) until analyzed.

In Example 3.10, note that consistent order is also used in sentences D and E for Teflon® and 100 ml.

■ *EXERCISE 3.3: REPEATING KEY TERMS AND KEEPING A CONSISTENT ORDER*

In the following example, key terms from paragraph 1 (protocol) are varied in paragraph 2 (results), so the relation between the two paragraphs is not easy to see.

1. Revise paragraphs 1 and 2, making the key terms the same in both paragraphs.

In addition, a topic is presented in paragraph 2 that does not appear in paragraph 1.

2. In your revision, present all topics and put them in the same order in both paragraphs.

The study protocol consisted of recordings of atrioventricular nodal and infranodal conduction times made during baseline, during right atrial overdrive pacing at progressively shorter coupling intervals, and during attempts to measure antegrade refractory periods by the extrastimulus technique.

There was no evidence of ventricular pre-excitation either during sinus rhythm or during atrial pacing. Atrioventricular nodal and infranodal conduction times were normal during sinus rhythm. Both during atrial overdrive and during measurement of antegrade refractory periods, atrioventricular nodal conduction time was suddenly prolonged.

Keeping a Consistent Point of View

In Chapter 2, we saw that the topic should be the subject of the sentence. Similarly, in a paragraph, if the topic of two or more sentences is the same, the subjects should be the same in all of those sentences. Having the same subject in two or more sentences that deal with the same topic is called keeping a consistent point of view.

Specifically, the point of view is consistent when the same term, or the same category of term, is the subject of successive sentences that deal with the same topic. The point of view is inconsistent when the topic is the same but the subjects of the sentences are different. An inconsistent point of view is disorienting to the reader.

Same Term.   Sometimes the same term should be the subject of successive sentences, as should be done in Example 3.11.

Example 3.11

*A*Propranolol had variable effects on the hypoxemia-induced changes in regional blood flow. *B*In the cerebrum, the increase in blood flow caused by hypoxemia was not significantly altered by propranolol. *C*However, in other organs, such as the gut and the kidneys, and in the peripheral circulation, propranolol caused a more severe decrease in blood flow than did hypoxemia alone.

In Example 3.11, all three sentences describe how propranolol (the independent variable) affected regional blood flow (the dependent variable), but only sentences A and C are written from the same point of view—the point of view of the independent variable. Sentence B is written from the point of view of the effect on the dependent variable.

The change in point of view is a problem for two reasons. First, a contrast is easiest to see if the two contrasting sentences (B, C) are written from the same point of view, that is, if the subjects of the two sentences are the same. Second, for the supporting sentences (B, C) to relate clearly to the topic sentence (A), they should be written from the same point of view (that is, they should have the same subject) as the topic sentence.

A consistent point of view in all three sentences makes this paragraph clearer and easier to read.

Revision

*A*Propranolol had variable effects on the hypoxemia-induced changes in regional blood flow. *B*In the cerebrum, propranolol did not significantly alter the increase in blood flow caused by hypoxemia. *C*However, in other organs, such as the gut and the kidneys, and in the peripheral circulation, propranolol caused a more severe decrease in blood flow than did hypoxemia alone.

Same Category of Term.   The subject does not always have to be the same word in order for the point of view to be consistent. Sometimes all that is necessary is the same category of word.

Example 3.12

The control injection of naloxone produced no significant changes in arterial blood pressure or heart rate. The arterial blood pressures and heart rates measured after 24 h of morphine infusion did not change significantly.

In Example 3.12, both sentences describe a cause and its effect, but the subject of the first sentence is the cause (control injection) whereas the subject of the second sentence is the variables affected (arterial blood pressures and heart rates). Thus, the point of view is inconsistent and the similarity is not easy to see. Both sentences should begin with the same category of term—the cause.

Revision A

The control injection of naloxone produced no significant changes in arterial blood pressure or heart rate. Twenty-four hours of morphine infusion produced no significant changes in arterial blood pressure or heart rate.

In the revision, the category of each subject is the same—the cause. Thus, the point of view is consistent and the similarity is easy to see. In addition, now that the point of view is consistent, it is easy to combine the two sentences:

Revision B

Neither the control injection of naloxone nor the 24-h morphine infusion significantly altered arterial blood pressure or heart rate.

As Example 3.12 (above) illustrates, keeping the point of view consistent is particularly important when you are making comparisons. Another example is given in Example 3.13. In this example, the authors describe others' findings from one point of view but then describe their own findings from the opposite point of view. As a result, it is difficult to tell whose findings the authors' findings agree with.

Example 3.13

Olsen et al. (22) concluded that series interaction was more important than direct interaction; Visner et al. (23), using a nearly identical preparation and protocol, concluded the opposite. We found that direct interaction was about one-half as important as series interaction in determining left ventricular volume at end diastole when the pericardium was on, and that the direct interaction effect decreased when the pericardium was removed.

Revision

Olsen et al. (22) concluded that direct interaction was less important than series interaction; Visner et al. (23), using a nearly identical preparation and protocol, concluded the opposite. We found that direct interaction was about one-half as important as series interaction in determining left ventricular volume at end diastole when the pericardium was on, and that the direct interaction effect decreased when the pericardium was removed.

In the revision, keeping a consistent point of view makes the similarity between the authors' work and Olsen et al.'s work easier to see.

To make the similarity explicit, and thus even easier to see, the authors could add an introductory phrase such as "Like Olsen et al.," or a general statement such as "Our results support the conclusion of Olsen et al." before the last sentence. But note that adding an introductory phrase or a general statement without keeping a consistent point of view would not work as well: "Olsen et al. (22) concluded that series interaction was more important than direct interaction; . . . Like Olsen et al., we found that direct interaction was about one-half as important as series interaction. . . ." Even though the similarity is announced, it is difficult to see because the point of view is not consistent.

Using "I" or "We."   It once was fashionable to avoid using "I" or "we" in scientific research papers on the grounds that these terms are subjective, whereas science is objective. But is science purely objective? Do not scientists make choices when designing experiments (when, how, how much)? Do not scientists define terms, make assumptions, have purposes, interpret results, make inferences? These are subjective actions. Thus, as the following examples illustrate, writing from the point of view of "I" or "we" is appropriate in a scientific research paper wherever judgment is exercised—generally, in the Introduction, Methods, and Discussion sections, and in the corresponding parts of the abstract.

Example 3.14

To determine the mechanism for the direct effect of contrast media on heart muscle mechanics, <u>this study</u> on heart muscles isolated from cats <u>was carried out</u>.

This sentence from an Introduction is dull and contains a dangling modifier (see Chap. 2; did the study or the authors determine the mechanism?).

Revision

To determine the mechanism for the direct effect of contrast media on heart muscle mechanics, <u>we carried out</u> this study on heart muscles isolated from cats.

Example 3.15

A nosocomial infection <u>was defined</u> as one that was clearly not present in the culture of any body fluid when the infant was admitted, although <u>it was recognized</u> that virtually all infant colonization, and therefore all infections, are nosocomial.

In this sentence from a Methods section, two acts of judgment are described: defining and recognizing. But who was making these judgments is not stated. Moreover, the author has gone out of his way to write the second point in a stiff, awkward, inelegant way: "it was recognized that." In contrast, "We recognized that" is direct, vigorous, and natural, and completely informative.

Revision

<u>We defined</u> a nosocomial infection as one that was clearly not present in the culture of any body fluid when the infant was admitted, although <u>we recognize</u> that virtually all infant colonization, and therefore all infections, are nosocomial.

Example 3.16

^A Acetylcholinesterase activity has been found in most ganglion cells of the myenteric and submucosal plexuses of the enteric nervous system, but differences have been found in the intensity of the acetylcholinesterase reaction, and ganglia have been classified accordingly (5). ^B Likewise, differences in the intensity of the acetylcholinesterase reaction <u>were found</u> in the ferret trachea. ^C However, the intensity of the reaction appeared to depend more on the ganglion cell's position and on the presence of overlying connective tissue than on acetylcholinesterase content. *D*Therefore, <u>no attempt was made</u> in this study to classify ganglion cells according to the amount of their acetylcholinesterase activity.

In sentence B of this paragraph from a Discussion section, it is not immediately obvious who found the differences in the ferret trachea. Upon reflection, the reader realizes it is the author of this paper, because this paper is about ferret tracheas. But reflection should not be necessary. Especially when you are discussing others' work in the same paragraph as your own, it is clearest to use "we" to identify your work. It would also be more natural to use "we" in sentence D.

Revision

*A*Acetylcholinesterase activity has been found in most ganglion cells of the myenteric and submucosal plexuses of the enteric nervous system, but differences have been found in the intensity of the acetylcholinesterase reaction, and ganglia have been classified accordingly (5). *B*Likewise, <u>we found</u> differences in the reactivity in the ferret trachea. *C*However, the intensity of the reaction appeared to depend more on the ganglion cell's position and on the presence of overlying connective tissue than on acetylcholinesterase content. *D*Therefore, in this study <u>we made no attempt</u> to classify ganglion cells according to the amount of their acetylcholinesterase activity.

Example 3.17

<u>It is concluded</u> that this method is a sensitive quantitative measure of lung interstitial fluid and can detect pulmonary edema and congestion in the dog lung before alveolar flooding occurs.

Revision

<u>We conclude</u> that this method is a sensitive quantitative measure of lung interstitial fluid and can detect pulmonary edema and congestion in the dog lung before alveolar flooding occurs.

The most controversial use of "we" is in the Methods section. The use of "we" in statements of judgment, as illustrated above, should not be controversial, but the use of "we" in the Methods section definitely is. The advantage of using "we" in Methods is that it makes for vigorous, readable writing because using "we" generally forces the author to use the active voice, which is inherently lively. The disadvantage of using "we" is that "we" is not usually the topic in Methods; rather, the variable or the technique is usually the topic. You cannot simultaneously have the advantage of "we" and avoid the disadvantage, so either using "we" or avoiding "we" in Methods is defensible. For an explanation and examples, see Chapter 5: Materials and Methods.

■ *EXERCISE 3.4: KEEPING A CONSISTENT POINT OF VIEW AND A CONSISTENT ORDER*

Example 1

Revise Example 1 so that the point of view is consistent.

AMortality in this series of patients was 90%. **B**Generally, survival in clinical series has been less than 20%. **C**The only exception to this is the experience of Boley (2), who reported a mortality of 46%.

Example 2

In Example 2, make both the point of view and the order of the details consistent.

AThe response produced by bradykinin alone usually consisted of a contraction followed by a longer lasting relaxation. **B**Adding indomethacin (2 μg/ml for 20–30 min) along with bradykinin reduced the magnitude of the relaxation to 7% of that induced by bradykinin alone. **C**The magnitude of the contraction, when one was present, was increased after treatment with indomethacin and bradykinin.

Example 3

Example 3 is difficult. To determine the best point of view in this example, ask yourself what the true topic is and make it the subject of the sentence. Also, put the action in the verb.

AThe greatest decrease in cardiac output in both groups occurred immediately after the injection of endotoxin. **B**Although both groups evidenced a recovery in output, the first group showed a greater return toward control values.

Putting Parallel Ideas in Parallel Form

Use Parallel Form for Parallel Ideas.   Parallel form is a subset of consistent point of view. For sentences to have a consistent point of view, the subjects of the sentences must be the same term or the same category of term. For sentences to be parallel, the entire pattern of one sentence must be the same as the pattern of the companion sentence(s). This use of parallel form for sentences within a paragraph is an extension of the use of parallel form for items in pairs or in series within a single sentence (see Chap. 2). In paragraphs, using parallel form for consecutive sentences is a standard pattern of organization. Parallel organization is particularly effective for presenting contrasting ideas, as shown in the last two sentences of Example 3.18.

Example 3.18

*A*The $\log_{10}$ function eliminated some waves. *B*The factor that determined whether a wave was eliminated or amplified was the divisor. *C*When the divisor was greater than the absolute value of the peak of a wave, the wave was eliminated. *D*When the divisor was less than the absolute value of the peak of a wave, the wave was amplified.

In Example 3.18, the last two sentences are parallel sentences that support the point made in the topic sentence (sentence B). Note that in the parallel sentences, the sentence patterns are the same: subject ("the divisor"), verb ("was"), completer ("greater than X," "less than X"); subject ("the wave"), verb ("was eliminated," "was amplified"). Furthermore, because these sentences describe a contrast, the terms used are opposites: "greater," "less"; "eliminated," "amplified."

Parallelism within a paragraph can be longer than two sentences, as illustrated in Example 3.19.

Example 3.19

*A*After fetal injection of naloxone, fetal arterial blood pH and P_{O_2} both decreased (from 7.39 ± 0.01 (SD) to 7.35 ± 0.02 and from 23.0 ± 0.5 to 20.8 ± 0.8 mmHg, respectively). *B*There was no change in arterial blood P_{CO_2}. *C*After maternal injection of naloxone, only fetal arterial blood P_{O_2} decreased (from 24.4 ± 0.8 to 22.2 ± 1.0 mmHg). *D*There were no significant changes in fetal arterial blood pH or P_{CO_2}.

The paragraph in Example 3.19 is organized into two parallel subtopics. The first subtopic (sentences A and B)—the effects of fetal injections—is parallel to the second subtopic (sentences C and D)—the effects of maternal injections. Within each subtopic, the first sentence is about the variables that changed; the second sentence is about the variables that did not change. Thus, sentences A and C (variables that changed) are written in one parallel form ("After fetal/maternal injection of naloxone, Q decreased"), and sentences B and D (variables that did not change) are written in another parallel form ("There was/were no change(s) in R").

As these examples show, using parallel form to organize sentences within a paragraph is the clearest way of presenting parallel ideas.

Make the Verbs Parallel.   An important factor for parallelism is that the verbs must be either the same (when the ideas are similar) or the opposite (when the ideas contrast). In Example 3.18, sentences C and D present contrasting ideas, and the verbs are appropriately opposites: "was eliminated," "was amplified." In Example 3.19, sentences A and C present similarities; so do sentences B and D. The verbs are therefore the same: "decreased" (A and C); "was," "were" (B and D).

Corollary: Do Not Use Parallel Form for Nonparallel Ideas. For parallel form to be an effective pattern of organization, it must be reserved only for parallel ideas. Nonparallel ideas should not be written in parallel form.

Example 3.20

To determine whether cholinergic or adrenergic nerves mediate secretion of fluids from tracheal submucosal glands, <u>we did</u> experiments on glands excised from ferrets. **To induce** secretion, <u>we stimulated</u> the tissue both electrically and pharmacologically. **To inhibit** secretion, <u>we added</u> XXXX to the bathing solution.

In this paragraph, three sentences are in parallel form (the pattern is infinitive + object, subject + verb + object). But the ideas are not parallel. The first sentence gives the overall purpose of the study and the general type of experiment done. The second and third sentences give specific purposes and procedures. Therefore, the ideas in the second and third sentences should be expressed in a different form.

Revision A

<u>To determine</u> whether cholinergic or adrenergic nerves mediate secretion of fluids from tracheal submucosal glands, we did experiments on glands excised from ferrets. <u>We induced secretion</u> by stimulating the tissue both electrically and pharmacologically. <u>We inhibited secretion</u> by adding XXXX to the bathing solution.

Revision A shows one way to revise this paragraph to avoid putting nonparallel ideas in parallel form. Note that the last two sentences, which express parallel ideas, are still in parallel form.

Revision B

We wanted to determine whether cholinergic or adrenergic nerves mediate secretion of fluids from tracheal submucosal glands. To do this, we studied the secretory responses to <u>electrical and pharmacological</u> stimulation of segments of ferret trachea in vitro <u>in the presence</u> and <u>in the absence</u> of <u>a specific nerve blocker</u> and <u>autonomic antagonists</u>.

In Revision B, the ideas of the second and third sentences have been reorganized so that parallel form is used only within the last sentence (see underlined words), not as a means of organizing the sentences. This is fine. The important point is that the two sentences, which do not give parallel information, are not in parallel form.

Signaling the Subtopics of a Paragraph

Signaling Subtopics Announced in the Topic Sentence. We saw at the beginning of this chapter that ideally a paragraph should begin with a topic sentence so that readers know what the paragraph is about before they read it. Similarly, each subtopic in the paragraph should be signaled as soon as that subtopic begins so that readers will know what the subtopic is before they start reading about it. The signals should be both visual and verbal. A new topic is signaled visually by a new paragraph and verbally by a topic sentence. A new subtopic within a paragraph is signaled visually by a new sentence and verbally by putting the name of the subtopic in a key term or a transition phrase at the beginning of that sentence. Signals of the topic and subtopics are illustrated in Example 3.21, which we first examined at the beginning of this chapter (Example 3.1).

Example 3.21

*A*There are **three different theories** put forward for the very slow relaxation of catch muscles of molluscs. *B***One theory** holds that catch is due to some unusual property of myosin in these muscles that produces a slow rate of detachment (12). *C*In this theory, paramyosin would have no special role beyond that of providing the long scaffolding on which the myosin is positioned as well as the mechanical strength for the large tensions developed. *D***The second theory** holds that tension is developed by actin-myosin interaction but is maintained by paramyosin interactions (13, 14). *E*Because the thick filaments are of limited length, interaction would have to occur through fusion of thick filaments (15). *F***A third theory**, to which I subscribe, pictures a structural change in the paramyosin core affecting the rate of breaking of myosin-actin links at the filament surface (5, 16).

In Example 3.21, the topic of the paragraph (three different theories) is signaled visually by the new paragraph and verbally by the topic sentence (A). The three subtopics are signaled visually by the new sentences B, D, and F, which are the first sentences that deal with each subtopic, and verbally by having the name of each subtopic at the beginning of that sentence: "One theory," "The second theory," "A third theory."

Signaling Subtopics = Signaling the Organization. In Example 3.21, note that the topic sentence implies that the paragraph will be organized by enumeration. That is, "there are three different theories" implies that the paragraph will describe each of the three theories in turn. This implied organization is carried out in the supporting sentences and is signaled by the key terms that name the subtopics: B, "One theory," D, "The second theory," F, "A third theory." Thus, by signaling the subtopics, you are also signaling the organization of the paragraph.

Signaling Subtopics Not Announced in the Topic Sentence. Even if the topic sentence does not name more than one topic, the paragraph might contain a subtopic, as in Example 3.22. In this case, it is especially important to signal the subtopic by naming the subtopic at the beginning of the sentence, since the topic sentence does not prepare us to expect any subtopics.

Example 3.22

*A***"Pulmonary" nerve endings** were relatively insensitive to phenyl diguanide (table 1, fig. 3B). *B*Of 25 **"pulmonary" nerve endings** tested, only 10 were stimulated when this drug was injected into the right atrium, and in only one of these did firing exceed 2.2 impulses/s. *C*(If the latter **ending** be excluded, the average peak frequency of the endings stimulated was only 1.7 impulses/s.) *D***The exception**, which fired with an average frequency of 17.4

impulses/s at the peak of the response, was encountered in the only dog in which right atrial injection of phenyl diguanide evoked reflex bradycardia within the pulmonary circulation time (latency 2.2 s). *E*Moreover, in this dog arterial pressure fell, whereas in all other dogs it rose, but only after sufficient time had elapsed for the drug to reach the systemic circulation.

In Example 3.22, the topic sentence at the beginning of the new paragraph names the topic of the paragraph in the first three words—"pulmonary" nerve endings—and then states the point: were relatively insensitive. The next two sentences (B, C) support this point. However, the last two sentences (D, E) are about a new subtopic—an exception that does not support the point. This new subtopic is signaled visually by starting a new sentence (D) and verbally by putting the topic, "the exception" (key term), at the beginning of the sentence.

Signaling the Organization (Subtopics) in Paragraphs That Have No Topic Sentence. Signaling the organization in paragraphs that have no topic sentence is tricky. The problem is that two signals are needed at the beginning of the paragraph—a signal of the topic of the paragraph and a signal of the first subtopic. It is impossible to put both signals first, so one of the signals will be weak, as shown in Example 3.23.

Example 3.23

*A***Blood flow to the serum-instilled lung** decreased **in the control experiments** to 20% of baseline values and did not change over 4 h (Figure 3). *B*In contrast, **after beta adrenergic agonists**, blood flow decreased less (to about 75% of baseline). *C*Furthermore, the blood flow recovered to baseline levels by 2 h, and at 4 h was even slightly above baseline. *D***After intravenous nitroprusside**, blood flow to the serum-instilled lung was similar to blood flow after beta adrenergic agonists.

In Example 3.23, the topic of the paragraph is blood flow to the serum-instilled lungs. The paragraph is organized according to the independent variable: sentence A, control experiments; B–C, beta adrenergic agonists; D, intravenous nitroprusside. The topic of the paragraph is signaled by putting the key term ("blood flow to the serum-instilled lung") at the beginning of the first sentence. Consequently, the signal of the organization of the paragraph ("in the control experiments") must come later in the sentence and therefore is weak, if not entirely useless. To function as a signal, the term or phrase must appear at the beginning of the sentence. However, if the author had put "in the control experiments" at the beginning of sentence A, the signal of the topic of the paragraph would have been lost. The solution is to add a topic sentence.

Revision

*A*Both beta adrenergic agonists and nitroprusside inhibited the decrease in pulmonary blood flow that occurred after instillation of serum. *B***After serum alone** (control), blood flow to the serum-instilled lung decreased to 20% of baseline values and did not change over 4 h (Figure 3). *C*In contrast, **after beta adrenergic agonists**, blood flow decreased less (to about 75% of baseline). *D*Furthermore, the blood flow recovered to baseline levels by 2 h, and at 4 h was even slightly above baseline. *E***After intravenous nitroprusside**, blood flow to the serum-instilled lung was similar to blood flow after beta adrenergic agonists.

Now that a topic sentence has been added, the topic sentence signals the topic of the paragraph and the introductory phrases at the beginning of sentences B, C, and E (boldfaced) signal the organization. In addition, because the subject of the topic sentence is the independent variable, the topic sentence implies that the paragraph will be organized according to the independent variable.

Signaling Parallel Subtopics.   When the subtopics in a paragraph are parallel, the signals of the subtopics should also be parallel. These parallel signals should indicate how the paragraph is organized. For example, in Example 3.23, the parallel signals of the subtopics are "in the control experiments," "after beta adrenergic agonists," and "after intravenous nitroprusside." Thus, this paragraph is organized according to the independent variable. In Example 3.18, the parallel signals are "When the divisor was greater. . . " and "When the divisor was less. . . ." The paragraph is organized according to the magnitude of the divisor. In Example 3.19, there are two levels of organization—one primary and the other secondary. The primary organization is which animal received the injection, and the primary organization is signaled by "after fetal injection of naloxone" (sentence A) and "after maternal injection of naloxone" (sentence C). Within each of these primary subtopics, the secondary organization is which variables changed. Variables that changed are described first (sentences A and C); variables that did not change are described second (sentences B and D). No signal is needed for the secondary organization here. However, if this paragraph were expanded by the addition of several more sentences on each subtopic, the secondary organization would need to be signaled, just as the primary organization is.

The Duration of a Signal.   When a subtopic is signaled at the beginning of a sentence, the signal holds until you change it. Thus, in Example 3.23, the subtopic of sentence B ("after beta adrenergic agonists") carries over to sentence C. That is, we know that recovery of blood flow to baseline levels took place after beta adrenergic agonists were given. Similarly, the topic of the entire paragraph—blood flow to the serum-instilled lung—holds throughout the paragraph. Even though the serum-instilled lung is not mentioned in sentences B and C, we understand that the paragraph is still talking about blood flow to the serum-instilled lung. Thus, signaling the topic and subtopics (that is, the organization) of a paragraph is a powerful tool for creating continuity in a paragraph.

Summary

- The topic of a paragraph can be signaled visually by beginning a new paragraph and verbally by stating the topic or the point in a topic sentence at the beginning of the paragraph.
- Subtopics within a paragraph can be signaled visually by beginning a new sentence and verbally by naming the subtopic in a key term or an introductory phrase at the beginning of the sentence.
- If the subtopics are parallel, the signals should be parallel and should indicate how the paragraph is organized.
- If the signal of a topic or subtopic is placed at the beginning of the paragraph or the sentence, it holds until a new signal appears.

■ EXERCISE 3.5: PARALLEL FORM AND SIGNALING SUBTOPICS

1. Parallelism in Two Sentences; Signaling Subtopics

a. *Rewrite the following paragraph from a Results section so that both the content and the form are parallel. (Thus, the point of view will be consistent; that is, the subjects of the sentences will be the same.) Add or omit content if necessary. One approach is to ask yourself what you expect after reading the first sentence and the first four words of the second sentence.*

b. *Signal the subtopics by putting either a key term or an introductory phrase that names the subtopic at the beginning of each sentence.*

c. *Below your revision, identify the signal of the subtopics and the point of view that you used. (The point of view = the subject of the sentence.)*

d. *Make the last sentence make sense.*

Note: Control conditions = before conversion.

In rat papillary muscle, caffeine (3 mM) converted load-sensitive relaxation (Fig. 1A, B) to load-insensitive relaxation (Fig. 1C, D). In cat papillary muscle, under control conditions (Fig. 2A, B), relaxation was sensitive to load. In contrast to the response in rat papillary muscle, the addition of 3 mM caffeine to cat papillary muscle (Fig. 2C, D) even at concentrations of 5 mM (Fig. 3A, B) or 10 mM failed to eliminate the load sensitivity of relaxation.

Signal of the subtopics: ───────────────────────────────

Point of view: ───────────────────────────────

2. Parallelism in More Than Two Sentences

In the paragraph below, sentences B and C are on one subtopic (tracheal segments fixed in Bouin's fixative) and sentences D and E are on another subtopic (tracheal segments fixed in 0.2% glutaraldehyde). Sentences B and D present parallel ideas and are written in parallel form. Sentences C and E also present parallel ideas, but they are not written in parallel form.

Revise so that sentences C and E are in parallel form.

ATracheal segments were placed either in Bouin's fixative for 24 h at room temperature or in 0.2% glutaraldehyde in 0.08 M cacodylate buffer (pH 7.5) for 1 h at 4°C. **B**Tracheal segments fixed in Bouin's fixative were dehydrated in graded ethanol solutions, cleared in alpha-terpineol, and embedded in paraffin. **C**Paraffin-embedded tissues were sectioned at 7 μm with a rotary microtome (American Optical). **D**Tracheal segments fixed in 0.2% glutaraldehyde were dehydrated in graded acetone solutions and embedded in araldite (Polysciences). **E**Thick sections (1 μm) were cut with an ultramicrotome (Porter-Blum MT-1).

3. Preserving Parallel Form

The paragraph below is the same as Example 3.19. The author now wants to include a statement about the maternal responses to naloxone. The maternal responses were that none of the variables changed after either fetal or maternal injections of naloxone. Revise this paragraph, adding the maternal responses without destroying the parallel form or the signals of the topics.

AAfter fetal injection of naloxone, fetal arterial blood pH and P_{O_2} both decreased (from 7.39 $\pm$ 0.01 (SD) to 7.35 $\pm$ 0.02 and from 23.0 $\pm$ 0.5 to 20.8 $\pm$ 0.8 mmHg, respectively). **B**There was no change in arterial blood P_{CO_2}. **C**After maternal injection of naloxone, only fetal arterial blood P_{O_2} decreased (from 24.4 $\pm$ 0.8 to 22.2 $\pm$ 1.0 mmHg). **D**There were no significant changes in fetal arterial blood pH or P_{CO_2}.

Using Transitions to Indicate Relationships

When you are writing a paragraph, you have a reason for putting one sentence after another. The reader needs to know what that reason is. In some cases the reason is obvious. For example, the second sentence of Example 3.22 obviously gives evidence for the assertion made in the first sentence: "'Pulmonary' nerve endings were relatively insensitive to phenyl diguanide (table 1, fig. 3B). Of 25 'pulmonary' nerve endings tested, only 10 were stimulated when this drug was injected into the right atrium, and in only one of these did firing exceed 2.2 impulses/s."

If the reason for putting one sentence after another is not obvious, you need to indicate the reason. The technique for indicating how sentences (or parts of sentences) are related is transitions. Transitions can be words or phrases.

Transition Words. Transition words are standard terms that indicate standard logical relationships. Examples include "therefore" and "thus" (conclusions), "because" and "since" (cause or reason), "for example" (example), "first" (sequence), "in addition" (addition), and "in contrast" and "however" (contrast). Note that transition "words" actually include standard phrases, such as "for example," "in addition," "in contrast," and even "on the other hand."

To see how important transition words are in guiding your understanding of sentences and paragraphs, read each of the following examples both with and without the underlined words.

Example 3.24

Relationship

Transition Words Within a Sentence

reason

The lymphocytes that infiltrate the alveolar walls in this rejection phase are likely to be conveyed by the blood, because they infiltrate all alveolar walls synchronously all over the lungs.

consequence

Both of these high-density-lipoprotein-associated proteins are initially synthesized as proteins and therefore undergo both co- and post-translational proteolysis.

concession

Although individual residues in the repeated-sequence blocks in the core have diverged, the patterns of amino acids are identical.

Transition Words Between Sentences

By widening our focus to the entire trachea, we were able to see that most ganglion cell bodies (72%) are located in the neural plexuses associated with the trachealis muscle and submucosal glands, and only a small proportion (28%) are located along the longitudinal nerve trunks. Furthermore, we were

addition

able to see that most of the ganglia in the superficial muscle and gland plexuses

conclusion

contain only 1–4 ganglion cell bodies (average, 2.8 ganglion cell bodies). Thus, previously reported ganglia along the longitudinal nerve trunk that contain 10–20 ganglion cell bodies are not typical of most tracheal ganglia.

Transition phrases. Transition phrases are nonprefabricated phrases that indicate either standard or nonstandard relationships between sentences. For example, to indicate cause-effect (a standard relationship), instead of the standard transition word "because," which would be used within a sentence, you can use a transition phrase such as "The reason is" or "This effect occurs because" at the beginning of a new sentence. An example of a nonstandard relationship that is indicated by a transition phrase is given in Example 3.25. The transition phrase is "in this theory."

Structure

A Topic sentence
B States first theory

C Explains a detail of B

D States second theory

E Explains a detail of D

F States third theory

Example 3.25 Transition Phrase in a Paragraph

A There are three different theories put forward for the very slow relaxation of catch muscles of molluscs. *B* One theory holds that catch is due to some unusual property of myosin in these muscles that produces a slow rate of detachment (12). *C* In this theory, paramyosin would have no special role beyond that of providing the long scaffolding on which the myosin is positioned as well as the mechanical strength for the large tensions developed. *D* The second theory holds that tension is developed by actin-myosin interaction but is maintained by paramyosin interactions (13, 14). *E* Because the thick filaments are of limited length, interaction would have to occur through fusion of thick filaments (15). *F* A third theory, to which I subscribe, pictures a structural change in the paramyosin core affecting the rate of breaking of myosin-actin links at the filament surface (5, 16).

In this paragraph, "in this theory" shows that sentence C explains a detail of sentence B. Without this transition phrase, it is difficult to tell how sentence C is related to sentence B. (Try reading sentences A–C without "in this theory.")

Other examples of transition phrases are given in the revision of Example 3.23 above ("after serum alone," "after beta adrenergic agonists," "after intravenous nitroprusside," which were called introductory phrases) and in Examples 3.27 and 3.28 in "Displaying Your Thinking" later in this chapter.

Placement of Transitions.   As illustrated in the examples above, transition words and phrases that link sentences should come at the beginning of the sentence. Putting the transition first indicates the logic of the idea that is to follow. Thus, before we read the sentence, we know that the sentence will present an additional idea ("furthermore"), a conclusion ("thus"), an explanation of a detail ("in this theory"), or whatever.

If you need to put both a transition and a signal of a subtopic at the beginning of a sentence, put the transition first. For example, "In fetal lambs, . . . However, in human fetuses, . . ."

■ EXERCISE 3.6: THE VALUE OF TRANSITIONS

Below are three versions of two sentences from a Methods section. For each version, state (1) what the logical relationship of the second sentence to the first sentence is and (2) how you know what the relationship is.

Version 1

The microspheres were prepared for injection as previously described (2). <u>They were then suspended</u> in 1 ml of dextran solution in a glass injection vial that was connected to the appropriate catheter and to a syringe containing 4 ml of saline.

Relationship:

How You Know:

Version 2

The microspheres were prepared for injection as previously described (2). <u>In brief, they were suspended</u> in 1 ml of dextran solution in a glass injection vial that was connected to the appropriate catheter and to a syringe containing 4 ml of saline.

Relationship:

How You Know:

Version 3

The microspheres were prepared for injection as previously described (2). <u>They were suspended</u> in 1 ml of dextran solution in a glass injection vial that was connected to the appropriate catheter and to a syringe containing 4 ml of saline.

Relationship:

How You Know:

■ *EXERCISE 3.7: THE MEANING OF SOME TRANSITION WORDS*

The sentences in the left-hand column illustrate clear, unambiguous uses of three common transition words—"and," "while," and "as." In the sentences in the right-hand column, these same words are used imprecisely and ambiguously. Supply precise, unambiguous transition words for the imprecise, ambiguous ones.

Clear, Unambiguous

a. No subject required chronic medication for asthma, _and_ no subject had had symptoms of a respiratory infection within 4 weeks of the beginning of the study.

b. We measured airway resistance and thoracic gas volume _while_ each subject sat in a constant-volume whole-body plethysmograph.

c. Asthmatic subjects develop bronchoconstriction after breathing sulfur dioxide in concentrations _as_ low _as_ 1 ppm at rest.

d. _As_ minute ventilation increases, oral ventilation increases faster than nasal ventilation.

Imprecise, Ambiguous

1. Nicotinic receptors have a widespread distribution in the peripheral nervous system, _and_ the response to nicotinic drugs should be interpreted with caution.

   Change _and_ to _____

2. The pH was 7.4 and the P_{CO_2} was 35 mmHg, _while_ the average P_{O_2} was 525 mmHg.

   Change _while_ to _____

3. High titer antibody to extractable nuclear antigen that is sensitive only to RNase is found uniformly in patients who have mixed connective tissue disease _while_ it is relatively uncommon in patients who have scleroderma or systemic lupus erythematosus.

   Change _while_ to _____

4. _As_ we found no changes in arterial blood gases or pH during continuous positive airway pressure up to 1.0 kPa, it is not likely that the change in respiratory rhythmicity during continuous positive airway pressure is an effect of chemoreceptor stimulation, as proposed by Kattwinkel et al. (5).

   Change _As_ to _____

TELLING THE STORY: STATING THE MESSAGE AND DISPLAYING YOUR THINKING

So far in this chapter, we have been concentrating on techniques for organizing sentences and for providing continuity in paragraphs. We also need to look at the story the paragraph tells.

Every paragraph not only presents specific details but also tells a story. The story weaves the details together and thus gives them meaning. The details are the trees. The story is the forest. The biggest problem in many scientific research papers is that the reader cannot see the forest for the trees.

We will examine this problem at three levels: the paragraph (this chapter), each section of the paper (Chaps. 4–7), and the paper as a whole (Chap. 12).

At all three levels, two components are needed for the story to be clear: a statement of the message and a display of the thinking that leads to the message. These components of the story are particularly important in paragraphs that present arguments, so that the reader will be able to identify the message and will be able to follow the thinking that leads to it. Below are some examples of stating the message and displaying thinking in paragraphs of argument.

Stating the Message

To be unmistakable, the message must be stated. In Example 3.26, which is a paragraph from a Discussion section, the author does not state the message but instead presents a catalog of details. Readers who want to know what message the author is trying to send have to figure it out for themselves.

Example 3.26

AThe final variable that can shift the pressure-dimension relation acutely is a change in temperature. **B**Rectal temperature was monitored in many dogs and tended to drift downward from 38°C to 36°C. **C**The greatest drift in temperature (to 36°C) occurred during the thoracotomy and then temperature usually remained stable. **D**Templeton et al. (38) reported greater cardiac muscle stiffness and greater diastolic pressure consistent with a leftward shift in the pressure-dimension curve at 33°C (P_{LVED}, 6.6 mmHg) than at 37°C (P_{LVED}, 1.8 mmHg). **E**The major increase in diastolic pressure came at temperatures below 35°C. **F**The authors believed that the elevation in diastolic pressure was mediated by changes in viscous rather than elastic properties. **G**However, [1]all recorded temperatures in the present study were greater than 35°C, [2]temperature was usually stable during the experimental protocol at 37°C, and [3]there was no evidence that viscous factors changed during maximal coronary blood flow.

When we get to sentence D, our eyes begin to glaze over. Although we can understand what sentences D–G are saying, we do not know why we are hearing them. What is the point of all this detail?

The revision makes the point clear, because the author states the point (the message). The details are unnecessary, so they have been omitted.

Revision

A Topic
  AThe final variable that can shift the pressure-dimension curve acutely is a change in temperature. **B**In our experiments, rectal temperature tended

^X *Message*
    +
    Thinking

to drift downward from 38°C to 36°C. ^CThe greatest drift in temperature (to 36°C) occurred during the thoracotomy and then temperature usually remained stable. ^X**This change in temperature probably did not shift the pressure-dimension curve,** since a leftward shift has been reported only at temperatures below 35°C (38).

In the revision, the point implied by sentence G of the original version is now stated (sentence X, boldfaced and underlined). It is wiser to state the message than to leave it for readers to guess, because they might guess wrong.

Note that the revised paragraph has two topic sentences—one stating the topic (sentence A: change in temperature) and the other stating the message (sentence X: that the change in temperature probably **did not shift** the pressure-dimension curve). Note also that the difference between a topic sentence that states a topic and a topic sentence that states a message is the verb (here, "did not shift.") That is, the message is in the verb.

Telling Your Own Story

Your primary allegiance when you write a paper is to telling your own story. Your allegiance is not to retelling someone else's story. In telling your story, select the points that you need from published papers and weave them in. You should rephrase the points in the way that will work best in your story. When rephrasing, be careful to represent the other authors' points in a way that the authors would accept; that is, do not distort their ideas. In the revision of Example 3.26 above, the statement at the end of sentence X ("since a leftward shift has been reported only at temperatures below 35°C") accurately represents the statement in the original example ("The major increase in diastolic pressure came at temperatures below 35°C.").

■ EXERCISE 3.8: STATING THE MESSAGE

In the paragraph below, which is from a Discussion section, the author does not state the message. Rather, he presents two sets of scientific details without indicating how they are related.

1. Revise this paragraph, indicating the relationship between the two sentences and thus stating the message of the paragraph. That is, make clear why the information in sentence 2 is being stated.

2. Underline the statement of the message in your revision. (The message is not "our results." It is how the two sentences are related.)

Our findings differ from those of Malik and Kidd (12), who found that the effect of the addition of carbon dioxide, studied over a period of 20 min, was to supplement the effect of hypoxia on pulmonary vascular resistance in spontaneously breathing dogs. Important differences in experimental design between the latter and the present studies are not only the species and the age of the animal studied, but also the duration of the periods of study.

Displaying Your Thinking

In addition to the message being stated, the thinking that led to the message must be displayed. Let the reader think along with you. Whatever steps are going through your mind should be put on paper so that the reader can see them too.

Displaying Thinking in a Short Argument

In Example 3.26, in addition to not stating his message, the author did not display his thinking. Instead, he recited a list of facts, some directly relevant to the topic (sentences D, E, G1, G2) and others less directly relevant (F and G3). We do not know how the author interprets these facts or what he wants us to think after we read them. This paragraph is a case of all trees and no forest.

In the revision, the message is stated (boldfaced and underlined) and the thinking is displayed (underlined). The message is the conclusion that change in temperature did not shift the pressure-dimension relation. The thinking that led to this message is the reason the author feels confident that this conclusion is right—because a leftward shift has been reported only at temperatures below 35°C.

Note that the crucial link between the conclusion and the display of thinking is a single transition word—"since." Without this transition word, we would not easily see how the two ideas in sentence X are related, that is, how the display of thinking is related to the conclusion. (Try reading the revision without the word "since.") Thus, "since" is crucial for clarity and for ease of reading. It lets the reader think along with the author and follow the argument.

Note also that the first three words of sentence B of the revision ("in our experiments") are a transition phrase that shows the movement of the story from a general phenomenon, stated in sentence A, to the specific findings of this study, stated in sentence B. This transition, which was missing in the original version, helps the reader follow the author's thinking.

Displaying Thinking in a Long Argument

Sometimes there is only one step in an argument, as in the revision of Example 3.26. Other times the display of thinking can run for several sentences, as in the examples below. In this case, the steps in the argument should form a linked chain, or line, of argument. The reader should be able to follow the argument easily as it moves from one step to the next. Making the chain of argument clear to the reader is particularly important in long arguments that do not follow standard patterns of organization (such as pro-con or parallel form), as in Example 3.27 below.

To display thinking in a long argument, the most useful techniques are topic sentences, transition words, and transition phrases. Used together, these techniques create the forest. In biomedical research papers, perhaps the most underused technique is transition phrases. Examples 3.27 and 3.28 illustrate how transition phrases can be used along with topic sentences, transition words, and other techniques of continuity to let the reader think along with you and follow your argument.

Structure of the Argument	Example 3.27	Techniques of Continuity
A Finding and implication		

A Like Karoum et al. (21), we estimated the half-life of ganglionic dopamine to be considerably less than 1 h, which indicates a very rapid rate of turnover.

B Topic sentence (speculation based on A) (message)

B Although measures of total dopamine turnover cannot distinguish between the rates of turnover associated with SIF cells and principal neurons, from our results we suspect that this rapid rate of turnover is accounted for primarily by precursor dopamine in principal neurons.

B Transition word; Key terms; Transition phrase

C Finding that supports B

C We based this suspicion on our finding that within 1 h after injection of the synthesis inhibitor α-MT, and 40 min after injection of the synthesis inhibitor NSD-1015, the ganglionic dopamine content had dropped by about 60%, leaving some 7 pmol of dopamine that was resistant to further significant depletion for at least 3 h.

C Transition phrase; Key terms

D Finding used to interpret C

D To interpret these data, we used Koslow's finding that approximately 40% of the dopamine in the rat superior cervical ganglion is stored in SIF cells (26).

D Transition phrase; Key terms

E Interpretation of C based on D

E Applying this figure to our measure of ganglionic dopamine (18 pmol/ganglion) would mean that about 7 pmol of dopamine is contained in SIF cells.

E Transition phrase; Key terms

F Topic sentence (speculation restated more specifically) (message)

F Therefore, we speculate that the 7 pmol of dopamine remaining 1 h after synthesis was inhibited represents SIF cell dopamine that is slowly turning over, whereas the 60% that is rapidly depleted represents precursor dopamine in principal neurons that is rapidly turning over.

F Transition word; Transition phrase; Key terms

B, F Consistent order

G Support for F

G This notion is consistent with reports which have shown that SIF cell catecholamines have a very slow turnover in the rat superior cervical ganglion (32, 41).

G "This" + category term; Transition phrase

In this paragraph, the structure, which does not follow a standard pattern, is clear because the author uses the techniques of continuity, particularly transition phrases, to display his thinking. The structure of the paragraph is as follows:

A states a finding and an implication of that finding (that the rate of dopamine turnover is rapid).

B is a topic sentence that presents a speculation about the source of the implication described in A.

C presents an experimental finding upon which the speculation stated in B is based.

D adds a piece of information that helps interpret C.

E uses D to spell out the implication of C.

F concludes by restating more specifically the speculation first stated in B.

G supports F with previous findings.

The message of the paragraph is stated in sentences B and F. Thus, like the revision of Example 3.26, this paragraph has two topic sentences: sentences

B and F. But in this paragraph, both topic sentences state points: sentence B states the point of the paragraph generally, and sentence F restates the point more specifically. In addition, sentence A can be viewed as a topic sentence that states the general topic of the paragraph (rapid rate of dopamine turnover).

The display of thinking rests on these topic sentences, on the transition phrases, and on other techniques of continuity.

The transition words and phrases that display thinking are as follows:

A. Like Karoum et al. (21), we estimated
B. Although . . . , from our results we suspect that
C. We based this suspicion on our finding that
D. To interpret these data
E. Applying this figure to our measure of ganglionic dopamine (18 pmol/ganglion) would mean that
F. Therefore, we speculate that
G. This notion is consistent with reports which have shown that

The other techniques of continuity used in Example 3.27 are as follows:

Repetition of key terms: dopamine (A, B, C, D, E, F); ganglionic/ganglion (A, C, D, E, G); turnover/turning over (A, B, F, G); rate(s) (A, B); rapid/rapidly (A, B, F); slowly/slow (F, G); SIF cell(s) (B, D, E, F, G); principal neurons (B, F); precursor (B, F); synthesis inhibitor/synthesis was inhibited (C, F); 7 pmol (C, E, F); depletion/depleted (C, F); superior cervical (D, G); rat (D, G).

"This" plus a category term: "this notion" (G).

Consistent order: SIF cells first; principal neurons second (B, F).

Note that thinking is displayed in every sentence of this paragraph, thus guiding the reader through the argument.

Here is another example of a paragraph in which thinking is displayed and the story is easy to follow.

Structure of the Argument	*Example 3.28*	*Techniques of Continuity*
A How the finding was obtained	*A* The picture of the architecture of the tracheal nerves and ganglia that we reconstructed was obtained by reacting the whole mount preparation for acetylcholinesterase activity. *B* It is possible that some axons did not stain and that the picture we obtained is not complete. *C* For example, El-Bermani (4), using methylene blue and silver techniques and the histochemical reaction for acetylcholinesterase to examine 10-μm sections of airways, found a discrepancy between the number of bronchial nerves stained with the classical techniques and the number which were acetylcholinesterase positive. *D* However, we do not think that such a discrepancy exists in our whole mount segments. *E* One reason is that acetylcholinesterase is widely distributed not only in cholinergic neurons but also in some noncholinergic neurons (16). *F* In addition, this enzyme is present in parasympathetic ganglion cells and in some cells of sympathetic and sensory gan-	
B Possible problem (topic)		*B Transition phrase; Key term*
C Support for B		*C Transition word; Key terms*
D Denial of problem		*D Transition word; Transition phrase; Key terms*
E, F Support for D		*E Transition phrase; Key terms*
		F Transition word; "This" + category term
		E, F Consistent point of view

G *Assertion of the validity of the finding (message)*

glia (16). **G**<u>We believe that</u> this widespread distribution of acetylcholinesterase in the nerves and ganglia of the airways and the fact that axons with acetylcholinesterase activity run in the same Schwann cell sheath as those without this activity (11) have enabled us to faithfully reconstruct the overall architecture of the nerves and ganglia of the ferret trachea.

G *Transition phrase; Key terms*

In Example 3.28, we can follow the author's thinking easily. The first reason is that the structure of the argument is clear. (Clear structure is the prerequisite for continuity, as we saw at the beginning of this chapter.) The organization of the argument in this paragraph is pro-con (or, in this case, "con-pro"). The author first argues against a possible objection to the validity of the finding and then argues for the validity. Specifically,

A presents a fact (how the finding the paper reports was obtained).
B states a possible problem with the validity of this finding.
C provides some support for the possible problem.
D denies the likelihood of the problem.
E and F provide support for this denial (reasons the problem is unlikely).
G concludes by asserting the validity of the finding.

The second reason we can follow the author's thinking is that the author uses topic sentences to state the topic (B) and the message (G). We could even say that this paragraph has three topic sentences: A states the general topic (the picture of the architecture of tracheal nerves and ganglia), B states the specific topic (the possibility that the picture of the architecture is incomplete), and G states the message (the belief that the picture is a faithful reconstruction of the architecture of the tracheal nerves and ganglia).

Third, the thinking in this paragraph is displayed every step of the way not only by topic sentences but also by transition phrases, transition words, and other techniques of continuity (repetition of key terms and consistent point of view). The transition phrases are "it is possible that" (B), "we do not think that" (D), "one reason is that" (E), and "we believe that" (G). Try reading the paragraph without the words "we believe that" to see how this transition phrase contributes to the display of thinking.

Sentences That Move the Story Forward. Not every sentence you write will move the story forward. That is, not every sentence will be a step in the argument. Some sentences will exemplify, amplify, or modify steps in the argument. In Example 3.27, sentences A–F move the story forward. Sentence G gives supporting evidence for the speculation in F. Although this sentence is not necessary for following the story (as you can see by reading the paragraph without sentence G), it is necessary for convincing the reader of the truth of sentence F and therefore should not be omitted.

The transition words and phrases and the other techniques of continuity that you use should make clear which sentences move the story forward and which sentences do not. In Example 3.27, the transition words and transition phrases in sentences B–F all show that the story is moving forward (see the transition words and phrases underlined in Example 3.27). The transition phrase at the beginning of sentence G ("this notion is consistent with reports which have shown that") indicates support rather than forward movement of the story. In general, supporting sentences do not move the story forward. Often supporting sentences are introduced by the transition word "for example."

The reason that it is important to know which sentences move the story forward is that these sentences display the thinking that creates the forest, the element that is so often missing from scientific research papers.

The sentences that move the story forward are not always easy to separate from the supporting sentences. This is the case in Example 3.28 because the supporting sentences supply key terms used in the other sentences: "discrepancy" in C is picked up in D; "distributed" in E is picked up in G. Still, the forward movement of this paragraph is in sentences B, D, and G (B: "it is possible that"; D: "however, we do not think that"; G: "we believe that"). Sentences C, E, and F are primarily supporting sentences that validate the points being made in sentences B, D, and G: C gives examples, which are signaled by the transition word "for example"; E and F give reasons for D. The reasons are signaled by the transition phrase, "one reason is that." Thus, even though this paragraph is tightly woven because of repetition of key terms, the reader can still tell which sentences move the story forward and what the function of the other sentences is.

Lively, Readable Writing.   Notice that "we" is used five times in Example 3.27 (sentences A, B, C, D, and F) and four times in Example 3.28 (sentences A, B, D, G), always in sentences that move the story forward. The use of "we" in these sentences gives us a sense of the scientist behind the science and brings life and personality to the display of thinking. As a rule, injecting yourself into your writing by using "we" and transition phrases that reveal your thinking makes writing lively and readable. These techniques work best when they reflect firm conviction and your confidence in what you know and what you think and when they are used along with the principles of word choice (Chap. 1) and sentence structure (Chap. 2), as in Example 3.28.

Summary

In the previous three examples we have seen that by stating your message and displaying your thinking you can ensure that you tell a story and do not lose the forest for the trees. The most useful storytelling techniques are topic sentences, transition phrases, and transition words. These techniques can also ensure clear movement between sentences that move the story forward (and thus create the forest) and those that do not.

Condensing

In addition to stating the message and displaying your thinking, it is important to avoid obliterating the message and the display of thinking with unnecessary detail. In Chapter 2 we saw that sentences should be short and not overloaded with information. Similarly, paragraphs should be as short as possible consistent with a clear, complete explanation, description, or argument. Take every opportunity to omit unnecessary detail and unnecessary repetition, whether it is a few words (as in Example 3.29) or several sentences (as in Example 3.26 above and Example 3.30 below).

Example 3.29

*A*We chose a period equal to three times the time constant because 95% of the change in anesthetic concentration within a compartment, and likewise 95% of the recovery from a compartment, should occur during this period. *B*These percentages are rough estimates of the amount distributed to and subsequently recovered from each compartment. *C*However, the distinct separation of these compartments (see above) means that most anesthetic eliminated from each compartment should occur during the periods we chose.

Revision

A We chose a period equal to three times the time constant because 95% of the change in anesthetic concentration within a compartment, and likewise 95% of the recovery from a compartment, should occur during this period. *B* Although these percentages are rough estimates, *C* the distinct separation of these compartments (see above) means that most anesthetic eliminated from each compartment should occur during the periods we chose.

In Example 3.29, repeating what the percentages are rough estimates of is unnecessary. The point is that the percentages are rough estimates. Adding the extra words focuses the reader's attention on something that is not the point and obliterates the display of thinking, making it difficult for the reader to see the logical connection between sentences B and C. Omitting the unnecessary words permits a closer link between the two sentences (which in the revision are two parts of one sentence) and thus makes the logical connection clear.

In Example 3.30, more extensive condensing is needed.

Example 3.30

A Mean pulmonary artery pressure and cardiac output did not change after instillation of serum alone or serum with epinephrine or terbutaline (Table 1). *B* Left atrial pressure fell slightly below baseline after all three treatments but the decrease was statistically significant only after epinephrine (Table 1). *C* Peak airway pressure increased slightly after all three treatments but the increase was statistically significant only for epinephrine and terbutaline (Table 1). *D* There was a significant increase in lung lymph flow and a significant decrease in the lymph-to-plasma protein concentration ratio after all three treatments. *E* Both the rise in lymph flow and the decrease in the lymph-to-plasma protein concentration ratio were greater after terbutaline and epinephrine than after serum alone (Table 2). *F* Arterial oxygen tension decreased after all three treatments, although it was always greater than 85 mmHg.

In Example 3.30, the message is lost because of the catalog of details and because of unnecessary repetition of "after all three treatments" in sentences B–D and F and of "the rise in lymph flow and the decrease in the lymph-to-plasma protein concentration ratio" in sentence E. In the revision, the details in sentences A–C have been omitted, and three sentences have been condensed into one. This condensing de-emphasizes the less important variables and allows the reader to notice the changes in the more important variables. In addition, the treatments are named at the beginning of the paragraph, thus signaling the topic of the paragraph, so they do not need to be repeated in every sentence. Also, a category term ("changes") is used in E to avoid repeating the details of what increased and what decreased, as was done in the revision of Example 3.8 above.

Revision

A After serum was instilled either alone or with one of the two beta adrenergic agonists, there were no important changes in hemodynamics or peak airway pressure (Table 1). *D* However, after all three treatments lung lymph flow increased and the lymph-to-plasma protein concentration ratio decreased.

E<u>Both of these changes</u> were greater after terbutaline and epinephrine than after serum alone (Table 2). *F*Arterial oxygen tension decreased, although it was always greater than 85 mmHg.

Now that the noise-to-message ratio is decreased, the message of the paragraph is clear.

■ *EXERCISE 3.9: DISPLAYING THINKING*

Below is the first paragraph of an Introduction. In this paragraph, the message is stated and the thinking is displayed. These statements form the argument.

1. *In the left margin, outline the structure of the argument and identify the* <u>message</u> *(as done in Examples 3.27 and 3.28). Caution: Although we have seen this* <u>type</u> *of paragraph before, the specific structure of this paragraph is not the same as the structure of any paragraph earlier in this chapter. To figure out the structure, decide what organization the topic sentence could imply.*

2. *In the right margin, identify the techniques of continuity used to link sentences (as done in Examples 3.27 and 3.28). Consider how these techniques focus on the structure of the argument.*

3. *Which sentences move the story forward?* _____

Structure of the Argument; Message

Techniques of Continuity

A_1Hypothermia is presently used to prevent myocardial damage during surgery requiring circulatory arrest, A_2but the effect of hypothermia per se on the myocardium is not clear. BSome studies in dogs have found that hypothermia causes myocardial damage. CIn those studies, subendocardial hemorrhages, calcified necrosis, and fatty degeneration were seen in the heart after 1–4 hours at body temperatures between 21 and 30°C (9, 10). DHowever, other studies in dogs and rabbits have not found myocardial damage under similar conditions of hypothermia (6, 8). ESimilarly, studies of patients who were hypothermic as a consequence of various medical disorders have found no evidence of permanent myocardial damage. FIn those patients, although serum activity of total creatine kinase MB isoenzyme was increased, there was no clinical or postmortem evidence of acute myocardial infarction (2, 7).

■ *EXERCISE 3.10: CONDENSING*

In the paragraph below, the point is hard to see because of the unnecessary repetition.

Revise this paragraph, omitting all unnecessary repetition and condensing the paragraph as much as possible.

Pulmonary artery constriction increased input resistance to 170% of control, and microvascular injury increased it to 215% of control (Fig. 7). Although mean input resistance was higher during microvascular injury than during pulmonary artery constriction, this difference was not significant ($P = 0.7$).

<table>
<tr><td>

SUMMARY OF GUIDELINES FOR PARAGRAPH STRUCTURE

</td></tr>
</table>

GENERAL

Paragraphs should be organized, should have continuity, and should tell a story.

SPECIFIC

Organization

Use topic sentences to state the topic or the message of the paragraph.
Put the topic sentence first, if possible.
Organize supporting sentences in a logical way that clearly supports the point made in the topic sentence.
Standard patterns of paragraph organization that occur frequently in scientific research papers include enumeration of specifics in the order of most to least important or vice versa, enumeration of specifics in the order announced in the topic sentence, pro-con, comparison and contrast, parallel structure, funnel, and chronological order.

Continuity

Do not skip steps.
Repeat key terms.
    Repeat key terms exactly, or use a category term plus "this" or "these."
    Repeat key terms early in the sentence.
    Use different terms for different meanings.
Keep a consistent order.
    Do not change the order of the items.
    Do not omit any items.
    Do not add any items.
    Do not interrupt the sequence of items with other information.
Keep a consistent point of view for similar ideas.
Use parallel form for parallel ideas.
Signal the subtopic (that is, the organization of the paragraph) at the beginning of the sentence.
Use transition words or phrases to indicate the logical link between ideas.

Telling the Story

State the message.
Display your thinking.
Use transition words and phrases to make clear which sentences move the story forward and which sentences do not.
Use "I" or "we" when displaying judgment.
Omit unnecessary detail.

OVERALL GUIDELINE

The goal is clarity.

SECTION II

THE TEXT OF THE BIOMEDICAL RESEARCH PAPER

In Section I, The Building Blocks of Writing, we saw how to choose words and how to arrange words in sentences and paragraphs. In Section II, we move to the next larger unit of thought—the sections of a biomedical research paper.

Principles for writing each section of a research paper are based on principles of paragraph structure. In addition, some specific principles of word choice and sentence structure are particularly relevant to various sections of the research paper and are included in the appropriate chapters.

Before turning to the principles for writing individual sections of the research paper, we need to understand the overall structure of a paper that reports original research results. Over the years, a standard four-part structure has developed. The four parts, or sections, are the Introduction, Materials and Methods, Results, and Discussion (Materials and Methods is also called Methods and Materials, and is often referred to simply as "Methods"). In addition to these four sections of the text, a research paper has a title, an abstract, references, and, usually, figures, tables, or both. These parts of the research paper will be dealt with in later sections of this book.

Separation of the text of a research paper into four individual sections has an attendant danger. The danger is that the story line can get lost. As a result, the reader cannot see the forest for the trees and does not get the message of the paper. To prevent these problems, the trick is to focus each section of the research paper on the question the research was designed to answer. Nothing is more important to the clarity of a research paper than focusing each part of the paper on the question.

To focus on the question, think of the main function of each section of the research paper in relation to the question, as follows:

Introduction:	States the question
Materials and Methods:	Describes experiments done or observations made to answer the question
Results:	Reports results found that answer the question
Discussion:	Answers the question

In addition, in each section of the paper, emphasize information that is directly relevant to the question. Subordinate or omit other information. The next four chapters explain how to emphasize information relevant to the question and thus ensure that the story line does not get lost.

The story line is not equally strong in all four sections of the research paper. It is strongest in the Introduction and the Discussion and weakest in Methods and Results. Thus, we can think of the text of a research paper as kind of sandwich: the outside parts (Introduction and Discussion) are primarily storytelling (and thus subjective); the inside parts (Methods and Results) are primarily descriptive (and thus more objective).

The outside parts (the Introduction and Discussion), although interrupted by the Methods and Results, form a single, continuous story. The Discussion picks up where the Introduction leaves off. Specifically, as we will see, the Introduction ends with a question and the Discussion starts with the answer. Thus, the shape of their story is somewhat like the top and bottom halves of an hourglass: the Introduction narrows to the question and the Discussion opens out from the answer. Methods and Results also form a sequential pair, but the shape of their story is different. The Results section is essentially parallel to part of the Methods section. For example, if Methods describes three series of experiments, Results describes three series of results, and in the same order as in Methods. Thus, the four sections of a research paper can be viewed as two pairs rather than as four separate parts.

The next four chapters explain how to keep the story going both in each of the four sections of the research paper individually and in the two pairs of sections. Each chapter is organized in five parts: functions, content, organization, length, and details.

CHAPTER 4

THE INTRODUCTION

FUNCTIONS

The Introduction has two functions. One is to awaken the reader's interest. The other is to be informative enough to prepare readers, whether or not they are specialists in your field, to understand the paper.

To awaken interest, an Introduction should be direct and to the point, it should be specific rather than vague and general, and it should be as short as possible consistent with clarity and informativeness. In addition, it should be written in a readable style (see Chaps. 1 and 2).

To be informative, an Introduction should follow the guidelines given below.

CONTENT FOR "RESULTS PAPERS"

A "results paper" is a paper in which you describe experiments you did and the new results you obtained.

Essential Content

The most important statement in the Introduction is the statement of the question. Before stating the question, the Introduction tells what is known or believed about the topic and what is still unknown or problematic. The Introduction also states what species and material were studied. When necessary, the Introduction can also include the experimental approach or the answer to the question.

If a study was retrospective, that is, if a question was asked after the data were gathered, the fact that the study was retrospective must be stated in the Introduction. For example, "Therefore, in this retrospective study, we determined. . . ." If a study was prospective, that is, if the experiments were designed and the data were gathered specifically to answer the question, that fact does not need to be stated. If a study was partly retrospective and partly prospective, each part should be identified.

References

The statements about what is known must include references (see sentence A in Example 4.1 below). The references should be chosen to reflect the key work that led to the question of your paper.

The number of references should be kept to a minimum. If a lot of work has been done on the topic, select papers describing the first, the most important, and the most elegant studies. Keep in mind that reference lists in papers you cite can lead readers to other references. You can also cite review articles.

Newness, Importance

Biomedical journals like to publish papers describing work that is "new, true, important, and comprehensible" (DeBakey, 1976). The Introduction is the place to make clear what is new about the work and why the work is important. The importance should be indicated if it is not obvious, particularly in papers submitted to general journals.

ORGANIZATION FOR "RESULTS PAPERS"

The Shape of the Introduction

The Introduction follows a standard pattern of organization—the funnel. That is, the Introduction narrows step by step from a starting point to a question. This step-by-step narrowing is the story the Introduction tells.

Known, Unknown or Problem, Question

The usual starting point of the Introduction is a topic sentence stating something known or believed, that is, something familiar to the readers. The known is often a recent addition to knowledge in the field, but it can also be a long-standing belief. The topic sentence stating the known indicates the general topic of the paper.

After the statement of the known comes either a statement of what is still unknown or a statement of a problem with what is known, for example, a problem with the way the known information was obtained. The statement of the unknown or the problem leads to the statement of the question. Thus, the Introduction funnels from (A) something that is known to (B) an unknown or a problem with what is known to (C) the question.

The Introduction can end with the statement of the question or can go on to state the experimental approach, the answer to the question, or both (see "The End of the Introduction" below).

Example 4.1 illustrates an Introduction composed of a brief funnel: one sentence each for the known, the unknown, and the question, followed by a brief overview of the experimental approach.

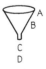

A *Known (general topic)*
B *Unknown*
    (specific topic)
C *Question*
D *Experimenal approach*

Example 4.1 Brief Introduction

AIt is known that several general anesthetics, including barbiturates, depress the bronchomotor response to vagus nerve stimulation (1, 7, 9). **B**However, the site of this depression has not been determined. **C**To determine which <u>site in the vagal motor pathway to the bronchioles is most sensitive to depression by barbiturates,</u> **D**we did experiments in isolated rings of ferret trachea in which we stimulated this pathway at four different sites before and after exposure to barbiturates.

Longer introductions also follow this funnel shape but expand it. For example, the Introduction in Example 4.2 has two statements of what is known (A, B); a sentence stating a problem with what is known (C); a sentence stating a solution and its importance (D); a sentence of details (E) expanding sentence D; a sentence stating the question (F), which is based on the solution stated in D; and a sentence stating the experimental approach (G).

Example 4.2   Longer Introduction

A Known

B Known
C Problem
*D Importance and implied
   solution*
E Details of D
F Question

G Experimental approach

*A*Previous investigations have demonstrated that metabolic alkalosis during exercise increases blood lactate concentrations substantially beyond the concentrations observed during exercise in the absence of metabolic alkalosis (8, 10, 16). *B*Conversely, metabolic acidosis decreases blood lactate concentrations. *C*However, for these investigations, alkali was ingested or infused, which is an artificial situation. *D*More important clinically is the effect of respiratory alkalosis that occurs during exercise in a variety of circumstances that involve increased respiratory drive. *E*These circumstances include interstitial lung disease and congestive heart failure. *F*The purpose of this study was to determine the effect of respiratory alkalosis during exercise on blood lactate concentrations. *G*We used a new biofeedback method by which ventilation, and thus arterial P_{CO_2} and pH, can be precisely adjusted independently of metabolic rate.

Newness, Importance

To make clear that your work is new, be sure that your question addresses an issue that you have said is unknown, as in Example 4.1 above. To make clear why the work is important, include a statement that implies or states the importance of the work. Three ways of stating the importance of the work are shown in Example 4.2 (sentence D) above and in Examples 4.3 (sentence A_2) and 4.4 (sentence A) below.

It is not always necessary to indicate the importance of the work. For example, in basic research, adding new knowledge is in itself important.

Stating the Question

The single most important statement in the Introduction is the statement of the specific question the research was designed to answer. The reason that the question is most important is that the entire paper depends on it.

The Question as Topic Sentence

The question sets up an expectation that the rest of the paper fulfills. Thus, the question serves as a super topic sentence for the entire paper. If the question is not stated, or is not stated clearly and specifically, readers do not know why the experiments were done or where the paper is headed. Instead of reading with an expectation in mind, the readers are groping toward an uncertain end point. So the question is important for the same reason that topic sentences are important, only more so. Whereas topic sentences work at the level of the individual paragraph, the question works at the level of the overall story that runs throughout the paper.

Inevitability of the Question

The question should follow inevitably from the previous statements of what is known or believed and what is still unknown or problematic. Thus, the topic of the question should be the same as the topic in the statement of what is known, and the question should be the question we would expect after reading the statement of what is unknown or problematic. The reason is that if you start the Introduction with a particular topic, we expect the paper to have something to do with that topic. Otherwise, why are you mentioning it? Similarly, if you say that something is unknown or problematic, we expect that your paper will try to resolve it. In fact, once you have stated the unknown (or the problem), you have no more choices: the unknown determines what the question must be. Thus, the question must follow inevitably from the unknown.

If we look again at Example 4.1, we can see that the question does follow inevitably from the previous statements. The question is, "Which site in the vagal motor pathway to the bronchioles is most sensitive to depression by barbiturates?" This question clearly derives from the statement of the unknown ("the site of this depression has not been determined"), which in turn clearly derives from the statement of the known ("several general anesthetics, including barbiturates, depress the bronchomotor response to vagus nerve stimulation").

In a paper that has two questions, both questions must follow inevitably from the previous statements. If the background information leading to the second question is omitted, as frequently happens, the reader does not know where the second question comes from.

Example 4.3   Missing Background for Question 2

A_1 *Known*
A_2 *Unknown; Importance*

B *Possible treatment*
C *Support for B*

D_1 *Question 1*

D_2 *Question 2*
D_3 *Experimental approach*

A_1 Because stasis of blood flow may be an important cause of hepatic arterial thrombosis in liver transplant patients (4), A_2 a prophylactic treatment that increases hepatic arterial blood flow might reduce the risk of thrombosis. B One possible treatment might be intravenous infusion of prostaglandin E_1. C This treatment is suggested by the finding that injections of prostaglandin E_1 directly into the hepatic artery increase hepatic arterial blood flow in cats (11) and dogs (12). D_1 Therefore, in this study, we asked whether a more distant infusion of a low dose of prostaglandin E_1, into a systemic vein, increases hepatic arterial blood flow and D_2 compared the efficacy of portal venous and systemic venous infusion D_3 by delivering prostaglandin E_1 as a continuous infusion into either the portal venous or the systemic venous circulation of young lambs.

In this example, the reader does not know why the authors compared the efficacy of portal venous and systemic venous infusion of prostaglandin E_1. In the revision, the necessary background information leading to this second question is added (sentence D, which states another possible treatment).

Revision

A Because stasis of blood flow may be an important cause of hepatic arterial thrombosis in liver transplant patients (4), a prophylactic treatment that increases hepatic arterial blood flow might reduce the risk of thrombosis. B One possible treatment might be intravenous infusion of prostaglandin E_1. C This treatment is suggested by the finding that injections of prostaglandin E_1 directly into the hepatic artery increase hepatic arterial blood flow in cats (11) and dogs (12). D Less direct injections of similar hepatic arterial vasodilators into the portal vein of cats also increase hepatic blood flow, though only one-half to one-third as effectively as the same doses injected into the hepatic artery (15). ^{E}Therefore, in this study, we asked whether a more distant infusion of a low dose of prostaglandin E_1, into a systemic vein, increases hepatic arterial blood flow and compared the efficacy of portal venous and systemic venous infusion by delivering prostaglandin E_1 as a continuous infusion into either the portal venous or the systemic venous circulation of young lambs.

Question Based on Suggestive Evidence

Sometimes the question is not stated immediately after the unknown or the problem. Instead, evidence suggesting a possible answer is stated. In this case, the question should follow inevitably from the suggestive evidence, as in Example 4.4.

Example 4.4 Question Based on Suggestive Evidence

^{A}*Known (Importance)*

^{B}*Known*

^{C}*Unknown*
^{D}*Support for C (possible factor refuted)*

^{E}*Another possible factor*
^{F}*Support for E (suggestive evidence)*

^{G}*Question; Experimental approach*

^{A}Since 1975 prostaglandins E_1 and E_2 (PGE_1, PGE_2) have been used to maintain the patency of the ductus arteriosus in infants who have congenital heart disease (1–6). ^{B}Although the fetal ductus is sensitive to the dilating action of PGE_1 and PGE_2 (7), the response of the ductus in the newborn to specific doses of these prostaglandins is variable (8). ^{C}The factors that regulate the responsiveness of the ductus to PGE_1 and PGE_2 are unknown. ^{D}One regulating factor that has been suggested is the infant's age (8); however, this factor is unlikely because the ductus is responsive to PGE_1 and PGE_2 even after many months of therapy (9, 10). ^{E}Another possible regulating factor may be the degree of constriction of the ductus arteriosus. ^{F}Support for this factor is that the ductus no longer dilates in response to PGE_1 and PGE_2 when it is fully closed (8, 9) but that the ductus does dilate when it is only partially constricted at angiography (11). ^{G}Therefore, we tested the hypothesis that the degree of constriction of the ductus arteriosus regulates the responsiveness of the ductus to PGE_1 and PGE_2 by doing experiments in newborn lambs.

In this Introduction, the known is stated in sentences A and B, and the unknown is stated in C. D states a possible answer and rejects it. E proposes a different answer. F gives suggestive evidence that supports the proposed answer. G then states a hypothesis (question) based on this suggestive evidence.

Degree of Specificity of the Question

In an earlier draft of Example 4.4, the author stated the question more generally. Instead of asking about the specific regulating factor that he suspected, he asked a general question: "Which factors regulate the responsiveness of the ductus arteriosus to PGE_2?" This general statement of the question would be appropriate if the question came immediately after the statement of the unknown (C). But since the question comes after one possible regulating factor has been refuted (D) and after another possible regulating factor has been suggested (E), a general statement of the question does not fulfill the expectation raised by the preceding funnel of statements of what is known and what is still unknown. A specific question is needed.

In contrast, in Example 4.1 the question is appropriately general. In Example 4.1, the author had no reason for suspecting that any particular site is sensitive to barbiturates. Thus, a general statement of the question immediately after the statement of the unknown is appropriate.

The point is that the statement of the question should be just as specific as the previous statements of what is known and what is unknown or problematic. The reason is that having the same degree of specificity in the question as in the previous statements ensures that the question follows inevitably from those previous statements and thus fulfills the expectation raised by the thinking that those previous statements display.

To ensure that the question is as specific as the previous statements, check that the key terms in the previous statements appear in the question. In Example 4.4, the key term "constriction"/"constricted" from sentences E and F does not appear in the general question originally posed ("which factors regulate . . . "), but it does appear in the specific question stated in sentence G. Thus, the specific question is more appropriate.

Identifying the Question

Sometimes the question is presented in the statement of the unknown. In this case, it is unnecessary to state the question again. Instead, at the beginning of the next sentence, you can simply identify the previous statement as the question by using a transition phrase, such as "to answer this question" or "to test this hypothesis," as in Example 4.5.

Example 4.5 Questions in "Unknown" Identified in the Next Sentence

*A*Known

*B*Known

*C*Unknowns
  (*Questions*)

D **Questions
  identified**;
  Experimental approach

AThe occurrence of a thermal transition in human serum lipoproteins depends on the triglyceride-cholesteryl ester ratio and the size of the lipoprotein particle (5). **B**The triglyceride-cholesteryl ester ratio is known to correlate negatively with the peak temperature of the thermal transition of intact low-density lipoprotein (3). **C**However, it is not yet known how low a triglyceride-cholesteryl ester ratio and how small a particle size are necessary for the occurrence of the thermal transition in triglyceride-rich lipoproteins from human serum. **D**To answer these questions, we assessed the triglyceride-cholesteryl ester ratio and the particle size in two classes of triglyceride-rich lipoproteins whose ratios of triglyceride to cholesteryl ester and whose particle size are between those of low-density lipoproteins and very low-density lipoproteins.

In this example from the end of an Introduction, the starting point (sentence A) states something known. The next sentence (B) states something more specific that is known. Sentence C states two unknowns, which are the questions this paper answers. Sentence D begins with a transition phrase identifying the statement of the unknowns as the questions ("To answer these questions. . . . ").

However, if, as in Example 4.1 above, the question is stated only partially in the statement of the unknown (as it is in sentence B), the entire question should be stated in the next sentence (as it is in sentence C). The reason is that the question is the focal point of the paper. Readers should not have to compose the question for themselves. The question should be stated for them in a single sentence.

Question Stated as a Purpose

The statement of the question often takes the form of a purpose. The form is, "To determine X, we. . . ." Thus, in Example 4.1: "To determine which site in the vagal motor pathway to the bronchioles is most sensitive to depression by barbiturates, we did experiments in isolated rings of ferret trachea in which we stimulated this pathway at four different sites before and after exposure to barbiturates."

Independent and Dependent Variables

Questions in biomedical research often include an independent variable and a dependent variable. An *independent variable* is the variable you set or manipulate at the beginning of the experiment. *Dependent variables* are the variables you observe or measure. For example, for the question in Example 4.1, "To determine which site in the vagal motor pathway to the bronchioles is most sensitive to depression by barbiturates," the independent variable is barbiturates and the dependent variable is depressed responsiveness of sites in the vagal motor pathway.

However, for descriptive questions, there is no independent variable. Thus, for the questions in Example 4.5, "how low a triglyceride-cholesteryl ester ratio and how small a particle size are necessary for the occurrence of the thermal transition in triglyceride-rich lipoproteins from human serum," there are no independent variables. The "dependent variables" are the triglyceride-cholesteryl ester ratio and particle size.

The Components of the Question

Thus, the statement of the question of a biomedical research paper should name the dependent variables and, when appropriate, should also name the independent variables. The statement of the question may also include the species or the population studied (see "Species and Material" below).

Linked Questions

In papers that ask more than one question, the second question sometimes depends on the answer to the first one. In this situation, the questions can be linked by "if so" or a similar phrase, as in Example 4.6.

Example 4.6 Linked Questions

This report describes experiments designed to determine whether exogenous arachidonic acid increases the release of prostaglandin E_2 from the ductus arteriosus and, <u>if so</u>, whether the exogenous arachidonic acid is the source of the prostaglandin E_2 released.

Signaling the Question

The sentence that states the question should begin with a signal of the question. The signal can take a variety of forms. Example 4.1 uses a short signal of the question: "To determine." This signal is often followed by a question word, such as "whether." In Example 4.1, the question word is "which" ("To determine which site"). Examples 4.2, 4.3, and 4.4 use other signals of the question: "The purpose of this study was"; "Therefore, in this study, we asked whether"; "Therefore, we tested the hypothesis that." Other signals used in examples later in this chapter are "This report describes experiments designed to determine whether"; "We asked whether"; "Therefore, our first objective in these studies was to determine whether"; "The present study was therefore designed to determine whether."

The verb used in the signal (if any) should be in the past tense except in signals such as "This report describes."

Telling a Story

The aim in the Introduction should be to tell a story. Each sentence should either move the story forward or support a sentence that does. For example, in Example 4.2 above, sentences A, B, C, D, F, and G move the story forward. Sentence E supports sentence D by mentioning two specific circumstances.

While telling the story, make sure that the continuity is strong. In particular, present all the key steps in the logical chain, repeat key terms, keep the point of view consistent where necessary, use transition words or phrases where necessary to show how a sentence relates to the sentence before it, thus displaying your thinking, omit unnecessary details (trees) that obscure or replace the story (forest). For example, in Example 4.2, thinking is displayed in sentences A, B, C, D, and F: "Previous investigations have demonstrated that," "Conversely," "However," "More important clinically is," "The purpose of this study was." This display of thinking guides the reader through the story of the paragraph.

The End of the Introduction

Experimental Approach

Sometimes the Introduction can end with a statement of the questions. However, often it is helpful for the reader to know the *experimental approach* to answering the question, especially if the approach is new, unusual, or complicated or if the study needs to be identified as having been done in vitro, retrospectively, or whatever. For example, in Example 4.1, the experimental approach makes clear that the study was done in vitro and states that four sites were tested.

The logical place for stating the experimental approach is after the statement of the question.

One convenient way to state the experimental approach is to attach it to the question in a sentence that begins with the question stated as a purpose, that is, in the form "to determine X, we . . . ," as was done in Example 4.1:

Question

Experimental approach

<u>To determine which site in the vagal motor pathway to the bronchioles is most sensitive to depression by barbiturates</u>, we did experiments in isolated rings of ferret trachea in which we stimulated this pathway at four different sites before and after exposure to barbiturates.

Note that the experimental approach gives an overview, not details of how or when some specific procedure was done. Specific details belong in Methods. The overview of the experimental approach belongs in the Introduction because this overview is part of the information needed to prepare the reader to understand the rest of the paper.

Indirect Experimental Approach

Sometimes the experimental approach is indirect. When this is the case, be sure that you make clear how the experiment you did provides an answer to the question you asked. For example, the experiment may assess an indicator or a reciprocal of the key variable. If you measured an indicator or a reciprocal instead of the variable itself, you need to indicate the relation between the two. The place to state this relation is either in the experimental approach at the end of the Introduction or in the Methods section (see Chap. 5).

Example 4.7 Identifying Indicators

Question

Experimental approach

We asked whether Basenji-Greyhound dogs have greater bronchial reactivity to hypotonic and isotonic aerosols than mongrel dogs do. We assessed bronchial reactivity by measuring both the increase in total pulmonary resistance after aerosol delivery and the increase in bronchial response to an acetylcholine aerosol.

Since there are many possible ways to measure bronchial reactivity, in Example 4.7 the author told what indicators of bronchial reactivity she measured. Stating the indicator is important for two reasons. One reason is that readers who are not specialists in the field cannot be expected to know that a particular variable (here both increase in total pulmonary resistance and increase in bronchial response to an acetylcholine aerosol) is an indicator of the phenomenon of interest (here bronchial reactivity). The other reason is that it is clearest for all readers to see a straightforward statement telling what indicator was chosen.

Species and Material

The *species* and the *material* studied (organ, tissue, cell line, molecule) must be stated in the Introduction. *Where* the species is stated depends on the kind of question you are asking. If the question is about a particular species, state the species in the question, as in Example 4.8.

Example 4.8 Question Limited to the Species Studied

A Unknown

B Question; Species

A Whether increased active transport of sodium induced by beta adrenergic agents increases lung liquid clearance in an intact adult animal is unknown. *B* Therefore, our first objective in these studies was to determine whether beta adrenergic agents increase lung liquid clearance in *anesthetized intact adult sheep*.

If the question is not limited to the species examined (usually because the species is serving as a model of a human condition), state the species in the experimental approach (as in Examples 4.1, 4.3, and 4.4). If the model is a new one, establish its validity. If the validity of the model has been established in published reports, the experimental approach can simply be a statement of what species you did the experiments on (Example 4.4).

For studies of human subjects, the species is frequently not stated in the question. However, terms used in the Introduction usually suggest that the species is humans. For example, in Example 4.2, suggestions that the species was humans are "during exercise" (sentence A), "important clinically" (D), and "interstitial lung disease and congestive heart failure" (E).

For studies of *specific* human populations, the population is always stated in the question, as in Example 4.9.

Example 4.9 Question Limited to a Subpopulation of Humans

The purpose of this study was to determine relative contributions of the inspiratory muscle groups to inspiratory pressure generation during non-rapid-eye-movement sleep in patients with occlusive sleep apnea.

The Answer to the Question

The Introduction may include the answer to the question (that is, the conclusion). Including the answer in the Introduction is not particularly necessary in short, uncomplicated papers. However, including the answer can be helpful and therefore is often advisable, particularly in papers that are unusually complicated. Here are two good ways to include the answer to the question.

One way is to state the answer instead of the question, in the form "we show that . . . , as in Example 4.10."

Example 4.10

In this paper, we show that X causes Y.

Another way to include the answer is to state the question and then state the answer briefly. The answer must come immediately after the question and must answer the question asked. To ensure that the answer answers the question asked, use the same key terms, the same verb (when appropriate), and the same point of view in the answer as in the question.

Example 4.11

We wanted to determine whether X or Z causes Y. We found that X causes Y.

In this example, the key terms X and Y are the same in the question and in the answer, the verb is the same ("causes"), and the point of view is the same (always cause to effect), not "We wanted to determine whether X or Z causes Y" (cause to effect) and then "We found that Y is caused by X" (effect to cause). Repeating key terms and the verb and keeping the point of view consistent make it obvious that the answer answers the question asked.

A detailed presentation of results is out of place in the Introduction. The reader is not prepared to hear them and is confused by the detail. If you want to state the answer to the question, do so, but do not state the results either instead of or in addition to the answer (see Exercise 4.2, Introduction 2).

Thus, the Introduction can sometimes end with a statement of the question(s). When necessary, the statement of the question can be followed by a statement of the experimental approach, a statement of the answer, or both.

CONTENT AND ORGANIZATION FOR "METHODS PAPERS"

A "methods paper" is a paper in which you describe a new method, apparatus, or material.

The Introduction of a methods paper, like the Introduction of a results paper, also begins with a statement of what is known, usually a method, an apparatus, or a material, or the reason that one is needed. The Introduction then states one or more problems or limitations of the existing method, apparatus, or material and ends by stating what the new method, apparatus, or material is and what its advantages are. The advantages should be the solution to the problem or limitation. An example of an Introduction to a methods paper is given in Example 4.12.

Example 4.12   Introduction for a Methods Paper

A Known: reasons a chamber is needed

B Problems with available chambers

C Problems with improvised chambers

D New chamber and its advantages

^AVarious types of physiological research require placing animals in a metabolic chamber for exposure to gases, collection of expired air, exposure to unusual atmospheric conditions such as hypoxia or hypobaric environments (6, 9), or measurement of oxygen consumption (1, 8). ^BAlthough equipment for such studies is commercially available, it is usually expensive, specialized for a single function, and applicable only for short-term studies with one animal. ^CImprovising with available laboratory equipment meets with variable success and often requires constant attention and repair. ^DWe now report a relatively inexpensive, reliable closed-circuit metabolic chamber that has proven useful for several research applications involving one or more animals housed for periods of hours or days.

In this Introduction, sentence A states the reasons a chamber is needed, sentences B and C state problems with available and improvised chambers, and sentence D introduces a new chamber that solves all of the problems of the previous chambers.

LENGTH

The Introduction should be as short as possible consistent with clarity and informativeness. The amount of background information needed for complete informativeness depends on how much the intended audience can be expected to know about the topic. For a typical journal article, one typewritten page (about 250–300 words) is often sufficient. When a longer Introduction is necessary, try to keep it to two typewritten pages (500–600 words).

One reason a longer Introduction may be necessary is that some component—the known, the unknown, the importance, or the experimental approach—may require explanation. Another reason may be that two different funnels are needed to funnel to two different but related questions. In this case, a danger is that the continuity between the two funnels will be weak. An example of an Introduction with two funnels is given in Example 4.13.

Example 4.13   A Long Introduction

A Known
B Problem

C Unknown

D–F Support for unknown

   D in another system
   E, F in this system (specific unknowns)

1 ^ASecretion of macromolecular glycoconjugates into the airways can theoretically happen from every epithelial cell type that lines the airways. ^BHowever, the study of macromolecular glycoconjugate secretion has been focused for many years mainly on cells that contain secretory storage granules (goblet cells, submucosal gland cells). ^CEssentially nothing is known about macromolecular secretion by airway surface epithelium from cells that do not contain granules (ciliated and brush border cells). ^DAlthough nongranulated cells from another organ, the rat intestine, have been shown by autoradiography to incorporate radiolabeled galactose and transfer it to apical surfaces (1), its further fate has not been investigated. ^ESimilarly, in airway surface epithelium of several species, although cytochemical methods have shown that acidic glycoconjugates are present on the surfaces of ciliated cells (and of other cell types) (2, 3), it has not been shown that this material is produced by the cell itself rather than being adsorbed from mucous cells or submucosal glands. ^FFurthermore, it has not been shown whether this material is secreted into the airways, what the mechanisms of secretion are, or what the composition of the secreted material is.

*G*Hypothesis
*H–K*Support
   *H*Finding
   *I*Interpretation

    *J*Evidence against I

    *K*Limitation of I

*L*Main questions

*M*Experimental approach

*N*Advantage of
   experimental approach

*O*Minor question

2 *G*One possible mechanism of secretion may involve bacterial proteinases. *H*Recently, bacterial proteinases were reported to increase secretion of radioactive sulfate-labeled, high-molecular-weight glycoconjugates from rabbit tracheal organ cultures (4). *I*Since rabbits lack submucosal glands, it was suggested that bacterial proteinases might stimulate mucin secretion from goblet cells during airway infection (4). *J*However, sulfate, a common marker for airway secretions in its radioactive form, is incorporated not only by epithelial cells that contain secretory granules but also by cells that do not contain secretory granules (5). *K*It is therefore difficult to conclude from which source(s) these sulfated macromolecules are being secreted.

3 *L*The present study was therefore designed to determine, first, whether airway epithelial cells that do not contain secretory granules are capable of elaborating and secreting sulfated macromolecules and, second, whether extracellular proteinases can affect this secretion, and if so, how proteinases from different sources vary in their secreting potency, in the subcellular site of secretion, and in the composition of the secreted products. *M*To answer these questions, we studied $Na_2{}^{35}SO_4$-labeled epithelial cells that were cultured from dog trachea and incubated with proteinases from bacteria, fungi, mast cells, or blood. *N*Because the cells in these cultures, unlike those in an intact tissue, do not contain secretory granules (6), this cell system enabled us to analyze secretion of sulfated products and the regulation of this secretion by extracellular proteinases without interference from sulfated secretions originating from intracellular secretory storage granules. *O*We also did preliminary experiments to establish the identity of secreted sulfated products.

    In this Introduction, paragraph 1 is a funnel that leads to the first question. But instead of posing the question here, the authors go on in paragraph 2 to develop another funnel based on one of the unknowns stated at the end of the first funnel. The second funnel leads to a second set of questions. In addition to having two funnels, this Introduction contains an extended explanation of an unknown (sentences D–F). Finally, the experimental approach is also extended by a sentence (N) that states the advantage of using the cell system chosen. Thus, this Introduction is long for three reasons: two funnels leading to related questions, extended explanation of an unknown, and extended explanation of the experimental approach.

    Despite its length, this Introduction has clear continuity from sentence to sentence and from paragraph to paragraph. As a result, the reader can easily follow the authors' thinking. A crucial display of thinking is the topic sentence at the beginning of paragraph 2 (sentence G). This sentence links paragraph 2 with paragraph 1 by picking up a topic from the end of paragraph 1 (one of the unknowns) and suggesting a possible answer. The rest of paragraph 2 argues in support of this suggested answer. Try reading this Introduction without sentence G to see why it is such an important link in the overall story.

    This Introduction also illustrates a technique for mentioning a question of minor importance: stating it in a separate sentence after stating the main questions. In paragraph 3 the main questions are stated in the first sentence (L) and the experimental approach to answering these questions is given in the next sentence (M). The experimental approach is then justified (N). Finally, almost like a postscript, the minor question is mentioned (O). Emphasizing the important question(s) and de-emphasizing the minor question(s) by putting them in separate sentences is a useful technique for focusing the reader's attention and orienting the reader to what to expect in the rest of the paper.

DETAILS

Verb Tense

In the Introduction, use present tense for statements that are currently true, such as what is known or believed and what is unknown. Use past tense for findings and for what you or others thought and did in the past.

The question is always stated in the *present* tense. Past tense should not be used. The reason is that the question should be about something that is true for all time, not just for the experiment you did. The signal of the question is generally in the *past* tense (see examples in "Signaling the Question" above).

Verb tenses are appropriately handled in Example 4.1:

(A) "It <u>is</u> known": still true, so present tense.
   "<u>depress</u> the bronchomotor response": still true, so present tense.
(B) "<u>has not been determined</u>": done in the past, so past tense.
(C) "<u>is</u> most sensitive": always true, so present tense. (This is the statement of the question.)
(D) "<u>did</u> experiments," "<u>stimulated</u> this pathway": done in the past, so past tense. (This is the statement of the experimental approach.)

Use of "I" or "We"

The use of "I" or "we" is appropriate in the Introduction to indicate the author's thinking. In particular, "I" or "we" is appropriate in signals of the question and in the experimental approach. Thus, in Example 4.4, the authors used "we" in the signal of the question: "Therefore, <u>we</u> tested the hypothesis that." In Example 4.5, the authors used "we" in the experimental approach: "To answer these questions, <u>we</u> assessed."

Modest authors can avoid using "I" or "we" if they prefer. One way to avoid using "we" while still identifying the thinking as your own is to use "our," as in Example 4.8: "Therefore, our first objective in these studies was." Another way to avoid using "I" or "we" is to talk about the study instead of about the authors, as in Examples 4.2 and 4.6: "The purpose of this study was to determine"; "This report describes experiments designed to determine." However, talking about the study depersonalizes the writing and makes it less lively.

Use of Others' Names

In general it is not necessary to use the authors' names when citing others' work in the Introduction. The story line will be clearest if you describe the science, not the scientists. So write the idea and then add the reference. Use the authors' names in the text only if you have a particular reason for doing so.

Word Choice: "If" and "Whether"

When stating a question, use "whether," not "if." For example, "We did experiments to determine <u>whether</u> beta adrenergic agents increase lung liquid clearance in anesthetized intact adult sheep." "Whether" implies alternatives: whether or not. Although "if" can also be used to imply alternatives, "if" is more commonly used in "if . . . then . . ." statements. For example, "If the temperature is too high, the cells will not grow."

Numbering Questions

Avoid using numbers to identify, for example, each of three questions. Normally, if you say that you studied three questions and then present them in a series, the reader can figure out which is question 1, etc. Use numbers only in situations in which the items might not be easy to identify.

If you must use numbers to identify items in a complex series, have no more than one set of such numbers in a paper.

SUMMARY OF GUIDELINES FOR INTRODUCTIONS OF "RESULTS PAPERS"

Funnel from what is known to the question.

> Tell a story. Start with the known (the topic). Move to the unknown or to a problem with the known. End with the question. Make sure that the question follows inevitably from the preceding sentences. If there are two questions, be sure to give background information leading to both questions. If necessary, also state the experimental approach. If you like, state the answer to the question.

> Make clear which sentences move the story forward.

> Make clear the function of sentences that do not move the story forward.

> Make sure that the continuity is strong. In particular, present all the key steps in the logic, repeat key terms, keep the point of view consistent where necessary, display your thinking by using transition words and phrases where necessary, omit unnecessary detail.

> Cite references that reflect the key work that led to the question of your paper.

> Keep the number of references to a minimum.

State the *question*.

> Make the question as *specific* as the previous statements funneling to it.

> Identify the question as the question if it is stated in a previous sentence (for example, in the unknown) by writing, "To answer this question," or something similar.

> Consider stating the question as a purpose and attaching it to the experimental approach ("To determine X, we . . .").

> Use "if so" or a similar phrase to join linked questions.

> Put a signal of the question at the beginning of the sentence.

> Be sure the question includes both the independent variable and the dependent variable, where appropriate.

> De-emphasize a minor question by stating it in a separate sentence after the main question.

> State the question in the present tense.

Be sure the *experimental approach* is evident.

> State it if necessary.

> Make sure that how the experiment answers the question is obvious. If you assessed indicators or reciprocals of the dependent variable, state the relationship between the indicator or reciprocal and the dependent variable.

State the *species*:

> In the question if the question is about the species.

> In the experimental approach if the question is not limited to the species examined.

State the *material* studied when appropriate.

State the *answer*:

> If it will help the reader follow the ideas in the paper, especially in long, difficult papers.

> Either in the form "we show that . . ." or as a question followed by the answer, using the same key terms, the same verb (when appropriate), and the same point of view.

Be sure that what is *new* about the work is evident.

Be sure the *importance* of the work is evident. State it if necessary.

Keep the Introduction *short*.

Aim to *awaken interest*.

■ *EXERCISE 4.1: CLEARLY WRITTEN INTRODUCTIONS*

1. *Check that the two Introductions below follow the guidelines in the Summary of Guidelines for Introductions. (Do not write this).*

2. *List the sentences that move the story forward.* _____

3. *In the right margin, outline the structure of the argument by writing the function of each sentence (as done in Examples 4.1–4.5, 4.12, and 4.13).*

4. *Do the questions follow inevitably from the preceding funnel of statements?*

   _____

5. *Circle the key terms that appear in the question. Also circle these terms in all earlier sentences.*

6. *Is the question stated in the present tense?* _____

7. *Where is the species stated—in the question or in the experimental approach?*

   _____

Structure

Introduction 1

*A*Measuring clearance from the lungs of micronic aerosols of technetium-99m-labeled diethylenetriaminepentaacetic acid (^{99m}Tc-DTPA) delivered into the lower respiratory tract is used to give an index of respiratory epithelial permeability. *B*When measured in upright normal subjects, the clearance of ^{99m}Tc-DTPA was reported to be faster in the upper regions of the lungs than in the lower regions (22). *C*Faster clearance in the upper regions of the lungs was also reported in upright smokers (17). *D*However, the authors did not correct their data for the radioactivity that recirculates after transfer from the lungs into the blood. *E*Therefore, we designed this study to determine whether the respiratory clearance of ^{99m}Tc-DTPA is different within lung regions after correction for recirculation of radioactivity and also to determine the influence of posture and smoking on the regional respiratory clearance of ^{99m}Tc-DTPA.

Introduction 2

1 *A*Preparative ultracentrifugational flotation (1) has long been the standard method for isolating lipoproteins. *B*Compositional analyses of the lipoprotein classes are predicated upon this form of isolation (2, 3), and most current metabolic and structural studies use lipoproteins that have been isolated by ultracentrifugation.

2   *C*Ultracentrifugational isolation, however, has been reported to cause structural changes in lipoproteins, specifically, the loss of apolipoproteins. *D*For example, in studies of both rat and human lipoproteins, a portion of the complement of apolipoproteins A-I and E (apo A-I and apo E) in serum was lost, as evidenced by its appearing at a density greater than 1.21 g/ml after ultracentrifugation (4–6). *E*Furthermore, the loss of apolipoprotein during ultracentrifugational isolation is greater than the loss caused by other isolation methods. *F*The loss of apo A-I from high-density lipoproteins during ultracentrifugational isolation, for example, can reach as much as 50% (7, 8).

3   *G*This study was undertaken to identify the ultracentrifugational factors that are responsible for the loss of apolipoprotein from human high-density lipoproteins. *H*The effects of four factors were studied: ionic strength, temperature, rotor configuration, and centrifuge tube material.

■ *EXERCISE 4.2: INTRODUCTIONS*

> *1. Based on the summary of guidelines for Introductions, <u>list the strengths and weaknesses</u> of each Introduction below. Support each strength and weakness with specific details.*
>
> *2. Assess how well each title fits its Introduction.*
>
> *3. <u>Rewrite</u> one or both of these Introductions, solving the problems you discovered in items 1 and 2.*

Introduction 1

HEAT STORAGE IN RUNNING ANTELOPES:
INDEPENDENCE OF BRAIN AND BODY TEMPERATURES

1 ^{A}The existence of camels, oryxes, gazelles, and other ungulates in hot deserts has long fascinated physiologists. ^{B}Unlike rodents, these animals are too large to burrow and cannot escape the desert sun. ^{C}Understandably, most of the work on temperature regulation of ungulates has been concerned with heat loads from the environment (6, 8, 10, 12, 16, 17, 19, 20, 23). ^{D}Internal heat loads, however, may pose thermal problems as great as or greater than the sun does. ^{E}Tremendous amounts of heat are produced when antelopes run at high speed. ^{F}Gazelles and eland have been clocked at 70–80 km/h (43–50 mph). ^{G}Using the recently developed relationship between body size and energetic cost of locomotion (22), we can calculate that a 15-kg gazelle running at 70 km/h would be producing heat at 40 times its resting metabolic rate. ^{H}These high bursts of speed are usually of short duration. ^{I}It seemed possible that antelopes might store rather than dissipate this heat.

2 ^{J}This study set out to answer two simple questions: (1) Does heat storage play an important role? and (2) If heat storage is important, do these animals possess unusual physiological mechanisms for coping with high body temperatures?

STRENGTHS   *WEAKNESSES*

Introduction 2

THE SEQUENCE OF EXPOSURE TO THE STIMULI DETERMINES THE EFFECT OF ALKALOSIS ON HYPOXIA-INDUCED PULMONARY VASOCONSTRICTION IN LUNGS FROM NEWBORN RABBITS

1 *A*Alveolar hypoxia causes pulmonary vasoconstriction. *B*To determine whether alkalosis or acidosis can increase or reduce hypoxia-induced pulmonary vasoconstriction, numerous investigators have studied the effects of alkalosis and acidosis on constriction of the pulmonary circulation in response to hypoxia (1–14). *C*Only a few of these investigators have studied the effect of alkalosis on hypoxia-induced pulmonary vasoconstriction in the lungs of newborn animals (10, 13, 14). *D*The results of these studies have been variable. *E*Alkalosis has been shown either to reduce or to have no effect on constriction of the neonatal pulmonary circulation in response to alveolar hypoxia.

2 *F*Understanding the effect of alkalosis on the neonatal pulmonary circulation and on the response of the pulmonary circulation to hypoxia is important because alkalosis, produced primarily by mechanical hyperventilation, is widely used in the treatment of newborns who have the syndrome of persistent pulmonary hypertension (15, 16). *G*Mechanical hyperventilation is often clinically effective in the treatment of these infants, but it is not clear whether the improvements are due to the alkalosis resulting from the therapy. *H*If alkalosis is responsible for the clinical improvement in these infants, it is possible that some of the deleterious effects of mechanical hyperventilation could be avoided by using alternative means of inducing alkalosis. *I*A clearer understanding of the effect of alkalosis on the constriction of the neonatal pulmonary circulation in response to hypoxia would aid in the management of these patients.

3 *J*The purpose of this study was to determine whether or not alkalosis reduces constriction of the neonatal pulmonary circulation in response to hypoxia by answering the following specific questions: 1) does alkalosis reduce pulmonary vascular resistance after it has increased in response to hypoxia, 2) does alkalosis reduce the ability of the pulmonary circulation to constrict in response to subsequent hypoxia, 3) does alkalosis introduced simultaneously with hypoxia reduce constriction of the pulmonary circulation, and 4) do both respiratory and metabolic alkalosis have the same effect on the pulmonary circulation and its response to hypoxia. ^{K}To answer these questions, we exposed isolated perfused lungs of newborn rabbits to alkalosis and alveolar hypoxia. ^{L}For each pair of lungs we used one of the following three sequences of exposure to the stimuli: 1) alveolar hypoxia followed by metabolic or respiratory alkalosis, 2) metabolic or respiratory alkalosis followed by alveolar hypoxia, or 3) simultaneous alveolar hypoxia with respiratory alkalosis. ^{M}We found that both metabolic and respiratory alkalosis reduced pulmonary vascular resistance that was elevated in response to hypoxia; neither metabolic nor respiratory alkalosis reduced constriction of the pulmonary vasculature in response to subsequent hypoxia; and simultaneous respiratory alkalosis and hypoxia significantly reduced pulmonary vascular constriction. ^{N}We conclude that the sequence of exposure to the stimuli determines the effect of both respiratory and metabolic alkalosis on hypoxia-induced pulmonary vasoconstriction in isolated, perfused lungs of newborn rabbits.

STRENGTHS   *WEAKNESSES*

CHAPTER 5

MATERIALS AND METHODS

FUNCTION

The function of the Materials and Methods section is to tell the reader what you did to answer the question posed in the Introduction, with sufficient detail and references to permit a trained scientist to evaluate your work fully or to repeat the experiments exactly as you did them.

CONTENT

The primary content of the Materials and Methods section consists of the following information:

Materials

Chemicals (drugs, culture media, buffers, gases)
What was examined (experimental materials, experimental animals, or human subjects)

Methods

What was done to answer the question (experimental protocol):
  Independent variable(s) (manipulations done to cause a change), if any
  Dependent variable(s) (changes measured or observed)
  Control(s) of independent variables
Why it was done (purpose)
How it was done (methods and apparatus of manipulation and of measurement and observation)
How it was analyzed (methods of analyzing the data, including statistical methods)

In addition to this primary content, the Methods section also includes preparation, assumptions, and definitions of indicators, as necessary.

The Methods section also includes references.

The Methods section does not include results. However, intermediate results, that is, results used in calculations done to obtain results that answer the question, can be included in the Methods section. Putting intermediate results in Methods is a better choice than putting them in Results because intermediate results are more relevant to methods than to results.

Sufficient detail includes the following:

Materials

Drugs

For drugs, state the generic name, manufacturer, purity, and concentration. If the drug is in solution, give the solvent, pH, temperature, total volume infused, and rate of infusion, if appropriate. State the amount of drug administered per kilogram of body weight and the duration of the injection. If the drug is placed in an organ bath or reservoir, calculate its concentration in fluid.

Culture Media, Buffers

For culture media and buffers, state the components and their concentrations. Also state the temperature, volume, and pH, if appropriate.

Gases

For gases, state the components and their concentrations. Also state the flow rate, if appropriate.

Experimental Materials

If you studied a molecule, cell line, tissue, etc., specify it.

Animals

For animals, state the species and weight, and also the strain, sex, and age, if they are important. Give details of sedation and anesthesia: agent used, amount, route, administration (single, repeated, or continuous), depth of anesthesia and how it was assessed. If anesthetics were not used, state the reasons. State that the research was approved by the appropriate committee at your institution.

Human Subjects

For human subjects, give enough information about age, sex, race, height, weight, state of health or disease, and specific medical and surgical management to be of use to researchers who want to compare your data with theirs or other people's, or to clinicians who want to see if your findings are applicable to their patients. Tell how the subjects were selected. State that the research was approved by the appropriate committee at your institution.

Methods

Protocol

The protocol is the sequence of procedures that make up an experiment. The protocol has two components: manipulations done to cause a change and measurements or observations made to assess the change. The variables manipulated and the variables measured or observed are often referred to, respectively, as the *independent* variable(s) and the *dependent* variable(s), though the variables measured or observed are not necessarily dependent on the variables manipulated.

The protocol also includes a description of the *control* experiments or procedures, that is, controls of the independent variable. Two common types of control are *baseline* measurements (that is, measurements made before the independent variable is manipulated) and *sham experiments* done on a separate group of animals without manipulating the independent variable (for example, one experiment in which a drug is administered and an exact parallel [sham] experiment in which the solvent without the active agent is administered).

Not all Methods sections have protocols. In some scientific disciplines (for example, human gross anatomy), no manipulations are done to cause a change, so only the measurements or observations made are described in the Methods section. In these disciplines, the experimental approach at the end of the Introduction is generally sufficient to give an overview of the experiment, so a description of the protocol is unnecessary.

In other scientific disciplines (for example, biochemistry), often several sequential experiments are done, and the outcome of one experiment determines what the next experiment will be. In these disciplines, the protocol is described in the Results section, not in the Methods section (see Chap. 6: Results, Example 6.16).

Purpose

It is not always obvious to the reader why you did certain procedures, so state the purpose of any procedure whose relation to the question or to the rest of the protocol is not obvious. In Example 5.1 below, the question being studied was "whether the bronchoconstrictor effects of low concentrations of SO_2 in asthmatic subjects vary when they breathe SO_2 by mouthpiece, by facemask, or by nose only, during exercise." In the protocol from their Methods sections, the authors first described the experiments they did to answer this question. They then described two other procedures, whose relation to the question was not obvious. Therefore, before describing each procedure, they stated its purpose. In addition, for the first procedure, they presented relevant background information. Giving background information and stating the purpose make clear how what you did helps to answer the question you asked.

Example 5.1 Purposes Stated

Background

The shape of the oral cavity in a person breathing through a mouthpiece may differ from that in a person breathing through the mouth without a mouthpiece, and therefore the amount of inhaled SO_2 penetrating to the airways may be altered. <u>To compare the airway response to SO_2 breathed through a mouthpiece with the response to SO_2 breathed without a mouthpiece,</u> we

Purpose

Procedure

had two subjects perform the exercise protocol while they were breathing 0.5 ppm SO_2 first by mouthpiece while wearing a noseclip and then by facemask while wearing a noseclip.

Purpose

<u>To verify that the bronchoconstrictor response to SO_2 was related to the concentration inhaled, regardless of the route of inhalation,</u> we constructed

Procedure

SO_2 dose-response curves from data on two subjects who breathed three different concentrations of SO_2 both through a mouthpiece and by facemask during exercise.

Note the use of a verb form to convey purpose: "To compare," "To verify" (in the underlined sentences).

Methods and Apparatus

The amount of detail needed when describing a method or an apparatus depends on how well known the method or apparatus is.

A well known method or apparatus need not be described. All that is needed is the reference, as in Example 5.2.

Example 5.2   Well Known Method

In these samples, lipids were extracted (Bligh and Dyer, 1959) for phosphorus determination (Bartlett, 1959) and for thin-layer chromatography (Poorthuis et al., 1976).

For a less well known method or apparatus, state the essential features and give the reference, as in Example 5.3.

Example 5.3   Less Well Known Method

Lamellar bodies were isolated according to a previously reported procedure (Baritussio et al., 1981). This procedure separates lamellar bodies into two populations that have different densities: light lamellar bodies, which are collected between 0.33 and 0.45 M sucrose, and dense lamellar bodies, which are collected between 0.45 and 0.58 M sucrose.

Similarly, if you modified a method or apparatus, state the essential features of the modification in addition to giving the reference. Also state the purpose of the modification, if knowing it would be helpful to the reader, as in Example 5.4.

Example 5.4   Modified Method

In lamellar bodies and other fractions obtained from the density gradient procedure, the amount of protein was determined (Lowry et al., 1951) using 1% sodium dodecyl sulfate (Eastman Kodak, Rochester NY) to reduce interference by lipids (Lees and Paxman, 1972).

In Example 5.4, the modification is "using 1% sodium dodecyl sulfate" and the purpose of the modification is "to reduce interference by lipids."

If a modification is trivial, it does not need to be mentioned.

For a new method or apparatus, present a complete description so that the reader can evaluate or use the method or apparatus with full understanding of how it works.

Analysis of Data

State how you calculated derived variables (such as pulmonary vascular resistance) either in Methods of Measurement and Calculation or in Analysis of Data.

State how you summarized your data. For this statement, provide the reader with information about both the magnitude of the data (what statisticians call a measure of central tendency) and the variability. What information you give to summarize the magnitude and the variability of your data depends on whether the data come from a normal distribution or a skewed distribution.

When the data seem to have been drawn from a normal distribution (or, at least, are distributed symmetrically about the mean), it is reasonable to use the mean and standard deviation (SD) to summarize the data. The mean provides a description of the overall magnitude of the data. The standard deviation provides a measure of the variability in the sample. People often use the mean and the standard error of the mean (SEM) (which equals the standard deviation divided by the square root of the sample size) to summarize data. But using the mean and the standard error of the mean is generally not a good way to summarize data for two reasons. One reason is that the standard error of the mean does not indicate the variability in the sample (as an estimate of the variability in the underlying population); rather, the standard error of the mean quantifies the uncertainty in the estimate of the true mean (that is, the mean of the underlying population). Another reason not to use the standard error of the mean to summarize data is that many readers do not know the difference between the standard error of the mean and the standard deviation. When these readers see a standard error of the mean, they misinterpret it as indicating the variability in the sample. To avoid the chance of this misinterpretation, it is clearest to use the mean and standard deviation (which does indicate the variability in the sample) to summarize data.

When the data appear to come from a skewed distribution (that is, an inordinate number of high or low values, compared to the mean), the mean and standard deviation do not provide an accurate summary of the data. In this case, you should report the median and the interquartile range (that is, the range between the 25th and the 75th percentiles).

For statistical analysis, state the statistical tests that you used and, for tests that are not well known, also give a reference to the report or book that describes the tests as you used them. Well known tests that do not need to be referenced include Student's t test, chi square, standard forms of analysis of variance, linear regression, correlation, and widely used nonparametric tests such as the Wilcoxon signed-rank test.

Except when using the simplest of statistical methods (such as the t-test), if you used a computer program to analyze your data, state which program (including version or release number) and which nondefault options you used. Provide a reference.

State which measurements the statistical tests you used compare with each other.

If the size of the sample analyzed for each comparison (n) is not obvious from the protocol, state the sample size in the Analysis of Data section.

State the P value at which you considered differences statistically significant. In addition, give specific P values in figure legends, footnotes to tables, or the Results section, where each P value can be linked with the relevant data.

To determine whether to accept or reject a hypothesis, a P value is not always sufficient. A difference can be statistically significant but biologically or clinically unimportant. For example, a difference can be statistically significant because the sample size is large rather than because a treatment has a large effect (see Glantz, pp. 174–175). Thus, it is often useful to assess the size of the difference in comparison with the variability in the data sample by calculating the 95% confidence interval (see Glantz, Chap. 7, and Gardner and Altman).

Example 5.5   Sample Analysis of Data Section

Data are summarized as mean ± SD.[1] To analyze the data statistically, we performed a one-way analysis of variance[2] for repeated measurements of the same variable.[3] We then used Dunnett's multiple range t test (10)[4] to determine which means were significantly different from the mean of the control periods.[3] We considered differences significant at $P < 0.05$.[5]

[1] *How the data were summarized*
[2] *Statistical test used (well known; no reference needed)*
[3] *Measurements that were compared*
[4] *Statistical test used (unfamiliar test; reference needed)*
[5] P *value at which differences were considered statistically significant*

Preparation

Preparation consists of procedures done before the experiments can be done. In physiology experiments, for example, preparation often includes anesthesia and insertion of catheters. For examples, see Example 5.14 and Exercises 5.1 and 5.2 at the end of this chapter.

Assumptions

If your experimental design is based on assumptions, state the assumptions and your reasons for believing that they are valid. If your reasons are lengthy, they can be presented in the Discussion (see Chap. 7, Example 7.10).

Indicators

If you assessed an indicator of a variable, make clear what variable it is an indicator of. For example, "We infused blood into the superior and inferior venae cavae at about 25 ml/kg over 2 min until <u>mean left atrial pressure, our indicator of preload</u>, increased by about 100%." Then in the rest of the Methods section, talk about mean left atrial pressure, not about preload. If you identified the indicator in the Introduction, you do not have to identify it again in Methods.

ORGANIZATION

Overall Organization of Topics Within the Materials and Methods Section

Organize Chronologically and by the Type of Information

The overall organization of the Materials and Methods section is essentially chronological. In addition, because Materials and Methods is a long section that presents several different types of information, Materials and Methods is divided into subsections according to the type of information. Below are two possible sequences of subsections, one for studies that involve manipulating an independent variable and the other for studies that have only dependent variables.

SCHEMATIC OUTLINES OF TWO "TYPICAL" MATERIALS AND METHODS SECTIONS

Possible Organization for a Physiology Paper	*Possible Organization for a Human Gross Anatomy Paper*
I. Surgical Preparation	I. Materials
II. Protocol	II. Preparation of Samples
A. Independent variables	III. Procedures for the Dependent Variables
B. Dependent variables	A. Procedure 1
C. Control series	B. Procedure 2
III. Methods	C. Procedure 3
A. Independent variables	etc.
B. Dependent variables	IV. Analysis of Data
IV. Analysis of Data	

For an example of a Methods section from a physiology paper in which the physiology outline is followed (except for III A) see Exercise 5.1 at the end of this chapter.

Describe the Protocol Early in the Materials and Methods Section

The protocol should be described early in the Methods section (usually right after the preparation) because the protocol gives the overview. The protocol is the framework against which the details of methods of measurement make sense. Without the protocol, the reader will know how you did each procedure but will not know how each procedure helps answer the question.

Make the Protocol Tell a Story

In physiology papers and other papers that have independent as well as dependent variables, the protocol is the part of the Methods section that continues the story begun in the Introduction. That is, the Introduction poses a question and the protocol tells what you did to answer the question. For the story to be clear, the protocol should be in a separate subsection and should be kept as simple and uncluttered as possible. To ensure that the story in the protocol is clear,

- Put other types of information in separate subsections (unless they are so brief that they will not unduly clutter the protocol).
- Omit unnecessary ("housekeeping") detail.
- Avoid repetition. For example, if one step appears two or more times, do not keep repeating it. Find a way to describe it just once.
- Provide an overview by describing the independent and dependent variables sequentially.

Organization Within Subsections

Within each subsection of Methods, organize topics either chronologically or in order of most to least importance. For preparation, chronological order is best. For the methods subsection, the organization depends on the type of information. If you have methods for both independent variables and dependent variables, describe the methods for the independent variables first (chronological order). If you measured both dependent variables that answer the question and dependent variables that monitor the animals' health, describe the methods for the dependent variables that answer the question first (most to least important).

Protocol

In the protocol, describe the independent variable first and the dependent variable second. That is, use chronological order—first what you did to cause an effect (independent variable) and then what effects you observed or measured (dependent variables). Often authors describe only the independent variable in the protocol. They describe dependent variables separately, in the methods of measurement. But methods of measurement tells, in detail, *how* you did the experiments. The point of including dependent variables in the protocol is to give an *overview of what you did to answer the question and in what order you did it.* For this overview to be complete, both the independent and the dependent variables must be included (see Examples 5.6 and 5.7 and the revision of Example 5.8 below).

Controls

Describe the controls in the most appropriate part of the protocol. Where a control is described depends on the length of the description and on the type of control. If the control can be described briefly (in a few words), it should be described along with the description of the main experiment, as in Example 5.6.

Example 5.6   Control Described Briefly With the Independent Variables

To determine the effect of beta-adrenergic agonists on clearance of liquid and protein from the lungs, we instilled into one lower lobe either <u>serum alone</u> (6 sheep),[1] serum mixed with terbutaline (10^{-5} M, Geigy, Summit NJ) (6 sheep), or serum mixed with epinephrine (5.5×10^{-6} M, Am Quinine, Shirley NY) (6 sheep),[2] and then measured the variables described in the general protocol.[3]

> [1] = *Sham control*
> [2] = *Independent variables*
> [3] = *Dependent variables*

If a control needs to be described at length (one sentence or more), it should be described separately. Where to describe a lengthy control depends on whether the control is a baseline or a sham experiment. A lengthy baseline control should be described before the main experiment is described (that is, at the beginning of the protocol), as in Example 5.7, because this is the actual sequence of events.

Example 5.7   Baseline Control Described at the Beginning of the Protocol

The effect of high frequency ventilation on the discharge of the three known types of pulmonary receptors was ascertained as follows. After a single afferent nerve fiber from a slowly adapting pulmonary stretch receptor, a rapidly adapting pulmonary receptor, or a pulmonary C-fiber was identified, <u>recordings were made for 1-2 min during normal controlled ventilation with the Harvard ventilator.</u>[1] The dog was then ventilated with the high frequency ventilator[2] and afferent nerve activity was recorded sequentially[3] at three mean airway pressures—low, intermediate, and high (approximately 0.5, 1.0, and 1.5 kPa, respectively)[2] —until a steady state was reached, usually 1-2 min.

1 = *Baseline*
2 = *Independent variable*
3 = *Dependent variable*

Note that in the description of the baseline, both the dependent variable (recordings of afferent nerve activity) and the independent variable (normal controlled ventilation) are included.

A lengthy sham control should be described after the main experiment (see Exercise 5.1, para. 5) because time sequence is not at issue; in fact, sham experiments and the main experiments are often done on separate days in random order. In addition, describing the sham experiment after the main experiment puts the emphasis on the main experiment, which is appropriate because the main experiment is what you did to answer your question.

For the same reason, quality controls, such as experiments done to check the validity of the independent variable, should be described after the main experiment.

Similarly, the description of baseline measurements should be kept as brief as possible. For example, instead of naming all the variables when describing the baseline measurements, use a category term and then name the variables either when describing the main experiment or, if necessary, separately, after describing the main experiment, as in the revision of Example 5.8.

Example 5.8   Baseline Control Described at Too Much Length

After a 30-min period of stabilization, baseline aortic, pulmonary arterial, left atrial, and vena caval pressures, heart rate, and cardiac output were recorded. Blood samples (1.0 ml) were collected from the pulmonary artery, ascending aorta, and coronary sinus for measurement of blood gases, hemoglobin oxygen saturation, and hemoglobin concentration. For measurement of blood flow, radionuclide-labeled microspheres of 15-μm diameter were then rapidly injected into the left atrium while reference blood samples were withdrawn from the ascending and descending aorta at a rate of 7 ml/min for 1.25 min. After these baseline measurements in room air, a gas mixture containing 9% oxygen in nitrogen was administered through the plastic bag, as described previously (4). After 45 min of hypoxemia, the measurements were repeated. During hypoxemia the presence of any significant right-to-left shunt through the foramen ovale or the ductus arteriosus was excluded by the indicator-dilution technique. Propranolol (0.5 mg/kg) was then administered intravenously, and after another 15 min, the measurements were again repeated. The lamb was then returned to room air and all measurements except microsphere injection were repeated at 15 and 30 min of recovery.

Revision

After a 30-min period of stabilization, baseline measurements were made in room air.*1* Then a gas mixture containing 9% oxygen in nitrogen was administered through the plastic bag, as described previously (4).*2* After 45 min of hypoxemia, variables were measured.*3* During hypoxemia the presence of any significant right-to-left shunt through the foramen ovale or the ductus arteriosus was excluded by the indicator-dilution technique. Propranolol (0.5 mg/ kg) was then administered intravenously,*2* and after another 15 min, measurements were again repeated.*3* The lamb was then returned to room air*4* and all measurements except blood flow were repeated at 15 and 30 min of recovery.*3*

The variables measured were as follows. Aortic, pulmonary arterial, left atrial, and vena caval pressures, heart rate, and cardiac output were recorded. Blood samples (1.0 ml) were collected from the pulmonary artery, ascending aorta, and coronary sinus for measurement of blood gases, hemoglobin oxygen saturation, and hemoglobin concentration. For measurement of blood flow, radionuclide-labeled microspheres of 15-μm diameter were then rapidly injected into the left atrium while reference blood samples were withdrawn from the ascending and descending aorta at a rate of 7 ml/min for 1.25 min.

> **1** = *Baseline*
> **2** = *Independent variable*
> **3** = *Dependent variables*
> **4** = *Recovery*

In the revision, the dependent variables are presented in a separate paragraph after the description of the protocol. Now that the sequence of baseline (1), independent variables (2), dependent variables (3), and recovery (4) that constitutes the protocol is uninterrupted, the reader can more easily see what was done to answer the question. (The question was whether blockade of beta-adrenergic receptors abolishes the deleterious response of newborns to acute, moderate hypoxemia.) Naming the dependent variables while describing the baseline (as in Example 5.8) overemphasized the baseline and interrupted the description of the protocol; the trees overshadowed the forest. Naming the dependent variables while describing the main experiment would also interrupt the description of the protocol. Thus, the best solution is to name the dependent variables separately, after the protocol, as in the revision.

In some studies, both a baseline and a sham control are used. Both should be clearly described (see Exercise 5.1, para. 5). To distinguish between the two types of control, even if you did not use both types in your experiments, call the baseline "baseline," not "control."

Relationship of Parts

Relate the Protocol to the Question It Answers

To ensure that the protocol relates clearly to the question it answers, you may need to restate the question before describing the protocol, as done in the first sentences of Examples 5.6 and 5.7 above. When there is more than one question, restate the appropriate question at the beginning of each protocol, so that the reader knows which protocol relates to which question. When restating the question, be sure to use the same key terms, the same verb, and the same point of view as in the original question. For example, if the question was

> "whether <u>nicotine receptors</u> **are involved** both in reflex stimulation of the central respiratory centers and in direct stimulation of the airway sympathetic ganglia,"

the beginning of the protocol for this question should read as follows:

> "To determine whether <u>nicotine receptors</u> **are involved** both in reflex stimulation of the central respiratory centers and in direct stimulation of the airway sympathetic ganglia, we blocked nicotine receptors and then assessed these variables while the dogs inhaled cigarette smoke."

Note that the question at the beginning of the protocol repeats the question exactly as it was stated in the Introduction: the key terms are the same, the verb is the same, and the point of view and the order of details are the same. Thus, the reader can easily recognize that this question is the same question asked in the Introduction.

Relate the Methods to the Results

For every result in the Results section there should be a method in the Methods section.

Relate the Parts Described in the Methods Section to Each Other

Be careful that the relation of parts is not lost by division of the Materials and Methods section into subsections. For example, if in the Surgical Preparation you say that you placed several catheters and in the Protocol you say that you injected drugs and measured various pressures, the reader is left to imagine which catheter was used for each procedure. Do not leave this (or anything else) to the reader's imagination: in one of the subsections state what each catheter was used for.

Signaling the Organization

Both visual and verbal signals can be used to indicate new topics in the Methods section.

Visual Signals

Visual signals include subtitles, new paragraphs, and new sentences. Subtitles can be used to indicate subsections of the Methods section. New paragraphs signal new topics within the subsections. New sentences signal subtopics within a paragraph.

Subtitles are unnecessary in short Methods sections. Similarly, a subtitle is not necessary before every paragraph of a Methods section. When used in long Methods sections, subtitles can be general, as in the outlines earlier in this chapter, or specific, describing the content of the subsection. For example, a paper on actin and the secretion of surfactant used the following specific subtitles in the Methods section:

> Animals
> Controls
> Stimulation with Isoproterenol
> Cytochalasin Treatment
> Analysis of Tissue Sections
> Lactate Dehydrogenase Activity

If subtitles are used, every section should have its own subtitle, and the subtitles should be parallel to each other. The following subtitles are not parallel: Surgical Preparation, Protocol, Microsphere Protocol, Analysis of Data, because "Protocol" is more general than "Microsphere Protocol." The subtitles were revised to be parallel as follows: Surgical Preparation, Pressure-Flow Relation Protocol, Microsphere Protocol, Analysis of Data.

Verbal Signals

Visual signals alone are rarely enough. Visual signals are for the eye. The brain also needs signals.

Verbal signals, for the brain, include topic sentences, transition phrases, and words. A topic sentence gives an overview of all the other sentences in a paragraph, as in Example 5.7 above and Example 5.9 below.

Example 5.9 Topic Sentence Signaling the Topic of the Paragraph

<u>The effects of intra-arterial pressure gradients on steady-state circumflex pressure-flow relations derived during long diastoles were examined in five dogs</u>. To obtain each pressure-flow point, we first set the mean circumflex pressure to the desired level and then arrested the heart by turning off the pacemaker. The pressure and the flow rate were measured after a steady-state was reached, usually within 2-3 s. In these experiments, one pressure-flow relation was derived in the absence of intra-arterial pressure gradients and the other in the presence of a gradient, when mean left main coronary arterial pressure was held constant at 100 mmHg.

A transition phrase stating the purpose of a procedure can signal the topic of a paragraph (as in Example 5.10 below) or a subtopic within a paragraph (as in the second sentence of Example 5.9 above). However, a purpose stated at the end of a sentence does not signal the topic (see sentences G and J of Example 5.14 below); the topic must be signaled at the beginning. Another example of a transition phrase signaling the topic is, "In the control series, ..."

Example 5.10 Transition Phrase Signaling the Topic of the Paragraph

<u>To prepare the enzyme solution</u>, the cells were first incubated in lipoprotein-deficient serum for 48 h. Then, after being washed with phosphate-buffered saline three times, the cells were harvested, suspended in 3 ml of phosphate-buffered saline, and homogenized in a glass-glass homogenizer by hand. The homogenate was centrifuged at $700 \times g$ for 10 min and the resultant supernatant was used as the enzyme solution.

In Example 5.10, the transition phrase at the beginning of the first sentence (underlined) signals that the topic of the paragraph is how the enzyme solution was prepared. The end of the first sentence gives the first detail of the preparation. The other two sentences give the remaining details of the preparation (in chronological order). Thus, the difference between a topic sentence and a transition phrase signaling a topic of a paragraph is whether the sentence gives an overview or only the first step.

Words, including verbs and key terms, can be used as signals of the topic of a paragraph or a subtopic within a paragraph. An example of a verb signaling a topic is "Dogs <u>were anesthetized</u>." The topic is anesthesia. An example of a key term signaling the topic is "The <u>respiratory rate</u> was adjusted to achieve an arterial P_{CO_2} between 30 and 40 mmHg." The topic is respiratory rate. Note that a key term signaling the topic is the same thing as making the topic the subject of the sentence, if the subject comes at the beginning of the sentence (see Chap. 2).

To signal the protocol, thus linking "what was done" to the question posed in the Introduction, either a topic sentence (see Examples 5.7 and 5.9) or a transition phrase stating the question as a purpose (see Example 5.6) can be used.

LENGTH

The Methods section should be as long as necessary to describe fully and accurately what was done and how it was done. However, Methods should be written in the fewest words possible and should not contain fussy detail. What constitutes fussy detail depends on what the readers of the journal to which you submit your paper can be expected to know.

DETAILS

Species

To ensure that the reader knows what species you studied, use the species name or the common name (for example, dog, cat) every time, not the general term "animal."

Verb Tense

Methods are reported in *past tense*, for example, "we <u>measured</u>," "catheters <u>were inserted</u>." (Also see examples above.)

However, to describe how data are presented in the paper, use present tense, because this information is still true. For example, "Data <u>are</u> summarized as mean ± SD."

Sample Size

When you have several different sample sizes (for example, for subgroups within a group), be sure that the numbers add up correctly throughout the Methods section (and throughout the paper). For example, if the Methods section begins by saying that experiments were done on 39 rabbits and later says that 25 rabbits were treated with one drug and 13 rabbits were treated with another drug, the reader wonders whether one rabbit was left untreated. Or if the Methods section says that 11 rabbits were prepared and then reports that 5 rabbits were used in the first protocol, 4 in the second protocol, and 6 in the third protocol, the reader wonders why 4 of the 15 were not prepared. If the author meant that 5 of the 11 were used in the first protocol, 4 of the 11 in the second protocol, and 6 of the 11 in the third protocol, that is the way to describe them: "4 of the 11," not "4."

Similarly, for studies of human subjects, make clear how the numbers of subjects relate to each other. For example, if 100 subjects were admitted to the study but 20 were disqualified, the total number studied is 80, not 100. Of these 80, if 30 were used in one protocol, clarify that the 30 were part of the 80, not in addition to the 80, by writing, "In 30 of the 80 subjects, we tested . . . " or "Of the 80 subjects, 30 were given . . . ." To indicate that in another protocol 30 different subjects were studied, write, "In 30 other subjects, we tested . . . " or "Thirty other subjects were given. . . ."

Information in Parentheses

In the Methods section, details are often placed in parentheses so that the flow of ideas in the sentence will not be interrupted. Some details that are commonly placed in parentheses are weights of animals or human subjects, concentrations, doses, manufacturers' names, and model numbers. For example, "Horse red blood cells (Colorado Serum Company, Boulder) were washed three times in 7 ml of 0.9% NaCl before use to remove preservatives." See also Example 5.12 below. If instead details are written before the noun, no parentheses are used. Compare "10 mg nitroglycerin" and "nitroglycerin (10 mg)."

Precise Word Choice

Use the verb that indicates precisely what you did: "measured," "calculated," "estimated." For example, "We <u>measured</u> heart rate and ventricular pressure and <u>calculated</u> maximal positive dP/dt." If you want to discuss measurements and calculations together, using one term that includes both, use "determined." For example, "We <u>determined</u> heart rate, ventricular pressure, and maximal positive dP/dt."

Avoid interchanging the following terms:

<u>Study</u>: A sustained, systematic inquiry into, or examination of, a phenomenon, development, or question
<u>Experiment</u>: A test done to examine the validity of a hypothesis (referred to as a study when the subjects are human)
<u>Series</u>: A set of two or more related experiments
<u>Group</u>: A number of experimental animals or human subjects treated similarly or having similar characteristics

One paper is equivalent to one study, but it can report many experiments, series of experiments, and groups of animals or subjects, as shown in Example 5.11.

Example 5.11

In this <u>study</u>, the <u>experiments</u> were organized into two <u>series</u>. In the first <u>series</u>, we measured the loss of 9-μm-diameter microspheres from the lungs; in the second <u>series</u>, we measured the loss of 9-μm-diameter microspheres from the left ventricular myocardium. Each <u>series</u> of <u>experiments</u> was performed on two <u>groups</u> of dogs, one <u>group</u> anesthetized with Innovar-Vet and a 75:25 mixture of nitrous oxide and oxygen and the other <u>group</u> anesthetized with halothane.

The Sound of Preparation Versus the Sound of Methods

Make preparation sound like preparation and make methods sound like methods. To do this, use the appropriate subject and verb. That is, make the topic the subject and put the action in the verb (see Chap. 2). In the preparation, the topics are such things as anesthesia and catheters, and the appropriate verbs are "was induced" and "were inserted." In methods of measurement, the topics are variables such as blood flow and total pulmonary resistance, and the appropriate verbs are "was measured" and "was calculated." Thus, the following sentence, which originally appeared in a preparation subsection, actually belongs in methods of measurement.

Example 5.12   A Methods of Measurement Statement

<u>Airflow</u> **was measured** by a differential transducer (Validyne MP45) connected to a heated pneumotachograph (Fleisch #1) located at the proximal end of the endotracheal tube.

If the author wanted to keep this sentence in the preparation, she would have to change the subject to "a differential transducer" and the verb to "was placed," as in Example 5.13.

Example 5.13   A Preparation Statement

<u>A differential transducer</u> (Validyne MP45) connected to a heated pneumotachograph (Fleisch #1) **was placed** at the proximal end of the endotracheal tube for measurement of airflow.

Note that the purpose of the differential transducer is mentioned at the end of the sentence in the preparation subsection so that the reader will know what variable the differential transducer measured.

Point of View

In the Methods section , the point of view can be either that of the experiment or that of the experimenter.

Point of view of the experiment: Blood samples were drawn.
Point of view of the experimenter: We drew blood samples.

If you choose the point of view of the experimenter, rather than the point of view of the experiment, many of your sentences will begin with "we." Beginning many sentences with "we" is obnoxious. Therefore, if you choose this point of view, keep the number of "we's" to a minimum and vary the beginnings of sentences so that very few begin with "we." To keep the number of "we's" to a minimum, put all the steps of a single procedure in one sentence.

<u>We</u> **dehydrated** the pellets, **cleared** them with propylene oxide, and **embedded** small pieces of each pellet in blocks of Spurr's resin.

To make the "we's" less prominent, vary the beginnings of the sentences. Begin some sentences with a word or a phrase indicating time sequence:

<u>After 30 s</u>, we centrifuged the samples.
<u>Then</u> we centrifuged the suspension as before.

Begin some sentences with the purpose:

<u>To prepare isolated surface layers for electron microscopy</u>, we resuspended the 0.1-ml pellets of packed, washed surface layers in 0.2–0.3 ml of buffer and pipetted this concentrated suspension into a 35-mm-diameter plastic culture dish partially filled with hardened epoxy resin that had been coated with polylysine.

Begin some sentences with a reason:

<u>Because these surface layers did not stick well to polylysine</u>, we processed them as small pellets.

Begin some sentences with a phrase subordinating the first step of a procedure:

<u>After fixing the surface layers for 0.5–2 h</u>, we rinsed them three times in glycine-free buffer and then post-fixed them in 1% OsO_4 in glycine-free buffer for 0.5–1 h.

Handling Point of View in the Methods Section

At the simplest level of sophistication, you can choose to write your entire Methods section from one point of view. If you choose the point of view of the experiment, this choice has the advantage of making the topic the subject of the sentence, thus emphasizing what is important (the method, the variable, etc.). The disadvantage is that most sentences will be in passive voice, which is dull. But since people read Methods to get precise information, the disadvantage of dullness is generally outweighed by the advantage of making the topic the subject. So choosing to write the Methods section from the point of view of the experiment is a defensible choice. The alternative, the point of view of the experimenter ("we"), is undeniably more lively because it usually requires the use of active voice. However, it sacrifices having the topic as the subject of the sentence. Also, using "we" is inappropriate if someone other than the authors (for example, a technician) actually did the work. In addition, if "we" is not carefully handled, it can be distracting. Nevertheless, if "we" is well handled, choosing to write the Methods section from the point of view of the experimenter is also a defensible choice. Since both points of view are defensible, choose whichever point of view you are more comfortable with.

At a higher level of sophistication, you can write some subsections from one point of view and other subsections from another point of view. For example, you can use "we" in the protocol, as in Example 5.6 above, but not in the methods of measurement, as in Example 5.4. An advantage of this choice is that subsections that are difficult to write from one point of view can be written from the other.

At the highest level of sophistication, you can choose one point of view for a given subsection but write some sentences from another point of view when you have a specific and obvious reason. For example, you can use the point of view of the experimenter ("we") for sentences that move the story forward and the point of view of the experiment for sentences that do not move the story forward, as in Example 5.14. The advantage is that the writing is smooth and clear.

What you want to avoid is changing back and forth from one point of view to another several times within one paragraph for no apparent reason.

Example 5.14 Handling Point of View in the Methods Section

AFive mongrel dogs, weighing 17.1 to 27.2 kg, were anesthetized with sodium pentobarbital (Nembutal, Abbott Laboratories, 25 mg/kg, i.v.), intubated, and ventilated with a positive pressure respirator (Model 607, Harvard Apparatus Co., Millis MA). **B**To maintain anesthesia during surgery and during the experiment, we gave additional doses of sodium pentobarbital (0.5–1.0 mg · kg^{-1} · h^{-1}). **C**We performed a thoracotomy through the fourth left intercostal space. **D**Through a 1- to 2-cm incision in the pericardium, we inserted a multiple-side-hole polyvinyl catheter and a 2 × 3 cm flat silastic balloon, which we placed at the level of the mid-left ventricle when the dog was supine. **E**The catheter and the balloon were used to measure pericardial pressure. **F**The catheter was also used to inject fluid into the pericardial cavity. **G**We sutured the incision in the pericardium watertight and placed a second flat balloon at the level of the first balloon on the outside of the pericardium in order to measure pleural pressure. **H**We led all three tubes through the thoracotomy incision. **I**Then we inserted a chest tube through a separate incision and advanced it behind the sternum about 20 cm towards the diaphragm. **J**We sutured both incisions and connected the chest tube to a suction line to remove the air from the chest.

This paragraph is written from the point of view of the experimenter except for two places: the first sentence (to avoid starting with "we") and the two sentences describing the purposes of the catheter and the balloon, which, unlike the other sentences in this paragraph, do not move the story forward. The author has made an effort to avoid starting every sentence with "we": of the 10 sentences, 3 start with nouns (underlined), 4 start with "we," and 3 avoid starting with "we" (underlined, italics). This paragraph could easily have been written without any "we's," but it would have been less lively.

Units of Measurement

The International System of Units (Système International d'Unités) (SI units) should be used. For a list of SI units and their abbreviations, see reference books, such as the CBE Style Manual (pp. 147–150), and articles in journals, such as Young's article in *Annals of Internal Medicine* (1987).

**SUMMARY OF
GUIDELINES
FOR METHODS**

FUNCTION

To provide enough detail and references to enable a trained scientist to evaluate or repeat your work.

CONTENT

Materials

Chemicals (drugs, culture media, buffers, gases).

Experimental materials (molecules, cell lines, tissues).

Experimental animals or human subjects.

Methods

Preparation, if necessary.

Protocol, when appropriate.
  Independent variables.
  Dependent variables.
  Controls.

Purposes of all protocols and all methods.

Methods and apparatus.

Analysis of data, including statistical analysis.
  How the data were summarized (for example, mean $\pm$ SD).
  Statistical tests used.
  Which measurements were compared.
  Sample size (n).
  P value at which differences were considered statistically
    significant.

Assumptions, if any.

Indicators, if any.

ORGANIZATION

Organize the Methods section chronologically and by the type of information.
  If your experiment required preparation of materials or animals, describe
    the preparation separately at or near the beginning of the Methods
    section.
  If your experiment followed a protocol, describe the protocol separately
    and early in the Methods section.
  Do not include methods of measurement in the protocol. Describe methods
    of measurement separately later in the Methods section.
  Two "typical" organizations for Methods sections are as follows:

Physiology	*Human Gross Anatomy*
Surgical Preparation	Materials
Protocol	Preparation of Samples
Independent variables	Procedures for Dependent Variables
Dependent variables	Procedure 1

Control series   Procedure 2
Methods   Procedure 3
   Independent variables   etc.
   Dependent variables   Analysis of Data
Analysis of Data

Within each subsection of the Methods section, organize topics either chronologically or from most to least important.

Make the protocol tell a story. For the story to be clear, the protocol must be

> Simple: Uncluttered by other kinds of information, unnecessary detail, or repetition.
> Complete: Describing both the independent and the dependent variables and all controls.
> All in one spot: Not scattered in various paragraphs.

Describe controls in the most appropriate part of the protocol.

> If a control can be described briefly, describe it along with the main experiment.
> If a control needs to be described at length, describe it separately.
>> Describe a separate baseline control as briefly as possible before describing the main experiment.
>> Describe a separate control series after describing the main experiment.

In studies of animals in which catheters were used, make clear, either in the preparation or in the protocol, which catheter was used for which purpose.

Provide signals of the organization so that the overview is clear. Use both visual and verbal signals.

> Visual Signals
>> Subtitles: To signal subsections in long Methods sections.
>> New paragraphs: To signal new topics.
>> New sentences: To signal new subtopics.
> Verbal Signals
>> A topic sentence gives an overview of the paragraph.
>> A transition phrase states a purpose that signals the topic of a paragraph or a subtopic within a paragraph.
>> Words signal the topic of a paragraph or a subtopic within a paragraph.

LENGTH

Make the Methods section as long as necessary to describe what you did but do not include unnecessary words or fussy detail.

DETAILS

Use the species name or the common name of the animal you studied (for example, dog, cat) throughout the Methods section. Do not use the general term "animal."

Write Methods in past tense.

Make relationships between sample sizes clear, for example by writing, "In 4 of the 11 rabbits" or "In 30 other subjects."

Distinguish between "measured," "calculated," and "estimated." Use "determined" when you need to describe two or more of these procedures together.

Distinguish between "study" and "experiment" and between "series" and "group."

Use the appropriate subject and verb when describing preparation and when describing methods so that preparation sounds like preparation and methods sound like methods. For example, "A differential transducer was placed for measurement of airflow" is a preparation statement and "Airflow was measured by a differential transducer" is a methods statement.

Use subjects and verbs that create the point of view that you prefer.

To focus on the topic, make the topic the subject.

To make the writing lively, make "we" the subject.

Use the International System of Units (SI units).

■ *EXERCISE 5.1: A CLEARLY WRITTEN METHODS SECTION*

1. *In the left margin of the Methods section below*
   a) *write the* <u>*topic of each paragraph*</u>*;*
   b) *identify the* <u>*protocol*</u> *that answers the question;*
   c) *in the protocol that answers the question, identify the* <u>*independent*</u> *and* <u>*dependent variables*</u>*, and all* <u>*controls*</u>*.*

2. *Is the protocol complete? _____ Is the protocol clear? _____*

3. *Is it easy to see how the protocol will yield the answer to the question? ___*

4. *Write the letters of*

   a. *All* <u>*topic sentences*</u> *_____,*

   b. *All sentences in which the topic of the paragraph is signaled by a* <u>*transition phrase*</u>*; underline the phrase _____,*

   c. *All sentences in which the topic of the paragraph is signaled by a* <u>*word*</u>*; underline or circle the word _____,*

5. *Is it easy to find the protocol that answers the question? _____*

6. *In the right margin, identify the* <u>*techniques of continuity*</u> *used between sentences within each paragraph.*

7. *Do you like the way point of view is handled (the use of "we")? _____*

8. *Why? _____*

The <u>question</u> this paper asks is, "Does stimulation of pulmonary C-fibers reflexively evoke increased secretion from tracheal submucosal glands?" To answer this question, the authors did experiments on segments of tracheas in dogs in which pulmonary C-fibers were stimulated by injection of capsaicin and then secretions from tracheal submucosal glands were measured.

Topic   *Techniques of*
                                                                     Continuity

Methods

Preparation

1 *A*Nine dogs (14–25 kg) were anesthetized with thiopental sodium (25 mg/kg i.v.) followed by chloralose (80 mg/kg i.v.). *B*Supplemental doses of chloralose (10 mg/kg i.v.) were given hourly to maintain anesthesia. *C*The dogs were paralyzed with decamethonium bromide (0.1 mg/kg) 10 min before measurements of tracheal secretion.

2 *D*The trachea was cannulated low in the neck, and the lungs were ventilated with 50% oxygen in air by a Harvard respirator (model 613), whose expiratory outlet was placed under 3–5 cm of water. *E*Percent CO_2 in the respired gas was monitored by a Beckman LB-1 gas analyzer, and end-expiratory CO_2 concentration was kept at about 5% by adjusting the ventilatory rate. *F*Arterial blood samples were withdrawn periodically and their P_{O_2}, P_{CO_2}, and pH were determined by a blood gas/pH analyzer (Corning 175). *G*Sodium bicarbonate (0.33 meq/ml) was infused i.v. (1–3 ml/min) when necessary to minimize a base deficit in the blood.

3 *H*The chest was opened in the midsternal line and a catheter was inserted into the left atrium via the left atrial appendage. *I*Catheters were also inserted into the right atrium via the right jugular vein and into the abdominal aorta via a femoral artery.

4 *J*A segment of the trachea (4–5 cm) immediately caudal to the larynx was incised ventrally in the midline and transversely across both ends of the midline incision. *K*The dorsal wall was left intact. *L*Each midline cut edge was retracted laterally by nylon threads to expose the mucosal surface. *M*The threads were attached to a stationary bar on one side and to a force-displacement transducer (Grass FT03) on the other. *N*The segment was stretched to a baseline tension of 100–125 g.

Protocol

5 *O*To stimulate pulmonary C-fiber endings, in each of the 9 dogs we injected capsaicin (10–20 μg/kg) into the right atrium. *P*Capsaicin was taken from stock solutions prepared as described elsewhere (4). *Q*At 10-s intervals for 60 s before and 60 s after each injection, we measured secretions from tracheal submucosal glands. *R*Injections were separated by resting periods of about 30 min. ^{S}As a control, in the same 9 dogs we measured secretion in response to injection of vehicle (0.5–1.0 ml) into the right atrium.

6 ^{T}Although capsaicin selectively stimulates pulmonary C-fibers from within the pulmonary circulation, it is likely to stimulate other afferent pathways, including bronchial C-fibers, once it passes into the systemic circulation (2, 5). ^{U}To verify that secretion in our experiments was not caused by systemic effects of capsaicin, we next measured secretion after injecting capsaicin (10–20 μg/kg) into the left atrium and again, 30 min later, into the right atrium of all 9 dogs.

7 ^{V}Finally, to verify that stimulation of pulmonary C-fibers was responsible for the secretions, we measured secretion in response to capsaicin (10–20 μg/kg into the right atrium) in the 9 dogs before and after blocking conduction in both of the cervical vagus nerves, which carry the pulmonary C-fibers, either by cooling the nerves to 0°C as described elsewhere (8) (4 dogs) or by cutting the nerves (5 dogs). ^{W}Before the first blocking experiment on each dog, we cut the recurrent and pararecurrent nerves so that the tracheal segment received its motor supply solely from the superior laryngeal nerves (14). ^{X}Consequently, when we cooled or cut the midcervical vagus nerves during an experiment, we could be certain that the changes in the tracheal responses were caused by interruption of the afferent vagal C-fibers.

8 ^{Y}As a further check on the effects of stimulating (and blocking) pulmonary C-fibers, in each of these protocols we also measured heart rate, mean arterial pressure, and isometric smooth muscle tension of the tracheal segment, which are known to be altered reflexively by stimulation of pulmonary C-fibers (3).

Methods of Measurement

9 *Z*The rate of secretion from submucosal gland ducts was assessed by counting hillocks of mucus per unit time as described elsewhere (8). *AA*Briefly, immediately before each experiment, the mucosal surface was gently dried and sprayed with tantalum. *BB*The tantalum layer prevented the normal ciliary dispersion of secretions from the openings of the gland ducts, so the accumulated secretions elevated the tantalum layer to form hillocks. *CC*Hillocks with a diameter of at least 0.2 mm were counted in a 1.2 cm^2 field of mucosa. *DD*To facilitate counting, the mucosa of the retracted segment was viewed through a dissecting microscope, and its image was projected by a television camera (Sony AVC 1400) onto a television screen together with the output from a time-signal generator (3M Datavision DT-1). *EE*The image and the time signal were recorded by a videotape recorder (Sony VO-2600) for subsequent playback and measurement of the rate of hillock formation.

10 *FF*Heart rate, mean arterial pressure, and isometric smooth muscle tension of the tracheal segment were recorded continuously throughout each experiment by a Grass polygraph. *GG*Heart rate was measured by a cardiotachometer triggered by an electrocardiogram (lead II). *HH*Arterial pressure was measured by a Statham P25Db strain gauge connected to the catheter placed in a femoral artery. *II*Isometric smooth muscle tension in the segment was measured by a Grass FT03 force displacement transducer attached to the lateral edge of the retracted segment, as described elsewhere (1, 14).

Statistical Analysis

11   *JJ*Data are reported as mean ± SD. *KK*To determine if there were significant differences in secretion before and after stimulation within each protocol, or significant differences in secretion between protocols, we performed two-way repeated-measures analysis of variance. *LL*When we found a significant difference between protocols, we performed the Student-Newman-Keuls test to identify pairwise differences. *MM*We considered differences significant at $P < 0.05$.

■ EXERCISE 5.2: CONTENT AND ORGANIZATION IN THE METHODS SECTION

Rewrite this Methods section where necessary after answering the following questions. In your revision, use "we." Avoid putting "we" at the beginning of the sentence.

1. In the left margin, (a) write the topic of each paragraph; (b) identify the protocol that answers the question; (c) in that protocol, identify the independent and dependent variables; (d) identify all controls.

2. Is it easy to see how the protocol will yield the answer to the question? ___

3. Write the letters of

   a. All topic sentences _____ ,

   b. All sentences in which the topic of the paragraph is signaled by a transition phrase; underline the phrase _____ .

4. Is it easy to find the protocol that answers the question? _____

5. In paragraph 2, counting each verb as one step, there are 12 steps. If you list these verbs, you will see a pattern of repeated steps. In your revision, avoid this repetition so that the overview of the experiment is clear.

6. Is the description of the baseline clear? _____ If not, clarify it in your revision.

7. Would you leave paragraph 4 where it is or put it earlier? _____ If earlier, where? _____ Why? _____

8. Is the purpose of any procedure in the protocol unclear? _____ If so, what? _____ Clarify it in your revision.

9. Is the sample size (n) clear? _____ If not, try to clarify it in your revision.

10. Does any information seem inappropriate to the Methods section? _____ If so, what? _____

    Where should this information go and why? _____

One question this paper asks is, "Does exogenous arachidonic acid increase prostaglandin E_2 production in the ductus arteriosus?"

The Results sections of this paper is Example 6.15 in Chapter 6: Results. Below is a part of the Methods section, which includes the protocol only for the question above. A diagram of the protocol is as follows:

Experiment

buffer	AA		AA + indo
90 min	90 min	30 min	90 min

Sham Control

buffer	buffer		buffer
90 min	90 min	30 min	90 min

Topic

Materials and Methods

Preparation of Ductus Arteriosus Rings

1 *A* After the pregnant ewes were given spinal anesthetics, breed-dated fetal lambs between 122 and 145 days of gestational age (term is 150 days) were delivered by cesarean section and exsanguinated. *B* The ductus arteriosus was removed from the lamb, dissected free of adventitial tissue, and divided into 1-mm-thick rings. *C* The rings were placed in glass vials containing 4 ml of buffer (50 mM Tris HCl, pH 7.39, containing 127 mM NaCl, 5 mM KCl, 2.5 mM $CaCl_2$, 1.3 mM $MgCl_2 \cdot 6\ H_2O$, and 6 mM glucose) at 37°C. *D* The preparation was allowed to stabilize for 45 min before experiments were begun.

Arachidonic Acid-induced Prostaglandin E_2 Production

2 *E* To determine whether exogenous arachidonic acid increases prostaglandin E_2 production, eight rings of ductus arteriosus **were placed** in fresh buffer and **incubated** at 37°C for 90 min. *F* After this, the buffer solution **was collected** for measurement of baseline prostaglandin E_2 production. *G* Next, the rings **were placed** in fresh buffer containing 0.2 µg/ml arachidonic acid (Sigma) (0.67 µM) and **incubated** for 90 min. *H* The buffer **was** then **collected** for measurement of prostaglandin E_2 and the rings **were washed** with fresh buffer for 30 min. *I* Finally, the rings **were placed** in fresh buffer containing 0.2 µg/ml arachidonic acid and 2 µg/ml indomethacin (Sigma) (5.6 µM) and **incubated** for 90 min. *J* After this incubation, the buffer solution **was collected** again for measurement of prostaglandin E_2. *K* The rings of ductus arteriosus **were blotted** dry and **weighed** (wet weight). *L* The mean weight was 22.1 ± 8.3 (SD) mg tissue per experiment.

3 *M* Recovery of prostaglandin E_2 from the buffer solution was calculated and prostaglandin E_2 content was measured as follows. *N* So that percent recovery could be calculated, ^{3}H-prostaglandin E_2 (6000 dpm, 130 Ci/mmol; New England Nuclear) was first mixed with the buffer solution from each incubation. *O* The solutions were then acidified to pH 3.5 with 1 N citric acid. *P* The prostaglandins were extracted with a mixture of cyclohexane and ethyl acetate (1:1) and purified in silicic acid microcolumns (4). *Q* Recovery was calculated by measuring radioactivity after extraction and comparing it to radioactivity measured before extraction. *R* Prostaglandin E_2 content was measured by radioimmunoassay (4) using a specific rabbit antiserum against an albumin-conjugated prostaglandin E_2 preparation. *S* Recovery of prostaglandin E_2 ranged from 50 to 70%. [T]Prostaglandin E_2 production is reported as pg/mg wet weight per 90 min incubation.

4   [U]In a control series of experiments, we measured prostaglandin E_2 production at the same 90-min intervals with the rings incubated in fresh buffer bubbled with oxygen.

5   [V]Stock solutions of indomethacin (16 mg/ml) and arachidonic acid (0.33 mg/ml) were prepared in ethanol each day. [W]The maximum concentration of ethanol in the incubation medium had no effect on prostaglandin E_2 production.

6   [X]Data are summarized as mean $\pm$ SD. [Y]To determine whether prostaglandin E_2 production differed among the three treatments, we analyzed the data with a single-factor repeated-measures analysis of variance. [Z]Then, to determine which treatment groups were different from the others, we conducted multiple comparisons with the Student-Newman-Keuls test. [AA]We considered differences significant at $P < 0.05$.

CHAPTER 6

RESULTS

FUNCTIONS

The Results section has two functions. One function is to state the results of the experiments described in the Materials and Methods section. The other function is either to present evidence (data) that supports the results or to direct the reader to figures or tables that present supporting evidence.

CONTENT

What to Include in the Results Section

The primary information in the Results section is results. However, not every result that you obtained from your experiments or observations needs to be reported in the Results section. The Results section should report only results pertinent to the question posed in the Introduction. Results should be included whether or not they support your hypothesis. Both experimental and control results should be included.

In addition to presenting results, the Results section can include data. However, most data, and in particular the most important data, should be presented in figures or tables, where the data are highly visible and easy to read.

Normally, the Results section does not include statements that need to be referenced, such as comparisons with others' results. However, if a brief comparison (one or two sentences) would not fit smoothly into the Discussion, it can be included in the Results section.

Results and Data

Results are different from data. *Data* are facts, often numbers, obtained from experiments and observations. Data can be raw (for example, all the phospholipid concentrations measured during an experiment), summarized (for example, mean and SD), or transformed (for example, percent of control). *Results* are general statements that interpret data (for example, "Propranolol given during normal ventilation decreased phospholipid concentrations").

Data can rarely stand alone. The result (= the message) must be stated. For example, what is the reader supposed to think after reading the two sentences of data in Example 6.1?

Example 6.1   Data but No Result

In the 20 control subjects, the mean resting blood pressure was 85 ± 5 (SD) mmHg. In comparison, in the 30 tennis players, the mean resting blood pressure was 94 ± 3 mmHg.

Are the data similar? Different? What is the point? The purpose of the Results section is to make the point clear. To make the point clear, state the result first and then present the data, as in Revision A below.

Revision A   Result Stated

The mean resting blood pressure <u>was higher</u> in the 30 tennis players than in the 20 control subjects (94 ± 3 (SD) vs. 85 ± 5 mmHg, $P < 0.02$).

In Revision A the point is clear: "was higher." Note that a P value for statistical significance is added to provide evidence that the difference was not likely to have occurred by chance. Also note that in other cases, the data may be presented in a figure or a table, as in Example 6.4 below, rather than in the text.

In addition to simply saying "was less than," "was greater than," "decreased," or "increased," you can, when appropriate, give a general idea of the magnitude of a difference or a change by using a percentage, as in Revision B.

Revision B   Result and General Idea of the Magnitude

The mean resting blood pressure <u>was 10% higher</u> in the 30 tennis players than in the 20 control subjects (94 ± 3 (SD) vs. 85 ± 5 mmHg, $P < 0.02$).

This statement of the result ("was 10% higher") gives a simpler and therefore clearer idea of the magnitude of the difference than do the data alone (94 ± 3 vs. 85 ± 5 mmHg).

Indicators and Variables

If you assessed an indicator of a variable, describe results for the indicator in the Results section. For example, if you assessed specific airway resistance as an indicator of bronchoconstriction, give results for specific airway resistance.

Accuracy and Consistency of Data

The data must be accurate. In addition, the data must be internally consistent. For example, if a value is given both in the Results and in the Discussion, the value should be the same in both places.

Statistical Analysis

For normally distributed data that have been analyzed statistically, report the mean and a statistic that estimates the variation from the mean [for example, the standard deviation (SD) or the range], and specify which statistic you are reporting. Also give the sample size (n) and the probability values for tests of statistical significance. (See the revisions of Example 6.1 above.)

For non-normally distributed data that have been analyzed statistically, report the median and the interquartile range (that is, the range between the 25th and the 75th percentiles).

When reporting results of statistical hypothesis tests, it is often useful to report 95% confidence intervals in addition to *P* values so that the reader is better able to judge the biological or clinical significance of the results (see Glantz, Chap. 7, and Gardner and Altman).

ORGANIZATION

Overall Organization

The Results section can be organized either chronologically or from most to least important.

Chronological Order

If the Methods section describes a chronological sequence of experiments, results in the Results section should be given in the same order, as in Example 6.15 at the end of this chapter. This principle expands a technique of continuity in paragraphs: keep a consistent order (see Chap. 3).

Materials and Methods	Results
Procedure 1	Procedure 1 → Result 1
Procedure 2	Procedure 2 → Result 2
Procedure 3	Procedure 3 → Result 3
etc.	etc.

Most to Least Important

Sometimes chronological order puts results that answer the question late in the Results section, where they are hard to find. In this situation, to emphasize results that answer the question, organize from most to least important. That is, put results that answer the question at the beginning of the first paragraph of the Results section or at the beginning of successive paragraphs starting with paragraph 1. Describe secondary results after describing the results that answer the question.

Organization Within Paragraphs

The biggest problem in many Results sections is that they lose the forest for the trees. The solutions are to organize information in each paragraph from most to least important and to subordinate control results, methods, figure and table citations, and data.

Organize From Most to Least Important

Within each paragraph in the Results section, organize information from most to least important. The most important information in a Results section is results, so a result should be in the first sentence of every paragraph. If explanatory details or data are needed, they should be presented after the result. Note that this is the recommended way of writing a paragraph: begin with a topic sentence stating the point; then give supporting sentences, organized to relate clearly to the point.

A Topic sentence (result)
B,C Supporting details
   (data)

Example 6.2   Result First, Supporting Details Second

   <u>*A*Two different patterns of phospholipid distribution were obtained depending on the bile samples.</u>   *B*The first pattern, which was the one most frequently observed, had a main peak of phospholipids in the range of 10^6 daltons and a shoulder in the range of 5×10^5 daltons.   *C*The second pattern had a main peak of phospholipids in the range of 5×10^5 daltons and a shoulder in the range of 10^6 daltons.

Note that this same strategy—stating the point and then giving the details—can be used in the last sentence, to indicate how the two patterns differ.

Revision

   *A*Two different patterns of phospholipid distribution were obtained depending on the bile samples.   *B*The first pattern, which was the one most frequently observed, had a main peak of phospholipids in the range of 10^6 daltons and a shoulder in the range of 5×10^5 daltons.   *C*<u>The second pattern was the reverse</u>, having a main peak of phospholipids in the range of 5×10^5 daltons and a shoulder in the range of 10^6 daltons.

The idea is to state the point so that the reader cannot miss it. In other words, if you want the reader to know something (here, that the second pattern is the reverse of the first pattern), state it; do not make the reader guess.

Subordinate Control Results

Control results sometimes need to be described first, for example, if the stability of the baseline needs to be established. However, control results, both for baseline and for control series, should be described along with or after experimental results whenever possible. For example, baseline data can sometimes be incorporated into a sentence describing the experimental results, as in Example 6.3.

Example 6.3   Experimental Result Incorporating Baseline Data

During the acute period of lipid infusion, lung lymph flow increased from 2.44 ± 0.32 (mean $\pm$ SD) to 4.00 ± 0.72 ml/h ($P < 0.05$).

   In this example, 2.44 ± 0.32 ml/h is the baseline value. To make the baseline value more noticeable, write "increased from *a baseline value of* 2.44...."
   Similarly, for a control series of experiments, the results can sometimes be incorporated into a comparison between experimental and control results, as in Example 6.4.

Example 6.4   Experimental Result Incorporating a Control Result

When either terbutaline or epinephrine was instilled along with serum into the air spaces, the excess lung water was significantly less than when serum alone was instilled (Fig. 1).

   In this example, the control series is described by "when serum alone was instilled," and the control data are given along with the experimental data in a figure.
   Alternatively, results for a control series can sometimes be reported after the results for the experimental series (see para. 1 of Example 6.15 at the end of this chapter).
   If baseline or control data are reported in a figure or a table, they do not usually need to be reported in the text.

Subordinate Methods

Do not use a methods statement as a topic sentence in the Results section. The topic sentences in the Results section should state results. In Example 6.5, the first sentence (topic sentence) states methods and the second sentence states results.

Example 6.5 Method as a Topic Sentence (Undesirable)

In three of the cats in the second series, the inhibitory effect of 1 μg isoproterenol was examined when baseline tension was induced exclusively by either cholinergic neurotransmission, exogenous acetylcholine, or exogenous 5-hydroxytryptamine. Injection of 1 μg isoproterenol evoked a differential inhibitory response, relaxation being greater when tension was induced by cholinergic neurotransmission or exogenous 5-hydroxytryptamine than by exogenous acetylcholine (Fig. 5).

In Example 6.5, since all of the methods details (except the number of cats) appear in the second sentence, the first sentence is unnecessary. A stronger way to begin this paragraph is to omit the first sentence and incorporate the number of cats into the second sentence. Thus, the paragraph includes methods but highlights results.

Revision

Injection of 1 μg of isoproterenol into 3 cats evoked a differential inhibitory response, relaxation being greater when tension was induced by cholinergic neurotransmission or exogenous 5-hydroxytryptamine than by exogenous acetylcholine (Fig. 5).

At least two techniques of sentence structure are available for including methods in sentences that state results. One technique is to make the method the subject of the sentence, as in the revision of Example 6.5 above and in Example 6.6B below. Another technique is to state the method in a transition clause and the result in the main clause, as in Example 6.6C.

Example 6.6 Including Methods Statements in the Results Section

A. Method as a Topic Sentence (Undesirable)

Method; Result We **administered** propranolol during normal ventilation. This beta-blocker **decreased** phospholipid (Fig. 1).

B. Method Subordinated as the Subject; Result in the Verb + Object

Method; Result Propranolol administered during normal ventilation **decreased** phospholipid (Fig. 1).

C. Method Subordinated in a Transition Clause; Result in Main Clause

Method; Result When propranolol was administered during normal ventilation, phospholipid **decreased** (Fig. 1).

The point is that in the Results section, the main verbs (boldfaced in the examples above) should describe results, not methods, so avoid sentences that state methods only, such as the first sentence in Example 6.6A. Having the main verb describe results is particularly important in the topic sentence.

Subordinate Figure and Table Citations

Do not use a figure legend or a table title as a topic sentence. Cite figures and tables (in parentheses) after statements that give results, preferably after the first result relevant to the figure or table.

Example 6.7   A Figure Legend Used as a Topic Sentence (Undesirable)

A summary of renal function data is presented in Fig. 2. Continuous positive airway pressure (7.5 cm H_2O) in newborn goats decreased urine flow, sodium excretion, and the glomerular filtration rate.

The first sentence is essentially a figure legend: Fig. 2. Renal function data. For a more powerful topic sentence, omit the figure legend and state the results. Cite the figure in parentheses at the end of the sentence that states the results.

Revision

Continuous positive airway pressure (7.5 cm H_2O) in newborn goats decreased urine flow, sodium excretion, and the glomerular filtration rate (Fig. 2).

The reason that a result is a more powerful topic sentence than is a figure legend or a table title is that a result states a point. In Example 6.7, the first sentence indicates only the topic of the paragraph—renal function data. The second sentence makes a point—that renal variables decreased, which is what the reader wants to know. Therefore, this sentence should be placed first, in the position of prominence, where the reader will find it readily. It should not be buried in the middle of the paragraph.

Furthermore, to use an entire sentence to direct the reader to the figure is wasteful. All that is necessary is to cite the figure in parentheses at the end of the sentence that states the result, as in the revision.

Finally, the result is a more powerful preparation for looking at a figure or table than a figure legend or table title is. The reason is that a result creates an expectation but a figure legend or table title does not. After reading a figure legend, the reader has no idea of what point to expect in the figure. In contrast, after reading a result, the reader knows exactly what point to expect and has only to agree or disagree with the point, not to hunt for it. For example, after reading Example 6.7 above, the reader would expect to find only renal function data, but after reading the revision, the reader would expect to find a specific result—decreases in all three variables. Having a clear expectation when looking at a figure is much more efficient than not knowing what you are supposed to see.

Subordinate Data

Data should not overwhelm results. In a Results section loaded with data, the reader loses the overview. Therefore, data should be kept to an absolute minimum in the Results section. Data that are presented in a figure or a table should not be repeated in the text, although one or two especially important values can be repeated for emphasis. Brief secondary data that do not warrant display in a figure or a table can be presented in the text by being placed within parentheses after the result.

Example 6.8 Data Overwhelming Results

Group 1: Serial Development of Alveolar Hypoxia Followed by Alkalosis.
The pulmonary artery pressure increased to 65 ± 21 (SD) % above baseline
during hypoxia but then decreased to $37 \pm 16\%$ above baseline when alkali
was infused into the lungs of 12 rabbits. Similarly, the pulmonary artery
pressure increased to $41 \pm 17\%$ above baseline during hypoxia but then decreased to $21 \pm 13\%$ above baseline when PI_{CO_2} was decreased (Fig. 2). Thus,
both metabolic and respiratory alkalosis decreased the pulmonary vascular
resistance after it had increased in response to hypoxia.

Group 2: Serial Development of Alkalosis Followed by Alveolar Hypoxia.
The baseline pulmonary artery pressure decreased from 9.4 ± 1.8 to 8.4 ± 1.5
cm H_2O when $NaHCO_3$ was infused and from 9.0 ± 2.1 to 7.9 ± 1.5 cm H_2O
when PI_{CO_2} was decreased in the lungs of 20 rabbits. The pulmonary artery
response to alveolar hypoxia at a pH of 7.35–7.42 was no different from the
response to alveolar hypoxia at a pH of 7.50–7.65 (Fig. 3). These results were
the same regardless of whether alkalosis was induced by decreasing PI_{CO_2} or by
infusing $NaHCO_3$ (Fig. 3). Thus, although both metabolic and respiratory alkalosis decreased baseline pulmonary resistance, they did not decrease constriction
of the pulmonary artery in response to subsequent alveolar hypoxia.

Group 3: Simultaneous Development of Alkalosis and Alveolar Hypoxia.
The pulmonary artery response to alveolar hypoxia was significantly lower at
a pH of 7.50–7.65 than at a pH of 7.35–7.42 in the lungs of 8 rabbits (Fig. 4).
Thus, simultaneous alveolar hypoxia and respiratory alkalosis decreased constriction of the pulmonary artery.

In this example, only the last sentence of each paragraph reports results.
The earlier sentences report data that are shown in figures and can therefore
be omitted, except for one sentence of baseline results and data. The data
should be in parentheses, as shown in Revision A.

Revision A

When metabolic or respiratory alkalosis was induced after hypoxia (12
rabbits), pulmonary artery constriction in response to hypoxia was reduced
(Fig. 2). In contrast, when metabolic or respiratory alkalosis was induced before
hypoxia (20 rabbits), pulmonary artery constriction in response to hypoxia was
not reduced (Fig. 3). However, baseline pulmonary arterial pressure decreased
(from 9.4 ± 1.8 to 8.4 ± 1.5 (SD) cm H_2O for metabolic alkalosis and from 9.0
± 2.1 to 7.0 ± 1.5 cm H_2O for respiratory alkalosis). When respiratory alkalosis
and hypoxia were induced simultaneously (8 rabbits), pulmonary artery constriction in response to hypoxia was again reduced (Fig. 4).

In the revision, results are prominent. However, the overview would be
clearer if repetition were avoided and similar results were reported together,
as in Revision B. (For this revision to work, metabolic and respiratory alkalosis
would have to be identified in the figures.)

Revision B

Pulmonary artery constriction in the 12 rabbits was reduced when alkalosis
was induced either after (Fig. 2) or during (Fig. 4) hypoxia, but not when
alkalosis was induced before hypoxia (Fig. 3). Baseline pulmonary artery pressure was altered only when alkalosis was induced before hypoxia, decreasing
from 9.4 ± 1.8 to 8.4 ± 1.5 (SD) cm H_2O for metabolic alkalosis and from 9.0
± 2.1 to 7.0 ± 1.5 cm H_2O for respiratory alkalosis.

Correlation Between Results and Methods

Check that for every result in the Results section there is a method in the Methods section. In Example 6.9, results are given not only for mean left atrial pressures but also for *changes* in mean left atrial pressure. But Methods did not say that changes in mean left atrial pressure were measured, so the reader is not prepared to hear about these changes. In the revision, a sentence is added to Methods to prepare for the results.

Example 6.9   Two Results but Only One Method

Methods

We monitored mean left atrial pressure and other hemodynamic variables and simultaneously performed transesophageal Doppler echocardiography of pulmonary venous flow and mitral inflow to determine whether pulmonary venous flow and mitral inflow velocities accurately estimate mean left atrial pressure.

Results

Doppler variables of pulmonary venous flow correlated more strongly with mean left atrial pressure and changes in mean left atrial pressure than did Doppler variables of mitral inflow (Table 2).

Revision

Methods

We monitored mean left atrial pressure and other hemodynamic variables and simultaneously performed transesophageal Doppler echocardiography of pulmonary venous flow and mitral inflow to determine whether pulmonary venous flow and mitral inflow velocities accurately estimate mean left atrial pressure. In addition, to assess whether changes in mean left atrial pressure in individual patients are accurately reflected by changes in pulmonary venous and mitral flow velocities, we performed transesophageal echocardiographic measurement during four 3-min study periods: after induction of anesthesia and intubation, after opening of the pericardium, after cardiopulmonary bypass, and after closing of the sternum.

LENGTH

Many authors think of the Results section as the heart of the paper, so they try to put the whole paper into the Results section—methods, figure legends, table titles, results, data, comparisons with the literature—in fact, everything except the Introduction. This temptation should be resisted. The Results section should be as brief and uncluttered as possible so that the reader can see the forest for the trees.

One exception occurs in scientific disciplines such as biochemistry, in which the outcome of one experiment determines what the next experiment will be.

In papers in these disciplines, the protocol is described in the Results section, not in the Methods section. Specifically, each set of results (except the first) is preceded by a brief description of why the experiment was done (purpose) and what the experiment was (protocol). These Results sections tend to be long, and the trees tend to obscure the forest. To limit this problem, keep detail (data) to a minimum, as in Example 6.16 at the end of this chapter.

DETAILS

Species and Material

The species and the material (tissue, cell line, etc.) should be mentioned at least once in the Results section, preferably in the first sentence.

Identifying Human Subjects

Do not use initials to identify study subjects. Use A, B, C, etc. if you refer to an individual subject. Use 1, 2, 3, etc. when you studied more than 26 subjects.

Verb Tense

Results are reported in *past tense*, because they are discrete events that occurred in the past. Examples are "Pulmonary artery constriction **was reduced**" and "Imidazole **inhibited** the increase in pulmonary arterial pressure induced by lipid infusion."

Comparisons

When comparing results, use "than," not "compared with." In particular, avoid ambiguous statements such as "X was increased compared with Y." Instead write "X was greater than Y," "X increased more than Y," "X increased but Y was unchanged," or whatever you mean (see Chap. 2, "Put Parallel Ideas in Parallel Form").

Precise Word Choice

Note the difference between *ability* and *actuality*:

Example 6.10   Ability versus Actuality

Ability: We **could not demonstrate** high-affinity, low-capacity DHE binding sites in heart particulates prepared from three adult sheep.

Actuality: **There were no** high-affinity, low-capacity DHE binding sites in heart particulates prepared from three adult sheep.

"Could not demonstrate" implies that binding sites may have been there, but the technique was not sensitive enough to detect them. "There were no" implies that no binding sites exist (so no method would be able to detect them). Know whether you are talking about ability or actuality, and choose your verb accordingly.

Note the difference between "did not increase" and "failed to increase." "Failed" implies an a priori expectation that the value *should* have increased.

"Did not" implies no a priori expectation. Generally, you should use the neutral description, "did not increase," when reporting results.

Qualitative words that describe magnitude are imprecise and therefore of little value when used alone. For example, what does "markedly" mean in "Heart rate increased markedly"? We need the data to be sure how big the increase was. If you use a qualitative word such as "markedly," go on to quantify it, either by citing a figure or a table or by reporting the data in the text. Actually, the best policy is to avoid qualitative words altogether in the Results section. Save qualitative words for the Discussion, for occasions when you need to emphasize the magnitude of a change or a difference.

"Significant" has become a code word for "statistically significant." Thus, "significantly" can no longer be used as a synonym for "markedly." If you say, for example, "Heart rate increased significantly," the reader expects statistical details to support that statement.

Statistical Details

The conventional way to write a mean and standard deviation or a mean and standard error of the mean is shown in Example 6.11.

Example 6.11   Mean and SD

48.7 ± 1.3 (SD) ml.

The standard way to write data that are being compared statistically is shown in Example 6.12.

Example 6.12   Statistical Details for Comparisons

Blood flow was redistributed more toward the right ventricle than toward the left ventricle (26.3 ± 2.9 (SD) vs. $19.5 \pm 1.5\%$ in 6 lambs, $P < 0.01$).

Note that five types of statistical information are presented: the mean ("26.3" and "19.5%"), the standard deviation ("2.9" and "1.5%"), identification of the statistic ("(SD)"), the sample size (n) ("in 6 lambs"), and the probability value of significance ("$P < 0.01$"). Generally, you should give all five types of statistical information. However, if a single statistic (for example, the standard deviation) and a single sample size (n) apply to all the data, then you can identify the statistic and the sample size the first time you give data, as in Example 6.12, and omit these details after that, as in Example 6.13.

Example 6.13   "(SD)" and n Omitted

Blood flow was redistributed more toward the right ventricle than toward the left ventricle (26.3 ± 2.9 vs. $19.5 \pm 1.5\%$, $P < 0.01$).

The statistic and the sample size should also be identified in the Methods section. For example, "Data are expressed as mean $\pm$ SD"; "The study protocol was performed on the remaining 6 lambs."

If in addition you report the confidence interval, Example 6.12 can be rewritten as follows:

Example 6.14   Confidence Interval Added

Blood flow was redistributed more toward the right ventricle than toward the left ventricle (26.3 ± 2.9 (SD) vs. $19.5 \pm 1.5\%$ in 6 lambs; 95% confidence interval for the difference = 3.8–9.8%, $P < 0.01$).

Some statisticians oppose using ± before the standard deviation or the standard error of the mean because it can be misinterpreted as a 95% confidence interval. The notation these statisticians recommend is "48.7 ml (SD 1.3)." Thus, Example 6.13 would become "Blood flow was redistributed more toward the right ventricle than toward the left ventricle (26.3% (SD 2.9) vs. 19.5% (SD 1.5), $P < 0.01$)." To decide which notation to use, consult the journal's instructions to authors.

When P values are given after data, as in Example 6.12, actual P values should be used both for differences considered significant (for example, $P < 0.01$) and for differences considered not significant (for example, $P > 0.75$). Writing "$P > 0.05$" is not helpful. Precise values allow the reader to interpret the data accurately. For example, a P value of 0.75 strongly implies absence of a statistically significant difference, but a P value of 0.06 probably does not. Contrary to popular belief, $P = 0.05$ is not a hard-and-fast cutoff point.

Finally, note that the sample size is not written "$n = 6$." The reason is that "$n = 6$" is unclear. Is it 6 lambs? Six experiments in one lamb? Six experiments in 4 lambs? So when describing the sample size, state not only the size of the sample (here, 6) but also what the sample is (here, lambs).

EXAMPLE OF A CLEARLY WRITTEN RESULTS SECTION

Example 6.15   A Clearly Written Results Section

The Results section below is a clearly written Results section from a paper containing two series of experiments. The purpose of the first series, as stated in the protocol, was "to determine whether exogenous arachidonic acid increases prostaglandin E_2 production" in fetal lamb ductus arteriosus. The purposes of the second series were "to determine whether the exogenous arachidonic acid is converted to prostaglandin E_2" and "to determine the amount of ^{14}C-arachidonic acid incorporated into tissue phospholipids." Subtitles were used for each series in the Methods. Part of the Methods section is given in Chapter 5 (Exercise 5.2).

Results

Arachidonic Acid-induced Prostaglandin E_2 Production

A Experimental result

1   *A*Incubation of rings of fetal lamb ductus arteriosus in arachidonic acid increased prostaglandin E_2 production to 3.5 times above baseline (Fig. 1). *B*This increase was blocked when the rings were incubated in arachidonic acid in the presence of indomethacin. *C*In the control series of experiments, prostaglandin E_2 production measured at the same 90-min intervals did not change (data not shown).

B,C Control results

Arachidonic Acid Conversion to Prostaglandin E_2

D Result (topic sentence)

2   *D*During incubation of rings of fetal lamb ductus arteriosus in ^{14}C-arachidonic acid, very little of the ^{14}C-arachidonic acid was converted to ^{14}C-prostaglandin E_2. *E*Only 0.048 ± 0.019 (SD) pg ^{14}C-prostaglandin E_2/mg wet weight tissue was measured. *F*This amount was less than 1% of the ^{14}C-arachidonic acid recovered from the incubation fluid and less than 1% of the immunoreactive prostaglandin E_2 measured.

E Data
F Comparison

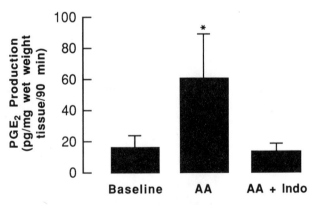

Figure 1. Production of prostaglandin E_2 (PGE$_2$) by rings of ductus arteriosus from fetal lambs. For each experiment, ductal rings from one lamb were incubated for 90 min each first in buffer alone (baseline), then in buffer containing arachidonic acid (AA), and finally in buffer containing arachidonic acid and indomethacin (Indo). Data are means $\pm$ SD of immunoreactive prostaglandin E_2 released into 4 ml of incubation fluid during each of eight experiments. *Significantly different from the other two values, $P < 0.01$.

G Result (topic sentence)
H Data

I Data

3 *G*These results are supported by the finding that very little of the ^{14}C-arachidonic acid was incorporated into tissue phospholipids (Table 1). *H*Only 1.8 ± 0.4% of the total ^{14}C-arachidonic acid recovered from the incubation fluid and from the tissue was found in the phospholipid fraction. *I*Equally small amounts of the label were found in neutral lipid and in the tissue fatty acid fractions (Table 1).

Strengths

Only results pertinent to the questions are reported.

Control results are included.

A general idea of the magnitude of the responses is given in sentences A ("3.5 times"), D ("very little"), and G ("very little"). Qualitative words describing magnitude ("very little," sentences D and G) are used here because the questions are about amounts; the data that quantify the qualitative words are given.

Most statistical information is given in the legend for Figure 1. In the text, only one piece of statistical information is given: the standard deviation is identified on first use (sentence E) to remind readers of what statistic is being presented.

The relation to the protocol is perfect. The results are in the same order as the three purposes stated in the protocol, and the results for each of the three protocols are in three separate paragraphs.

Results that answer the question are at the beginning of successive paragraphs, so they are easy to find.

Paragraphs 2 and 3 give data that support the results. Thus, the results in paragraphs 2 and 3 are topic sentences.

Controls, methods, and figure and table citations are subordinated.

Sentence A: Methods are subordinated as the subject of the sentence ("Incubation of rings of fetal lamb ductus arteriosus in arachidonic acid"); results are given in the verb and object ("increased prostaglandin E$_2$ production to 3.5 times above baseline"). The figure citation is subordinated in parentheses at the end of sentence A, the first sentence that states a result.

Sentences B, C: Control results are given after experimental results, the same order as used in Methods (see Exercise 5.2, paras. 2 and 4).

Sentence D: Methods are subordinated in a transition phrase ("During incubation of rings of fetal lamb ductus arteriosus in ^{14}C-arachidonic acid"); results are given in the subject and verb ("very little of the ^{14}C-arachidonic acid was converted to ^{14}C-prostaglandin E$_2$").

Sentences G and I: The table citation is subordinated in parentheses at the end of the sentence.

Most data are omitted from the Results section because they are shown in the figure and table.

The Results section is admirably brief.

The species and material studied are stated at the beginning of each subsection.

Results are reported in past tense.

The comparisons (sentences F, I) make a point rather than just reporting the data.

Continuity between paragraphs 2 and 3 is excellent because the thinking is displayed at the beginning of sentence G ("These results are supported by the finding that...").

EXAMPLE OF A RESULTS SECTION DESCRIBING BOTH PROTOCOL AND RESULTS

Example 6.16   A Results Section Describing Both Protocol and Results

This Results section is from a biochemistry paper in which a sequence of seven experiments was done. Because the outcome of one experiment determined what the next experiment would be, the protocol (in boldface) is presented paragraph by paragraph in the Results section rather than in a separate protocol in the Methods section, where several "if so's" would have been necessary. In addition, the results are interpreted at each step in preparation for the next experiment (in italics). Thus, this Results section is composed of three types of information: protocol, results, and interpretation of results. Note that details are kept at a minimum for each of these components. Thus, the display of thinking stands out, and the reader can follow the story.

The question this paper asks is, "Are the signal transduction mechanisms for activation of phospholipase C by the potent mitogens thrombin and PDGF in vascular smooth muscle cells different from each other?"

Results

1   Thrombin (1 U/ml) rapidly increased production of IP_3, IP_2, and IP in a sequential manner. The increases in IP_3 and IP_2 were transient, reaching a peak at 30 s and 60 s, respectively, and declining to near prestimulatory values within 5 min (Fig. 1). In marked contrast to thrombin, PDGF (7.5 nM) caused a sustained increase in all three metabolites for 6 min of stimulation. Consistent with the time course for IP_3 production, thrombin caused a transient increase in intracellular $[Ca^{2+}]$, whereas PDGF caused a sustained increase (Fig. 2). *The different time courses of the increases induced by thrombin and by PDGF raise the possibility that the signal transduction mechanisms for these two mitogens might be different.*

2   **To study the signal transduction mechanism for the two mitogens, we used pertussis toxin, which modifies the function of some G proteins.** Pertussis toxin significantly blunted the thrombin-induced increases in IP_3 (Fig. 1) and intracellular $[Ca^{2+}]$ (Fig. 2), *indicating a role for a G protein in thrombin-induced cellular responses.* In contrast, pertussis toxin did not affect the PDGF-induced increases in either IP_3 (Fig. 1) or intracellular $[Ca^{2+}]$ (Fig. 2).

3   **To ask whether the pertussis toxin-insensitive mechanism for PDGF also involves a G protein, we examined the effect of GTPγS, a stable GTP analog, on IP_3 release in saponin-permeabilized vascular smooth muscle cells. GTPγS has been shown to potentiate many G protein-mediated responses by direct activation of the G protein (15-17).** We found that in permeabilized vascular smooth muscle cells, GTPγS increased IP_3 release synergistically with both thrombin and PDGF (Fig. 3). *Thus, like thrombin, PDGF requires a G protein for activation of phospholipase C.*

4   **Because guanosine 5'-O-(2-thiodiphosphate) (GDPβS) attenuates G protein-mediated cellular responses by competing with GTP for binding (18), we tested GDPβS.** *In support of the notion that a G protein is involved in the signal transduction for PDGF*, GDPβS blunted PDGF-induced IP_3 release in permeabilized cells (Fig. 4). *Thus, whereas thrombin uses a pertussis toxin-sensitive G protein as a signal transducer to activate phospholipase C in vascular smooth muscle cells, PDGF appears to use a pertussis toxin-insensitive G protein.*

5   Next we tested the protein kinase C stimulator, phorbol 12-myristate 13-acetate (PMA), which blunts G protein-mediated activation of phospholipase C in some systems (19). In vascular smooth muscle cells, we found that PMA strongly inhibited thrombin-induced, but not PDGF-induced, IP_3 release (Fig. 5). PMA did not affect basal release of IP_3 (200 vs. 215 cpm/dish). Consistent with its effect on IP_3 release, PMA blunted thrombin-induced, but not PDGF-induced, Ca^{2+} mobilization (Fig. 6). *This effect of PMA requires functional protein kinase C,* since PMA did not inhibit thrombin-induced Ca^{2+} mobilization in cells that were made deficient in protein kinase C activity (data not shown).

6   Since PMA has been suggested to act on several targets, including the binding of a hormone to its receptor, we performed receptor-binding studies using ^{125}I-thrombin to see if thrombin receptors are the target of PMA. Acute PMA treatment did not affect either the dissociation constant (K_D) for thrombin or the maximal binding (B_{max}) for thrombin (Fig. 7). *Thus, PMA must act by interfering with one or more events distal to the binding of thrombin to its receptor.*

7   Another possible target for PMA action is the G protein itself. To investigate this possibility, we examined the effect of PMA on GTPγS-induced inositol phosphate release. GTPγS caused a progressive release of inositol phosphate, which was inhibited by 55% by PMA treatment (Fig. 8), *suggesting that PMA inhibits thrombin-induced cellular responses by affecting the function of the G protein directly.*

In this Results section, protocol 1 (in para. 1) raises the question about whether the signal transduction mechanisms for thrombin and PDGF are different. Protocol 2 begins to identify a difference by finding a pertussis toxin-sensitive G protein for the thrombin mechanism but not for the PDGF mechanism. Protocol 3 finds a pertussis toxin-insensitive G protein for the PDGF mechanism. Protocol 4 confirms this finding. Protocol 5 provides further evidence that the mechanisms are different: PMA affected the thrombin mechanism but not the PDGF mechanism. Protocols 6 and 7 pursue the PMA effect on thrombin. Protocol 6 shows that the PMA target is an event distal to the binding of thrombin. Protocol 7 shows that the target is the G protein.

Thus, this Results section shows how to display thinking and keep the overview clear while describing both protocol and results in a Results section in which the results of one protocol lead to the next protocol.

SUMMARY OF GUIDELINES FOR RESULTS

FUNCTIONS

To state the results of the experiments described in Materials and Methods.

Either to present data that support the results or to cite figures or tables that present data.

CONTENT

Report only results pertinent to the question.
    Include results whether or not they support your hypothesis.
    Include control results.

Keep data to a minimum in the text. Present most data, in particular important data, in figures and tables.

Present data after stating the result they support, not instead of stating the result.

Give a clear idea of the magnitude of a response or a difference by reporting percent change or the percentage of difference rather than by quoting exact data.

If you assessed an indicator of a variable, describe results for the indicator.

Be sure that data are accurate and internally consistent.

For normally distributed data that have been analyzed statistically, report the mean and a statistic that estimates the variation from the mean (for example, the standard deviation) and specify which statistic you are reporting. Also give the sample size (n) and probability values for tests of statistical significance. For non-normally distributed data that have been analyzed statistically, report the median and the interquartile range.

OVERALL ORGANIZATION

Organize the Results section either chronologically or from most to least important. For most to least important, put results that answer the question(s) at the beginning of the Results section or at the beginning of paragraph 1 and successive paragraphs.

ORGANIZATION WITHIN PARAGRAPHS

Organize information in each paragraph of the Results section from most to least important. State a result at the beginning of each paragraph. If explanatory details and data are necessary, put them in supporting sentences after the result.

Subordinate controls by describing control results along with or after experimental results whenever possible, not before experimental results.

Subordinate methods, for example by making them the subject of the sentence or by putting them in a transition clause.

Subordinate figure and table citations by putting them in parentheses after a sentence stating a result, usually the first result relevant to the figure or table.

Subordinate data by putting them in parentheses after the result. If data are presented in a table or a figure, do not repeat them in the text.

CORRELATION BETWEEN RESULTS AND METHODS

Check that for every result in the Results section there is a method in the Methods section.

LENGTH

Keep the Results section brief and uncluttered so that the reader can see the forest for the trees.

If the outcome of one experiment determines what the next experiment will be, describe the protocol in the Results section, and keep details to a minimum so that the trees do not overshadow the forest.

DETAILS

Mention the species and the material studied at least once in the Results section, preferably in the first sentence.

Use A, B, C, etc., to identify individual human subjects, or 1, 2, 3, etc., for more than 26 subjects.

Report results in the past tense.

When comparing results, do not use "compared with." In particular, avoid ambiguous comparisons such as "X was increased compared with Y."

Distinguish between "could not" and "did not" and between "did not" and "failed to."

Quantify qualitative terms such as "markedly."

Use "significant" and "significantly" for statistical significance.

Write means and standard deviations in the form "48.7 ± 1.3 (SD) ml." Use a similar form for means and standard errors of the mean.

For statistical comparisons, if a single statistic (for example, standard deviation) and a single sample size (n) apply to all the data and are identified clearly in the Methods section, do not repeat these details each time you give data; mention them only the first time.

If probability values are given in figures or tables, do not give them in the text.

Give actual P values both for significant and for nonsignificant differences.

Do not write "$n = $." Specify not only the sample size but also what the sample is (for example, "in 16 rabbits").

■ *EXERCISE 6.1: AN UNCLEAR RESULTS SECTION*

1. Considering principles of writing Results and principles of paragraph structure (see Chap. 3), which is the best paragraph in this Results section? ___ Why? _____

2. <u>Rewrite</u> paragraph 1 or 6. For paragraph 1, avoid repetition and condense as much as possible so that we can see the forest. For paragraph 6, make clear what the contrast is (sentences Z and AA) and condense the paragraph.

3. In your revision, do not use "compared to" when writing comparisons (see Chap. 2, "Put Parallel Ideas in Parallel Form").

The <u>question</u> this paper asks is, "Are nitrogen and sodium balance and sympathetic nervous activity (assessed by measuring blood pressure and norepinephrine concentration after postural changes) improved when obese subjects eat a pure protein diet rather than a mixed carbohydrate and protein diet?" Each of the seven subjects was on each diet for 21 days.

Results

1 *Substrate and Hormone Levels*

*A*Figure 1 shows the mean serum and urinary ketone acids and changes in the plasma concentration of insulin in subjects receiving the two diets. *B*Blood ketone acids during the pure protein diet reached a plateau at a level twice that reached after the carbohydrate-containing diet. *C*Total blood ketone acids on Day 21 were 1.94 ± 0.23 mmol on the protein diet and 1.08 ± 0.12 mmol on the mixed diet ($P < 0.001$). *D*Daily urinary excretion of ketone acid increased by Day 21 to 50.9 ± 12.5 mmol per 24 hours for the protein diet and 10.2 ± 2.9 mmol per 24 hours for the mixed diet ($P < 0.02$). *E*Plasma insulin, which had a basal level of 32 ± 6 μU per milliliter ($32 \pm 6 \times 10^{-2}$ IU per liter) with the protein diet and 29 ± 5 μU per milliliter ($29 \pm 5 \times 10^{-2}$ IU per liter) with the mixed diet, had a threefold greater decline when carbohydrate was eliminated [-14 ± 5 μU per milliliter ($-14 \pm 5 \times 10^{-2}$ IU per liter)] on Day 21 ($P < 0.05$). *F*There were no significant changes in the plasma concentration of glucagon with either diet. *G*Mean plasma glucose was significantly greater on Day 21 of the mixed diet [76 ± 2 mg per deciliter (4.2 ± 0.11 mmol)] than it was after the protein diet [71 ± 2 mg per deciliter (3.9 ± 0.11 mmol)] ($P < 0.005$).

2 *Nitrogen Balance*

*H*Figure 2 shows the average daily nitrogen balance for each diet regimen. *I*Mean daily nitrogen balance in subjects receiving the mixed diet, $-2.6 \pm$

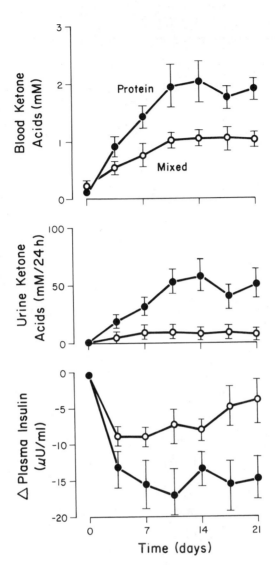

Figure 1. Blood ketone acids, urine ketone acids, and changes in plasma insulin during ingestion of a 400-kcal protein diet and a 400-kcal mixed diet (50% protein and 50% carbohydrate).

0.4 g per day, was not significantly different from that observed after the pure protein diet, -2.1 ± 0.9 g per day. *J*With both diet regimens, nitrogen balance was more negative during the first week (-4.6 ± 0.3 g per day on the mixed diet and -4.9 ± 0.5 g per day on the pure protein diet) than during the last week (-1.6 ± 0.3 g per day on the mixed diet and -1.0 ± 0.6 g per day on the pure protein diet). *K*However, the responses were not significantly different with the two diets during the first or last week ($P > 0.1$). *L*To determine whether protein diets result in better nitrogen balance if given for more prolonged periods, one subject was given each diet for a 5½ week period. *M*As shown in Figure 3, daily nitrogen balance during the mixed diet was similar to that observed during the pure protein diet. [N]Although the protein diet resulted initially in a greater negative nitrogen balance, beyond two to three weeks the net nitrogen losses were comparable, and they became zero after four to five weeks of each diet regimen.

3   *Sodium and Other Mineral Balances*

[O]Figure 4 compares the total cumulative sodium balance observed for each subject during the mixed-diet and protein-diet periods. [P]The mean cumulative sodium loss during protein consumption, -382 ± 117 mmol, was significantly greater than that observed with the mixed diet, -25 ± 105 mmol ($P < 0.02$). [Q]In contrast, there were no significant differences in other mineral balances between the two diets (protein diet vs. mixed diet: potassium, 21 ± 51 mmol vs. 13 ± 33 mmol; calcium, -159.5 ± 9.5 mmol vs. -136 ± 9 mmol; magnesium, -14 ± 3.5 mmol vs. -7 ± 2.5 mmol; phosphorus, -145 ± 50 mmol vs. -127 ± 26 mmol).

4   *Weight Loss*

[R]Total weight loss resulting from a pure protein diet, 10.2 ± 1.0 kg, was 20% greater than that seen after the mixed diet, 8.0 ± 0.8 kg ($P < 0.02$). [S]However, the calculated weight loss attributable to fluid losses with the protein diet, 2.5 ± 0.8 kg, was significantly greater than that with the mixed diet, 0.2 ± 0.7 kg ($P < 0.02$). [T]Consequently, the estimated nonfluid weight loss with the protein diet, 7.7 ± 0.2 kg, was no different from that with the mixed diet, 7.8 ± 0.1 kg.

5   *Blood Pressure*

[U]Blood-pressure values measured with the patient supine did not change significantly from control (prediet) levels with either the pure protein diet ($119 \pm 5 / 72 \pm 4$ vs. $114 \pm 2 / 69 \pm 2$ mmHg) or the mixed diet ($114 \pm 3 / 71 \pm 3$ vs. $114 \pm 2 / 69 \pm 3$). [V]However, with the pure protein diet the mean maximal fall in systolic blood pressure after standing, 28 ± 3 mmHg, was significantly greater than that with the mixed diet, 18 ± 3 mmHg ($P < 0.02$). [W]The exaggerated postural decline in systolic blood pressure during pure protein consumption was accompanied by an increase in adverse symptoms as determined from the daily questionnaire. [X]Although only one of the seven subjects reported symptoms of postural hypotension while receiving the mixed diet, all seven subjects noted such symptoms while on the pure protein diet.

6 *Plasma Norepinephrine*

[Y]The plasma levels of norepinephrine before and after each diet, measured with the subject supine and standing, are illustrated in Figure 5. [Z]The rise in plasma norepinephrine in response to standing with the hypocaloric mixed diet was no different from that observed before initiation of diet therapy. [AA]In contrast, the norepinephrine levels measured with the subject supine and after the subject had stood for 2 minutes were significantly lower after the protein diet than before the initiation of diet therapy. [BB]However, after subjects had stood for 5 and 10 minutes, the rise in plasma norepinephrine was comparable to that observed in the prediet period.

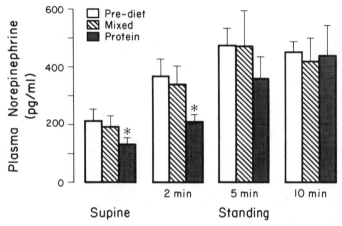

Figure 5. Plasma norepinephrine levels in the basal, supine state and after 2, 5, and 10 minutes of standing in obese subjects in the prediet (control) study and after 21 days of the mixed diet and the protein diet. The plasma norepinephrine levels measured with the patient supine and standing were virtually identical in the prediet (control) study and are consequently combined in this figure. *P* values refer to significance of difference as compared with the prediet values (paired t-test).

■ *EXERCISE 6.2: RESULTS*

On separate paper, <u>rewrite</u> the following Results section. In your revision,

1. Find the best way to begin.

2. Emphasize <u>results that answer the question</u>.

3. Make the Results section as <u>brief</u> as possible by omitting <u>unnecessary detail</u> and <u>unnecessary repetition</u>.

4. Clarify the <u>complete response to hypoxia</u>.

The <u>question</u> this paper asks is, "Is the decrease in ventilation during hypoxia reversed by naloxone?" Four subjects completed the 1.2 mg protocol. Three of the 4 completed the 10 mg protocol.

<u>Abstract</u>. During hypoxia, ventilation immediately increases due to peripheral chemoreceptor stimulation, but between 5 and 15 min later this response fades. We believe that this decrease in ventilation during hypoxia might originate in the central nervous system. <u>If this decrease in ventilation during hypoxia is mediated by endogenous opioid peptides, for example, endorphins, it should be reversed by naloxone.</u> We tested this hypothesis in 4 men. Each subject breathed an inspired oxygen concentration of 30% for 10 to 15 min followed by 50 min of isocapnic hypoxia (end-tidal P_{O_2} = 45 mmHg; end-tidal P_{CO_2} = control hyperoxic level). After 15 min of hypoxia, naloxone (1.2 or 10 mg) was injected intravenously, and ventilation was observed for 16 to 36 min after the injection. The gradual decrease in ventilation was unaltered by either naloxone or placebo. We conclude that naloxone has no effect on the decrease in ventilation in hypoxic adults and therefore that hypoxia-induced decreases in ventilation in adults are not mediated by endogenous opioid peptides.

Results

1 AChanges in minute ventilation in the group of 4 subjects who had been given 1.2 mg of naloxone are shown in Fig. 2. BThe results for each subject were analyzed statistically to determine whether naloxone altered the ventilatory response to hypoxia. CThe data were processed as a sequence of 4-min segments, each segment being represented as a mean and standard deviation of ventilation. DThe data from different experiments in an individual were aligned at the onset of hypoxia (as in Fig. 2) and the first segment started when ventilatory depression was established, but before naloxone was injected. EThe segments were numbered sequentially and scored for the presence of naloxone in each experiment. FA three-way analysis of variance was performed on ventilation, time (segment number), and presence of naloxone. GIn all 4 subjects, ventilation was not dependent on naloxone and was dependent on time ($P < 0.05$). HThe typical response is illustrated in Fig. 2. IThe results of experiments with 1.2 mg of naloxone are 1) ventilation gradually fell over about 50 min of hypoxia and 2) when 1.2 mg of naloxone was administered after 15–35 min of hypoxia in 4 subjects, no detectable increase of ventilation occurred.

2 ^{J}Changes in minute ventilation in the 3 subjects who were given 10 mg of naloxone or placebo are shown in Fig. 3. ^{K}In each subject we compared minute ventilation (mean $\pm$ SD over 200 s of breathing) before naloxone or placebo was given to minute ventilation after naloxone or placebo was given. ^{L}The latter values were obtained 20 (TW) or 30 (SK, PF) min after the injection. ^{M}We found that minute ventilation remained significantly decreased after administration of either naloxone or placebo in each subject ($P < 0.05$). ^{N}Grouping the data according to naloxone or placebo, we found that naloxone did not have a significant effect on ventilation ($P > 0.05$). ^{O}The results of experiments with 10 mg of naloxone are 1) ventilation gradually fell over about 50 min of hypoxia and 2) when 10 mg of naloxone or placebo was given after 20 or 30 min of hypoxia, this gradual reduction of ventilation was unaltered.

3 ^{P}The initial increase in minute ventilation with hypoxia was different in magnitude for each subject. ^{Q}Mean change (% $\pm$ SD) from resting level was 131 ± 61.2 ($n = 9$), 245 ± 121.4 ($n = 8$), 57 ± 11.2 ($n = 9$), and 401 ± 55.7 ($n = 5$) in subjects SK, TW, PF, and JS, respectively. ^{R}There was no significant correlation between the initial increase in minute ventilation and resting end-tidal P_{CO_2} (Fig. 4).

4 ^{S}Three subjects maintained their minute ventilation above resting level throughout hypoxia. ^{T}In subject PF minute ventilation decreased significantly, from a control value of 7.8 ± 0.91 to 7.2 ± 1.14 L/min (mean $\pm$ SD, $n = 9$) after 30 min of hypoxia, while end-tidal P_{CO_2} increased by 0.3 ± 0.2 mmHg (mean $\pm$ SD, $n = 9$, $P < 0.05$) during this period (no CO_2 inhalation needed). ^{U}In one experiment of SK, minute ventilation decreased from 9.8 L/min (resting level) to 9.6 L/min after 30 min of eucapnic hypoxia.

5 ^{V}End-tidal P_{O_2}, end-tidal P_{CO_2}, and arterial S_{O_2} during these experiments are summarized in Table 1.

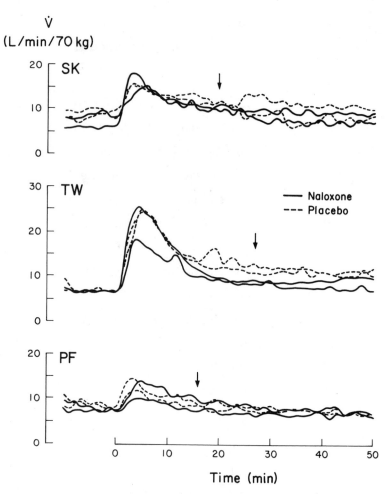

Fig. 3. Ventilation during hypoxia in 3 healthy men given 10 mg of naloxone or placebo. ↓ = time of injection.

CHAPTER 7

DISCUSSION

FUNCTIONS

The main function of the Discussion is to answer the question(s) posed in the Introduction. Other important functions are to explain how the results support the answers and how the answers fit in with existing knowledge on the topic.

CONTENT

The Discussion includes the answers to the questions posed in the Introduction and any accompanying support, explanation, and defense of the answers. In addition, the Discussion includes explanations of any results that do not support the answers; indications of the newness of the work; explanations of discrepancies with others' results; explanations of unexpected findings; explanations of limitations of the methods, of weaknesses in the study design, or of the validity of assumptions; and indications of the importance of the work.

Answering the Questions

The answers should answer the questions exactly as they were asked, using the same key terms, the same verbs (when appropriate), and the same point of view. The verb should be in present tense. For example, if the question was "Does sympathetic stimulation increase norepinephrine synthesis in rat superior cervical ganglia in vivo?" the answer would be either "This study shows that sympathetic stimulation *increases* norepinephrine synthesis in rat superior cervical ganglia in vivo" or "This study shows that sympathetic stimulation *does not increase* norepinephrine synthesis in rat superior cervical ganglia in vivo." Permuting the key terms or the verb or changing the point of view would make the answer more difficult to recognize.

The Population the Answer Applies To

The answer should be limited to the appropriate population. When stating the answer for studies of human subjects, you should generalize from the sample you studied to the population from which it came. For example, if you studied preterm infants who had respiratory distress syndrome, your answer will apply to all preterm infants who have this syndrome. However, your answer may not apply to *full-term* infants who have this syndrome or to preterm infants who have *other* syndromes, so "in preterm infants who have respiratory distress syndrome" must be included in the answer. For experiments done on animals, the answer will apply either to the animals or to some or all humans, depending on the question you asked. Thus, in the example under "Answering the Questions" above, the question was about rats, so the answer applies to rats. If your animals were serving as a model of a human condition, then the answer will apply to humans with that condition.

Correlation of Questions and Answers

If there is more than one answer in the Discussion, there should also be more than one question in the Introduction. The Discussion should not include an answer to a question that was never asked. For example, in a paper that asked what specific hormonally regulated proteins could be identified in second trimester human fetal lung, two answers were given. One answer identified proteins regulated by three classes of hormones. The other answer identified type II cells and fibroblasts as the cellular sources of two of these classes of hormones. But there was no question about cellular sources. To prepare the reader for the second answer, a second question had to be added to the Introduction: "What are the cellular sources of the hormonally regulated proteins?" If the author considers the second question and answer minor, they can be omitted from the abstract and the title, but if an answer appears in the Discussion, there must be a question for it in the Introduction.

Supporting the Answer

Sometimes the answer to the question is short and simple—merely a statement of the chief result. For example, for the question "to determine surface tension within alveoli at total lung capacity," the answer was "In this study we found that, at 37°C, alveolar surface tension at total lung capacity is 29.7 ± 5.6 (SD) mN/m." In this case, no supporting results are needed. However, the authors did defend their answer by comparing it with other published values (see Example 7.5 below).

Supporting the Answer by Stating Results

Usually the answer is not the same as the results. Rather the answer is a generalization based on the results, either directly or indirectly. Therefore, to convince the reader that the answer is valid, state the relevant results after stating the answer. Also cite a figure or a table if seeing specific data would help the reader. Do not assume that the reader has memorized the results or will search through the Results section, figures, and tables to find the results that support the answer. The purpose of the Discussion is to weave that story together for the reader.

Examples 7.1 and 7.2 show two ways to link results to the answer they support. Example 7.1 uses transition phrases. Example 7.2 uses a topic sentence and transition words.

Example 7.1   Transition Phrases to Link Results to Answers

The experiments presented here show that cloned human tumor necrosis factor α inhibits the expression of *MYC* in the human promyelocytic leukemic cell line HL-60 selectively and that it does so by decreasing the rate of synthesis of MYC mRNA. <u>Evidence that the inhibition of *MYC* gene expression is selective is that</u> expression of mRNA for reference proteins HLA-A, -B, and -C was not inhibited. In fact, transcription of HLA-A, -B, and -C mRNA was slightly increased (Fig. 5). <u>Evidence that the rate of synthesis of MYC mRNA</u>

decreases is that the half-life of degradation of MYC mRNA remained unchanged in cells treated with cloned human tumor necrosis factor α (Fig. 4) and that in nuclear "run on" assays, cloned human tumor necrosis factor α decreased the rate of *MYC* gene expression.

In this example, two answers are stated in the topic sentence, and the results supporting them are introduced by transition phrases that repeat key terms from the topic sentence. For another example of a transition phrase linking results to the answer they support, see Example 7.14 below.

Example 7.2   Topic Sentence to Link Results to the Answer

The hemodynamic data obtained in this study indicate that in the open-chest living dog a waterfall effect occurs in the large pulmonary veins where they exit from the surface of the lungs. Its presence has been demonstrated in two ways. First, the finding that upstream intrapulmonary venous pressures were influenced by changes in downstream extrapulmonary venous pressure at high but not at low downstream pressures is consistent with the concept of a pulmonary venous waterfall effect between the two measuring sites. Second, we found that under conditions of physiological flow when the downstream pressure of the pulmonary veins was zero, there was a short segment where the vein was leaving the lung in which intravascular pressure changed sharply from a positive upstream to zero downstream pressure.

In this example a topic sentence and transition words link the results to the answer.

Results Supporting the Answer Versus a Summary of Results

Using the appropriate results to support the answers, as done in Examples 7.1 and 7.2, is different from beginning the Discussion with a summary of the results. The difference is the difference between lining up pieces of a puzzle in a row (summary of results) and fitting the pieces together into a picture (answer supported by relevant results). The purpose of the Discussion is to present the picture so that we see that the results support the answer and are convinced that the answer is valid. The writing techniques that create a picture are topic sentences, transition phrases, and transition words.

Giving Credit to Yourself and Others

If others' results help support your answer, mention those results, and cite the appropriate references. Neither overplay nor underplay your own or others' contributions. If others' work clinches your point, say so. Conversely, if your work is the missing link that pulls together a lot of loose threads, say that too. Be neither too modest nor too boastful. Example 7.3 illustrates one way of giving appropriate credit to yourself and others.

Example 7.3   Giving Credit to Yourself and Others

By using whole mounts stained histochemically for acetylcholinesterase, we have reconstructed an overall picture of the architecture of the nerves and ganglia of the ferret trachea. This reconstruction, which incorporates and confirms the separate observations of previous investigators (6, 9, 11, 14, 24), includes several new observations that provide a more complete understanding of the tracheal innervation.

In this example, the first sentence of the Discussion states the answer. The second sentence gives credit to others and also makes clear what the authors' contribution is.

Explaining the Answer

In addition to stating the answer and supporting it with results, you may need to explain the answer. For example, why is the answer reasonable, or how does it fit in with previously published ideas on the topic? An example of an explanation of how the answer fits in with previously published ideas is given in the second and third paragraphs of Example 7.4.

Example 7.4   Explaining the Answer

1   In this study, we have found a second example of clustering for two members of the large collagen gene family and have demonstrated physical linkage between genes that have the same function—encoding both chains of a single collagen type. Specifically, we have conclusively localized the human α2 type IV collagen gene to the distal long arm of chromosome 13 by two independent methods. Hybridization to DNA from rodent-human hybrids with different deletions of chromosome 13 assigned the α2(IV) locus to the segment 13q22→terminus. Mapping by the chromosomal in situ technique allowed more refined sublocalization to the distal q33→q34 region. This region also contains the α1(IV) locus (30), as shown diagrammatically in Fig. 5.

2   These results thus lend further credence to our earlier suggestion that one might expect to find clustering of several collagen members and dispersion of others in a fashion analogous to the globin pattern (36). In that pattern, two separate multigene clusters containing the α and β globin genes are present on chromosomes 16 and 11, respectively (43–45). At both loci, the genes are tightly linked and contiguous.

3   The arrangement of the collagen genes that we report here is also reminiscent of the histones, since clusters of different histone genes map to at least three human chromosomes (46). For the histone gene family, we previously hypothesized that an ancestral site existed that gave rise to the present clusters distributed among multiple chromosomes by means of mechanisms involving recombination (36). A similar situation now emerges for the collagen gene family.

In this example, the first paragraph states the answer to the question and supports the answer with the results. The next two paragraphs explain how the answer (clustering of collagen genes) fits in with previously published ideas (clustering of globin genes and of histone genes).

Defending the Answer

If other possible answers have been proposed for the question you asked or if other answers are easy to imagine, you should explain why your answer is more satisfactory than those other answers. When defending your answer, you need to explain both why your answer is satisfactory and why others are not. That is, you must argue both for your answer and against the others. Only by giving both the pro and the con arguments can you make your answer convincing. An example of a pro-con defense of an answer is given in Example 7.5.

Example 7.5 Defending the Answer

In this study, we found that, at 37°C, alveolar surface tension at total lung capacity is 29.7 ± 5.6 (SD) mN/m. We believe that this value, which we determined by a direct technique, is accurate because it is close to the known equilibrium surface tension of about 25 mN/m for extracts containing pulmonary surfactant (10, 11). However, higher surface tensions have been suggested by other investigators, who did surface balance studies of lung extracts. Their values range from 31 to 50 mN/m (7, 8, 12). But deducing values for alveolar surface tension from lung extracts in surface balances is uncertain, because the actual concentration of surface-active agents at the alveolar surface is not known (5, 13). We suspect that the concentration of surface-active agents in lung extracts as usually assessed in surface balances might be lower than those in alveoli at total lung capacity and that if higher concentrations were used, surface tension values deduced from surface balance studies might be closer to equilibrium values.

In this example, the first sentence states the authors' answer (a surface tension value obtained by a direct technique) and the second sentence defends it by comparing it with the known value at equilibrium. This is the "pro" part of the pro-con argument. The rest of the paragraph presents the "con" argument. It argues that different answers are not likely to be accurate because the method used may not be measuring the same quantity. If we accept both the pro and the con arguments, we are willing to accept the authors' answer.

Explaining Conflicting Results

In addition to stating, supporting, explaining, and defending your answer as necessary, also mention any results you got that do not support your answer, and explain them as best you can. An example of such an explanation of conflicting results is given in the last three sentences of Example 7.6 below ("However, . . . ").

Example 7.6 Explaining Conflicting Results

The main finding of the present study is that β-adrenergic blockade does not impair performance of maximal or submaximal exercise at high altitude. As expected, treatment with the β-blocker propranolol substantially decreased heart rate at high altitude. However, contrary to our hypothesis, propranolol-treated subjects were able to maintain levels of oxygen uptake during maximal and submaximal exercise as great as those in placebo-treated subjects. This finding cannot be attributed to increased arterial oxygen saturation or hemoglobin concentration, since values for propranolol-treated subjects were no different from those for placebo-treated subjects. Rather, it appears that oxygen uptake was maintained by increasing stroke volume.

In this example, the third sentence states a finding that conflicts with the answer to the question. The fourth sentence rules out one possible explanation, and the fifth sentence proposes another possible explanation.

Establishing Newness

The newness of your work should be established in the Introduction by the statement of what is unknown. If you want to remind the reader of the newness of your work, one way to indicate newness is to contrast the point you are making with what was known before, as in Example 7.7, which is the first two sentences of a Discussion.

Example 7.7   Establishing Newness

Partial cDNA clones have been reported for mouse (38–40), rat (41, 42), and human (24) β-glucuronidase. In this study, we report the complete sequence of the full-length cDNA for human β-glucuronidase.

In this example, newness is indicated by the contrast between "partial" in the first sentence and "full-length" in the second sentence.

Avoid claiming priority ("This is the first report of . . . "). It is possible that the same or very similar work has been reported in the literature of another country either in English or in another language. If you feel strongly that you must claim priority, word your claim cautiously. For example, you might say, "To our knowledge, this is the first report of . . . ."

Explanation of Discrepancies

At the opposite extreme from others' results that agree with yours and support the answer to the question are others' results that should agree but do not. Such discrepancies need to be explained as best you can. An example of an explanation of a discrepancy is given in Example 7.8.

Example 7.8   Explanation of a Discrepancy

Apparent discrepancies between our human growth hormone values and those of earlier studies may be due to differences in study design. In our study, all subjects worked at the same relative intensity (60% $\dot{V}O_{2max}$), which meant different absolute work loads because of the subjects' different levels of cardiorespiratory endurance and body fatness. Moreover, the intensity was constant for 60 min. Earlier studies that reported lower training responses differed from this study design in one of three ways: controls and trained subjects were working at the same absolute work loads or relative intensity was not defined (12, 22, 27); the protocol was continuous and had progressive increases in work load, so intensity and duration were not separated (1, 12, 29); or resting human growth hormone values were higher in the pretraining than in the post-training protocol (12).

Explanation of Unexpected Findings

Unexpected findings can range from minor to exciting. In a few cases they are more exciting than the original question and take over the paper (see Exercise 7.1). When describing an unexpected finding, state at the beginning of the paragraph that the finding was unexpected (or surprising) and then explain it as best you can, as in Example 7.9.

Example 7.9   Explanation of an Unexpected Finding

A surprising finding was that in dogs treated with isoproterenol, oxygen extraction ratios during severe hypoxia were low. The ratios we found were less than 50%, whereas ratios in untreated dogs range from 80 to 90% (4). We suggest two possible explanations of why extraction of oxygen from skeletal muscle was not further increased to minimize the oxygen deficit in the isoproterenol-treated dogs. First, blood flow may have been directed through thoroughfare, nonnutritive channels during β-adrenergic stimulation rather than through nutritive channels, thereby decreasing the ability of the tissue to take up oxygen. Second, some metabolic autoregulatory stimulus may have dictated the amount of oxygen used during hypoxia so that when blood flow was increased, oxygen extraction was decreased in proportion to decreased metabolic needs. If these explanations are correct, they imply that the oxygen deficit is linked not only to oxygen delivery but also to some tissue signal originating at the cellular level.

Limitations of the Methods, Weaknesses in Study Design, Validity of Assumptions

If your methods have limitations or if your experimental design is weak or is based on any assumptions, you should state what the limitations, weaknesses, or assumptions are and explain why the limitations, weaknesses, or assumptions are acceptable. If the explanation is brief (one or two sentences), it can be stated in the Methods section. If the explanation is longer (one or two paragraphs), or if the limitation, weakness, or assumption is likely to affect your results seriously, the explanation should be included in the Discussion. If possible, explanations of limitations of methods, weaknesses in study design, or the validity of assumptions should be woven into the story (see Example 7.19 below). An example of an explanation of the validity of an assumption is given in Example 7.10.

Example 7.10 Explanation of the Validity of an Assumption

One assumption we made for the measurement of the pulmonary capillary filtration coefficient (K_f) was that isolating the lungs did not injure pulmonary vessels. This is a reasonable assumption, because we minimized lung ischemia by removing the lungs rapidly (within 5 min). In addition, the baseline K_f values in our study are low and agree with other reported K_f values (33). Finally, we have found that lungs isolated and perfused in a similar manner are stable for 3 h (unpublished observation).

In this example, the author first states what the assumption is and then gives three reasons that the assumption is reasonable.

Establishing Importance

The importance of the work is sometimes obvious from its newness—for example, if the cause of a disease was unknown and you are reporting the cause. Similarly, in basic research newness is usually sufficient evidence of importance. But if importance needs to be established, that can be done either in the Introduction (see Chap. 4) or in the Discussion. In the Discussion, importance can be established by describing applications or implications of the answer or by stating speculations based on the answer. Applications, implications, and speculations are often used as an ending of a Discussion (see "How to End the Discussion" below).

ORGANIZATION

To ensure that your Discussion is organized rather than rambling, think of the Discussion as telling a story, and focus the story on the question you asked in the Introduction. To tell a story, give your Discussion the three standard parts of a story—a beginning, a middle, and an end.

The <u>beginning</u> of the Discussion (that is, the first paragraph or more) should state the answer to the question and support the answer with results. Beginning with the answer is the best way to focus your story on the question.

The <u>middle</u> of the Discussion should discuss topics in the order of most to least important to the answer.

The <u>end</u> of the Discussion (that is, the last paragraph) should conclude either by restating the answer to the question or by making a special point, or both.

The guidelines below explain how to tell a story in the Discussion. The most important of these guidelines are to state the answer to the question at the beginning of the Discussion, to organize the other points in the order of most to least important, to use a topic sentence at the beginning of every paragraph to state the point, and to link the point of each paragraph to the point of the previous paragraph.

How to Begin the Discussion: Answer the Question

Begin the Discussion with the answer to the question, followed immediately by support for the answer. The reason for beginning with the answer to the question is that the beginning of the Discussion is a position of prominence and therefore should be used for the most important idea. In the Discussion, the most important idea is the answer to the question. The reason the answer is the most important idea is that the answer fulfills the expectation created by the statement of the question in the Introduction and by the statements in Methods and Results of what you did to answer the question and what you found that answers the question. Thus, the answer to the question is the culmination of the paper. It deserves the most prominent position in the Discussion—the beginning.

Signaling the Answer

At the beginning of the sentence that states the answer, put a signal that it is the answer. Signals of the answer include "This study shows that . . . ," "Our results indicate that . . . ," "In this study we found that . . . ," and the like. Signaling the answer is important because without a signal the answer could be mistaken for something already known. For example, does this sentence from the beginning of a Discussion state the answer to the question or something already known? "Polymorphonuclear leukocytes can now be induced to release a number of varieties of granule-poor anucleate fragments (cytoplasts), each with its own uses for the study of leukocyte function." To make clear that this sentence states the answer, add a signal. For example, "*In this study, we have created* polymorphonuclear leukocytes that can be induced to release a number of varieties of granule-poor anucleate fragments (cytoplasts), each with its own uses for the study of leukocyte function."

Stating the Species or the Study Population

The species or the study population must be included in the sentence stating the answer, just as it was in the sentence stating the question in the Introduction. State the species or study population in the answer if the question was about that species or population (as in Example 7.15 below) but in the signal of the answer if the question was general (as in Example 7.11). For humans, the species is often left unstated (see Examples 7.12–7.14).

Examples of Ways to Begin the Discussion

State the Answers to the Questions. The most straightforward way to begin the Discussion is to state the answers to the questions.

If your study dealt with one question, begin the Discussion by answering that question. Put a signal before the answer. Mention the species in the signal or in the answer, whichever is appropriate. Be sure the answer answers the question you asked.

Example 7.11 One Answer

This study in *newborn goats* demonstrates that continuous positive airway pressure (7.5 cm H_2O) **can impair** renal function in newborns.

In this example, the sentence begins with a signal of the answer (not underlined) and ends with the answer (underlined). The species (italicized) is named in the signal because the answer is not limited to that species. The answer matches the question stated in the Introduction: "The purpose of this study was to further define the effects of continuous positive airway pressure on renal function in newborns." The key terms are the same (continuous positive airway pressure, renal function, newborns) and the point of view is the same (cause to effect).

If your study dealt with two questions, you can begin the Discussion by answering both of the questions, as in Example 7.12, or you can answer only one question at the beginning of the first paragraph and the other question at the beginning of a later paragraph, preferably the second paragraph. The only information that should be given between the two answers is results supporting the first answer. Put a signal before each separate answer. Answer the questions in the same order as they appear in the Introduction.

Example 7.12 Two Answers

Our experiments show that cigarette-smoke-induced bronchoconstriction **is** much more severe than previously reported and *that* this bronchoconstriction **is mediated** principally by extravagal mechanisms.

This sentence answers both of the questions posed in the Introduction. It begins with one signal for both answers ("Our experiments show that") and then repeats "that" before the second answer to signal that it is also an answer. The species is not mentioned because the species studied was humans. The questions as stated in the Introduction were "We reassessed the severity of cigarette-smoke-induced bronchoconstriction. . . . We also determined the mechanism of cigarette-smoke-induced bronchoconstriction." Because the answers use the same key terms (underlined), it is clear that the answers answer the questions asked.

If your study dealt with three or more questions, beginning the Discussion by stating the answers to all the questions may sound too much like a summary. When you have several questions, it is generally best to answer only the first question or only the important questions in the first paragraph of the Discussion. Answer the other questions at the beginning of later paragraphs. You can restate all the answers together in the last paragraph of the Discussion, which is the best place for a summary.

Restate the Question(s) and Then State the Answer(s). Instead of beginning the Discussion with the answer, you can put a one-sentence restatement of the question before the answer. Restating the question before stating the answer is less abrupt of a beginning than is stating only the answer. If you restate the question in the Discussion, be sure that the question and the answer use the same key terms, the same verbs (when appropriate), and the same point of view. In addition, be sure that the question stated in the Discussion matches the question stated in the Introduction.

Example 7.13 Question and Answer

The question addressed by the present study was whether the chemical stimuli <u>hypercapnia</u> and <u>hypoxia</u> affect the magnitude of the <u>abdominal expiratory neural activity</u> in the absence of any changes in proprioceptive afferent activity from the lungs and chest and abdominal walls. The main finding of the study **is** that progressive hyperoxic <u>hypercapnia</u> and isocapnic <u>hypoxia</u> both **increase** <u>abdominal expiratory neural activity</u> while concurrently decreasing expiratory duration. For hypercapnia, the increases in the variables related to the magnitude of the abdominal neurogram and arterial P_{CO_2} were linear, whereas for hypoxia the increases were hyperbolic.

In this example, the question and answer use the same key terms and the same point of view (cause to effect). In addition, the question restated in the Discussion matches the question stated in the Introduction: "The aim of the present study was to determine whether <u>hypercapnia</u> and <u>hypoxia</u> affect the magnitude of the <u>abdominal expiratory neural activity</u> in the absence of any changes in proprioceptive afferent activity from the lungs and chest and abdominal walls." The results that support the answer are given immediately after the answer is stated and are signaled by transition phrases that repeat key terms: "For hypercapnia, . . . for hypoxia. . . ."

If you restate the question at the beginning of the Discussion, go on immediately to state the answer. Do not, for example, launch into a long review of your experimental approach. If you state the experimental approach, keep it brief. The longer the answer is delayed, the more difficult it is for the reader to find the answer. Since the answer is the most important information in the Discussion, it should be presented in the most prominent place—the very beginning of the Discussion. In Example 7.14, the answer is delayed until the third and fourth sentences, which is about as long a delay as is tolerable.

Example 7.14 Question and Delayed Answer

What <u>makes</u> an <u>initiator</u> tRNA an <u>initiator</u> and not an elongator? In an attempt to answer this question, we removed from *E. coli* $tRNA_2^{fMet}$ two of the features common to all prokaryotic initiator tRNAs, isolated and characterized the mutant tRNAs, and studied their function in protein synthesis in vitro. We found that what <u>makes</u> an <u>initiator</u> tRNA an <u>initiator</u> is not the T-1 mutation, because this mutation had no effect on protein synthesis (Fig. 1). Rather the $_{CCC}^{GGG}$ sequence conserved in the anticodon stem of both prokaryotic and eukaryotic initiator tRNAs is important for initiation. In our experiments, as one, two, and all three of the G · C base pairs were altered to those found in *E. coli* elongator methionine tRNA, the activity of the mutant tRNAs in protein synthesis initiation decreased progressively, a mutant with all three G · C base pairs altered being the least active (Fig. 3). The effect of the mutation was at the step of initiator tRNA binding to the ribosomal P site (Table 2).

In this example, the first sentence restates the question and the second sentence states the experimental approach to answering the question. The third and fourth sentences state the answer. The third sentence begins with a signal of the answer, then states a rejected answer using the same key terms, the same verb, and the same point of view as in the question, and ends with the reason for rejecting that answer. The fourth sentence states the accepted answer. Signaling the answer, repeating the key terms and the verb, and keeping the same point of view in the third sentence are especially important because of the sentence of experimental approach that intervenes between the question and the answer. Although the fourth sentence changes the point of view and the verb, it is clear that this is the answer because "rather" signals a contrast with the third sentence, which stated the rejected answer. The last two sentences of this paragraph present results that support the answer; the results are signaled by "In our experiments."

Provide a Brief Context and Then State the Answer. Providing a brief context is another way of avoiding an abrupt beginning of the Discussion. The context must accurately restate a point made in the Introduction and must be brief. One or at most two sentences are enough. If the context is extended to three or more sentences, the effect is to have a second Introduction. Two Introductions are at best unnecessarily repetitious and at worst conflicting and therefore confusing to the reader: which Introduction is the way the author really wants us to view this paper? Since the Introduction and the Discussion form a paired unit in a scientific research paper, keeping the context brief is the best way to give the sense that the Discussion picks up from where the Introduction left off.

Example 7.15 Context and Answer

Previous investigators suggested that drainage of liquid from the lungs of fetal rabbits begins at birth (1, 2) and is inhibited by cesarean section (2). Our results show that drainage of fetal lung liquid in rabbits begins before birth and depends on the experience of labor, not on the mode of delivery.

In Example 7.15, the first sentence is context. The second sentence states the answers to the questions. The first answer closely parallels the first part of the context, making it easy to see the difference between what was previously suggested and the conclusion of this study.

Although restating the question and providing context are more sophisticated ways to begin the Discussion than simply stating the answer to the question, the best way to begin the Discussion is usually the simple way—by stating the answer. Answers stated at the beginning of the Discussion are easiest for the reader to find and have the most impact.

Examples of Ways Not to Begin the Discussion

Do Not Begin the Discussion with a Summary of the Results. The place for a summary of the results is the Results section. In fact, the Results section *is* a summary of the results. If you find that you have written a long Results section and are tempted to put a summary of the results at the beginning of the Discussion, consider omitting the long Results section and using the summary of the results as the Results section instead.

Do Not Begin the Discussion with Secondary Information. Secondary information belongs later in the Discussion, after the answers to the questions have been stated.

Example 7.16 Beginning with Secondary Information (Undesirable)

The small but significant loss of plasma volume during the last 10 min of the normoxic rest period is difficult to explain.

The question stated in the Introduction was "to determine if the efflux in plasma volume during hypoxic submaximal and maximal exercise in the supine posture can exceed the maximum 15–22% reported for normoxic conditions." From this question we expect the beginning of the Discussion to state whether the efflux in plasma volume exceeded 22% in hypoxic subjects during exercise. Instead, we hear about a minor unexpected finding (loss of plasma volume in normoxic subjects at rest). This beginning is disorienting.

Example 7.17 Beginning with Secondary Information (Undesirable)

The results of the endurance time for the sustained isometric exercise at different contraction levels were consistent with previous reports (4, 25).

Instead of beginning by answering the question, this Discussion begins with information of secondary importance—comparison of a few of the results with previous findings. (The question was to determine "the endurance time during exercise consisting of sustained isometric contractions, intermittent isometric contractions, and dynamic contractions.") It is a shame to throw away the beginning of the Discussion on secondary information. Secondary information belongs in the middle of the Discussion, after the answers to the questions have been stated.

How to Continue the Discussion: Provide a Chain of Topic Sentences

Organizing the Topics

Once you have answered the questions, the problem is how to continue the Discussion. The most useful guideline is to move from most to least important topics. Importance is determined by the relation of the topic to the answer to the question. For example, in a results paper, support, explanation, and defense of the answer should come before any other topics.

Two or more paragraphs often have the same relation to the answer (for example, supporting the answer), so these paragraphs should be grouped together in one section of the Discussion. Thus, the Discussion is usually a series of sections, each containing one or more paragraphs. Just as the sections should be organized from most to least important, so the paragraphs within each section should be organized from most to least important. An example of a Discussion in which the topics and paragraphs are organized according to their importance is Example 7.31 at the end of this chapter.

Importance is somewhat subjective and relative. Thus, different coauthors of a paper might organize the same topics differently. Even the same author might organize the topics differently at a later time, depending, for example, on what other papers have recently been published.

Telling the Overall Story

It is not enough to organize topics and paragraphs from most to least important. In addition, you must indicate to the reader what the logic of the organization is: why is the second topic second and the third topic third? Thus, the topic sentence of the paragraph must indicate not only the point or topic of the paragraph but also the relation of the paragraph to the previous paragraph(s) (and thus to the answer to the question). That is, in addition to telling a story within each paragraph, you should use topic sentences to weave an overall story through the Discussion.

There are two ways of using topic sentences to weave an overall story through the Discussion. One way is to present an overview from the beginning (overview technique); the other way is to present one step at a time (step-by-step technique). In the overview technique, the author uses a topic sentence at the beginning of each section to announce the topic or the point of the section and then uses both a transition and a topic sentence at the beginning of each paragraph within the section to move from one paragraph to the next. Thus, the reader knows in advance what to expect in the next two or more paragraphs. The step-by-step technique works differently. Here the author uses a topic sentence at the beginning of one paragraph to announce one step in the story, another topic sentence at the beginning of the next paragraph to announce the next step, and so on, paragraph by paragraph. The paragraphs are linked by repetition of key words. The reader does not know what to expect in advance but is thinking along with the author, one step at a time.

The advantage of the overview technique is that it makes the story of the Discussion easy to follow. The advantage of the step-by-step technique is that it is interesting because it gives a sense of being there while the story is unfolding. However, to be successful, the step-by-step technique must be well handled. Specifically, the repetition of key terms must be clear so that the reader does not lose the thread of the story.

Using Topic Sentences to Tell the Overall Story

These two ways of proceeding in a Discussion use topic sentences at different levels of organization and of different types than we have examined so far.

Topic Sentences Used in the Overview Technique.   The overview technique uses topic sentences at two levels: the section and the paragraph. A section topic sentence announces the topic or the point of a section of a Discussion and in this way indicates the overall organization of the Discussion: section I is about X topic. To link the steps of the story within each section, a transition topic sentence is used at the beginning of each paragraph. A transition topic sentence is a topic sentence that contains a transition word, phrase, or clause at or near the beginning of the sentence. Examples of a section topic sentence and transition word topic sentences are given in Example 7.18.

Example 7.18   Section Topic Sentence and
Transition Word Topic Sentences

1   *A*<u>Several hemodynamic effects of chromonar could shift the diastolic pressure-dimension curve acutely</u>.   *B*<u>*One*</u> is an increase in heart rate, which could shift the diastolic pressure-dimension curve to the left by either of two mechanisms. (etc.)

2   *C*<u>*A second* hemodynamic effect</u>, afterload, can also shift the diastolic pressure-dimension curve. (etc.)

3   *D*<u>A *third* effect that can acutely shift the pressure-dimension curve to the</u>
<u>left</u> is ischemia. (etc.)

4   *E*<u>*The final* hemodynamic effect that can shift the pressure-dimension curve</u>
<u>acutely</u> is change in temperature. (etc.)

In this example, the section topic sentence (sentence A) announces the topic of the next four paragraphs. The paragraph topic sentences (sentences B, C, D, and E) each contain a transition word at the beginning of the sentence: "One," "A second," "A third," "The final." Thus, these are transition word topic sentences.

Keeping the Story Going Within a Section of the Discussion.   To keep the story going within a section of a Discussion, stronger transitions are needed in the topic sentences of later paragraphs than in the topic sentence of the first paragraph. There are two ways to make a transition stronger. One way is to repeat more key terms from the section topic sentence, as in Example 7.18 above. The other way is to use a transition phrase or a transition clause instead of a transition word, as in Example 7.19 below.

In Example 7.18 above, the first paragraph topic sentence (sentence B) uses only a transition word ("One"). This brief transition is sufficient to keep the story going because the paragraph topic sentence comes immediately after the section topic sentence. But paragraph 2 is farther from the section topic sentence, so a stronger transition is needed. In this topic sentence (sentence C), two key terms are repeated ("hemodynamic" and "effect") in addition to the transition word ("A second"). The topic sentences of paragraphs 3 and 4 use even stronger transitions in their topic sentences. They each repeat six key terms (D, "effect," "acutely," "shift," "pressure-dimension," "curve," and "left"; E, "hemodynamic," "effect," "shift," "pressure-dimension," "curve," and "acutely") in addition to their transition words (D, "A third"; E, "The final"). By repeating more key terms, these transition topic sentences keep reminding us of what the story is about, and the transition words indicate where we are in the story.

Keeping the Story Going Between Sections of a Discussion.   In addition to keeping the story going within each section of the Discussion, you must keep the overall story of the Discussion going between sections. For this purpose, use a transition phrase or a transition clause at the beginning of the topic sentence for each new section. A transition phrase or a transition clause is stronger than a transition word because a transition phrase or clause summarizes the topic or the point of the previous section before stating the topic or the point of the next section. In Example 7.19, a transition phrase at the beginning of paragraph 5 joins the section on limitations of the method (paras. 1–4) to the section on advantages of the method (para. 5). The transition phrase summarizes the topic of the previous section (limitations) and the rest of the sentence announces the topic of the next section (advantages).

Example 7.19   Section Topic Sentence and
Transition Phrase Topic Sentence

1   *A*<u>The imprecision we detected in the precursor-product relationship could</u>
<u>have arisen from limitations of the method.</u> *B*<u>*One* limitation</u> is experimental
variability. (etc.)

2 *C*<u>*Another* limitation of our method</u> is contamination of materials. (etc.)

3 *D*<u>*A third* limitation of our method</u> is that recovery of materials is incomplete. (etc.)

4 *E*<u>*A fourth* limitation of our method</u> is that the assumptions used for defining compartments may not be justified. (etc.)

5 *F*<u>*Despite these limitations*, our method of data analysis has advantages over those previously used to calculate surfactant turnover times.</u> *G*Unlike the method of Zilversmit et al. (8), it uses the specific activity-time data and readily reveals departures from ideal precursor-product relationships. *H*Unlike curve-peeling methods, it accounts for continued input of tracer and avoids the up to 200-fold overestimation of turnover time caused by neglecting continued tracer input.

In this example, the first sentence in paragraph 1 (sentence A) is a section topic sentence for paragraphs 1–4. The paragraph topic sentences for paragraphs 1–4 each use a transition word ("One," "Another," "A third," "A fourth") to indicate where we are in the story. In addition, to keep reminding us of what the story is about, the topic sentences for paragraphs 2–4, which are farther from the section topic sentence, repeat more key terms than the topic sentence for paragraph 1 does ("limitation of our method" vs. "limitation").

Paragraph 5 starts a new section. The topic sentence for paragraph 5 is a stronger transition topic sentence than those in paragraphs 1–4. It begins with a transition phrase to summarize the topic of paragraphs 1–4 ("Despite these limitations") and then states the point of paragraph 5 ("our method of data analysis has advantages over those previously used to calculate surfactant turnover times"). This transition phrase topic sentence keeps the overall story of the Discussion going by indicating a major junction in the story. If only a transition word ("nevertheless") had been used or, worse, if no transition had been used, the story of the Discussion would have been harder to follow. (Try reading Example 7.19 with "Nevertheless" or no transition in place of "Despite these limitations.")

Furthermore, together with the section topic sentence (sentence A), the transition phrase topic sentence at the beginning of paragraph 5 tells the overall story of the Discussion. From reading these two topic sentences, we see that the overall story has two steps: A. "The imprecision we detected in the precursor-product relationship could have arisen from limitations of the method." F. "Despite these limitations, our method of data analysis has advantages over those previously used to calculate surfactant turnover times." The step about limitations is dealt with in a section composed of four paragraphs and has five topic sentences: a section topic sentence and a paragraph topic sentence in paragraph 1 and paragraph topic sentences in paragraphs 2, 3, and 4; the step about advantages is dealt with in a section composed of one paragraph.

Finally, note that the explanation of the limitations of the method is woven into the story of the Discussion. The limitations are presented as possible reasons for the imprecision in the precursor-product relationship.

An even stronger transition topic sentence is the transition clause topic sentence. A transition clause topic sentence functions in exactly the same way as a transition phrase topic sentence does. But a transition clause is more powerful than a transition phrase because a transition clause contains a verb. An example of a transition clause is given at the beginning of paragraph 2 (sentence L) in Example 7.20.

Example 7.20   Section Topic Sentence and
Transition Clause Topic Sentence

1   *A*This study in rats shows that **perfusion** and **ventilation** of transplanted lungs are decreased independently by the reimplantation response. *B***Perfusion** is decreased by stenosis of the pulmonary artery anastomoses and by hilar stripping of the lung. *C*Stenosis of the pulmonary artery appears to be more important. *D*The evidence is that stenosis of the anastomosis of the pulmonary artery resulted in very low perfusion of the lung immediately after it was transplanted (Fig. 2). *E*This finding is in accordance with results of studies in dog lung transplants which showed that stenosis of vascular anastomoses increases vascular resistance of the transplanted lung (23, 24), which would decrease perfusion. *F*Hilar stripping of the lung also decreased perfusion, but this effect was only mild and transient (Fig. 2). *G*In the literature some authors concluded from reimplantation studies in dogs that hilar stripping of the lung causes permanently abnormal values of pulmonary vascular resistance and perfusion (25). *H*However, our results clearly support the conclusion of other authors that it is not hilar stripping (26, 27) but rather imperfect vascular anastomoses (23, 24, 28) that permanently decrease perfusion in the transplanted lung. *I*It is not clear how hilar stripping induces the transient decrease in perfusion. *J*Blood vessels might be compressed by perivascular edema, which was present for some days after hilar stripping. *K*However, this does not appear to be a satisfactory explanation of the perfusion decrease because the edema resolved rapidly, but the perfusion remained decreased for two weeks.

2   *L*Whereas **perfusion** is decreased by stenosis of the pulmonary artery anastomoses and by hilar stripping, **ventilation** of the transplanted left lung is decreased for some days after transplantation because of interstitial and alveolar edema resulting from transplantation ischemia and from hilar stripping. *M*Edema was observed in the bronchus during transplantation (Table IV), in histologic sections (Fig. 6A), and on chest radiograms (Fig. 4A). *N*The increased density of transplanted lungs on chest radiograms is the most common phenomenon of the reimplantation response described in primates (9, 29) and dogs (8, 20, 30). *O*Our conclusion that edema results from transplantation ischemia is clear from our finding that edema formation increased proportionally to the duration of transplantation ischemia (Fig. 3, Table IV), confirming previous findings in dogs (30). *P*However, pulmonary edema also developed in the absence of ischemia of the lung after hilar stripping (Figs. 3 and 5). *Q*Although the extent of the edema was mostly less than that caused by transplantation ischemia, its histological pattern was the same. *R*So it seems likely that pulmonary edema is caused by hilar stripping injury of the lung and is aggravated by ischemia. *S*This interpretation is in accordance with previous findings from our laboratory which showed that bilateral hilar stripping, when combined with ischemia of the lungs for at least one hour, decreased arterial oxygen tension (27).

In this example, a transition clause topic sentence is used at the beginning of paragraph 2. The transition clause (italicized) summarizes the point of the first paragraph. The topic sentence (not italicized) states the point of the second paragraph. This transition clause topic sentence reminds us of where we are in the story. If only a basic topic sentence (sentence L, not italicized) without the strong transition clause (sentence L, italicized) had been used, the reader would have started losing the forest, because the previous paragraph contains a lot of detail ("trees"). Try reading these two paragraphs without the transition clause (sentence L, italicized).

Thus, transition phrases or clauses are particularly useful at major junctions in the overall story of a Discussion. They are also useful to return the reader to the overall story after an interruption or after any long paragraph containing a lot of details that might make the reader lose the thread of the story, as in Example 7.20. For other examples of transition clause topic sentences, see Exercise 7.1.

Topic Sentences Used in the Step-By-Step Technique. The step-by-step technique for proceeding in a Discussion uses only paragraph topic sentences, not both section topic sentences and paragraph topic sentences as the overview technique does. The topic sentences used in the step-by-step technique do not include transitions. To provide continuity from paragraph to paragraph, key term topic sentences are used. In key term topic sentences, each topic sentence repeats a key term picked up from the previous paragraph and makes a new point about that key term. In Example 7.21, key term topic sentences are used at the beginning of paragraphs 2–5. (A paragraph from the Introduction for this Discussion is given in Chap. 3, Example 3.1.)

Example 7.21 Key Term Topic Sentences

1 *A*The present picture of the thick filament assembly in catch muscles of molluscs derives from the notion of a common plan for all myosin filaments (20). *B*Squire (21) proposed the first detailed packing models for such **structures** using a scheme of overlapping myosin molecules. *C*In his models, the overlapping myosin molecules make up planar ribbons (about 35 Å thick) that wrap into cylinders. *D*The filament diameters would be directly related to the number of molecules around the circumference. *E*The core could be hollow or could contain paramyosin. *F*The basic assumption in this model is that identical myosin molecules are equivalently related and specifically bonded in various thick filament arrays. *G*Wray (22) has recently developed related models involving the formation of myosin cables or ropes (about 40 Å in diameter) consisting of about three overlapping molecules twisted together, which are then grouped to form tubes of various diameters. *H*In both types of model, thick filaments of different diameters—found in different animals—would be built on the same basic plan. *I*In both types of model also, myosin-myosin interactions dictate assembly of the filament, and it is not possible in either type of model for the myosin heads arrayed at the surface to be in contact also with the paramyosin core.

2 *J*I suggest that the thick filaments of catch muscles might be **constructed** in a different way: myosin could form a surface layer, or **lattice**, only one molecule thick. *K*Paramyosin-myosin interactions rather than myosin-myosin interactions would control both the assembly of the filament and the state of the myosin at the surface. *L*This notion extends a picture we derived some 10 years ago from inspection of filament sizes and protein composition (5, 16). *M*Our preliminary measurements of both red and white portions of the adductors of clam muscles indicated that the "rod portion of myosin would be at least sufficient to cover the paramyosin surface completely" (5). *N*We then stated, "It is possible that there is a relatively constant surface area per myosin molecule in all paramyosin-containing muscles" (5). *O*In fact, our conclusion was based on a happy combination of incorrect biochemistry and wrong arithmetic. *P*Since that time further measurements of protein composition show even higher proportions of paramyosin in these catch muscles (7, 8). *Q*In contrast, most other types of muscle have higher proportions of myosin. *R*The important point, which appears to have been overlooked, is that the surface area per myosin molecule is relatively constant but different for two main classes of thick filament—those with and without very large paramyosin cores. ^{S}Only for thick filaments with large paramyosin cores might the surface layer be a **lattice** only one molecule thick.

3 ^{T}<u>How might this **lattice** be **organized**</u>? ^{U}It is an interesting fact that although the length of paramyosin is about 1275 Å, this molecule assembles into fibers with a "gap-overlap" arrangement having an axial repeat of 725 Å (23). ^{V}A simple staggering of small groups (or subfilaments) of paramyosin molecules arranged with this specific gap-overlap packing generates the characteristic "checkerboard" array of nodes seen in the core of catch muscle thick filaments by electron microscopy. (etc.)

4 ^{W}<u>In principle a variety of schemes might be advanced that relate these</u> **organizational** <u>notions to recent biochemical and pharmacological studies of</u> <u>the catch mechanism</u>. ^{X}A plausible picture can be developed based on the work of Achazi (19), who has suggested that a serotonin-stimulated increase in cAMP (28–30) mediates the dephosphorylation of paramyosin (see also ref. 31). ^{Y}One might picture that. . . . (etc.)

5 ^{Z}<u>Some predictions arise from these speculations</u>. ^{AA}For example, ... (etc.)

In this example, the first sentence of paragraph 2 (sentence J) is a key term topic sentence. It picks up the key term "structures" from paragraph 1, sentence B, and suggests a different type of structure. (The key term "structures" from paragraph 1 is repeated in the verb "constructed" in paragraph 2.) Similarly, the topic sentence of paragraph 3 picks up the key term "lattice," whose existence is proposed in paragraph 2, sentence J, and introduces a new topic—how the lattice might be organized. After the possible organization is described in paragraph 3, paragraph 4 begins with another key term topic sentence, which picks up the key term "organized" from paragraph 3 and goes on to relate the organization of the lattice to biochemical and pharmacological studies. Then, after a speculative explanation of one scheme that relates the lattice organization to other studies (in para. 4), paragraph 5 begins with a key term topic sentence that bases some predictions on these speculations. Although the word "speculation" does not appear in paragraph 4, the concept of speculation is clear from "might be advanced" and "A plausible picture can be developed" at the beginning of paragraph 4. Thus, this Discussion proceeds entirely by using key term topic sentences.

A Question as a Topic Sentence.   Note that the topic sentence in paragraph 3 is a question. Using a question as a topic sentence can provide interesting variety, but only if not overused. Usually one question as a topic sentence in a Discussion is enough. Two or more questions as topic sentences rapidly become gimmicky and seem contrived, not appealing. Having no questions as topic sentences is perfectly OK.

Combined Transition + Key Term Topic Sentences.   If we look back at Examples 7.18, 7.19, and 7.20, we can see that frequently both a transition and a repeated key term are used at the beginning of a topic sentence to keep the story going. In Example 7.18, both a transition word and key terms from the section topic sentence are used in topic sentences C, D, and E. In Example 7.19, both a transition word and a repeated key term are used in topic sentences B, C, D, and E. In F, which is a transition phrase topic sentence, a key term from the section topic sentence ("limitations") is repeated in the transition phrase. Similarly, in Example 7.20, the transition clause topic sentence at the beginning of paragraph 2 repeats the key terms "perfusion," "ventilation," "transplanted," "lung," and "decreased." In fact, transition phrases and transition clauses almost inevitably repeat key terms. Thus, the strongest storytelling topic sentences are a combination of a transition topic sentence and a key term topic sentence.

Chain of Topic Sentences. If section topic sentences and transition topic sentences or key term topic sentences are used at the beginning of every paragraph of a Discussion to tell the story, they form a chain of topic sentences. Thus, the reader should be able to read the first sentence or two of every paragraph and see the outline of the overall story of the Discussion. If instead each topic sentence deals only with the topic of its own paragraph without using a transition or repeating key terms, the Discussion will be a sequence of independent topic sentences, like beads without a string running through them to hold them together. The result is all trees and no forest. Because Examples 7.20 and 7.21 above use a chain of topic sentences, the outline of the story is clear.

OUTLINE OF EXAMPLE 7.20

OUTLINE OF TOPICS	*TYPE OF TOPIC SENTENCE*
I. The factors that decrease perfusion and ventilation during the reimplantation response (paras. 1–2)	I. Section topic sentence (sentence A)
A. Factors that decrease perfusion (para. 1)	A. Paragraph topic sentence (Key term topic sentence) (sentence B)
1. Stenosis of vascular anastomoses—most important (sentence C)	
2. Hilar stripping—less important (sentence F)	
B. Factor that decreases ventilation: interstitial and alveolar edema (para. 2)	B. Paragraph topic sentence (Transition clause topic sentence) (sentence L)
1. From transplantation ischemia (sentence O)	
2. From hilar stripping (sentence P)	

In the outline of Example 7.20, note that a transition clause topic sentence is used at the major junction (B) to summarize the point of paragraph 1 (section A) and then state the point of paragraph 2 (section B).

OUTLINE OF EXAMPLE 7.21

  I. Picture of the thick filament assembly (para. 1–2)
    A. Past—planar ribbons (para. 1)
    B. Proposed—lattice (para. 2)
 II. Organization of the lattice (para. 3)
III. Speculative relation of the lattice organization to biochemical and pharmacological studies (para. 4)
IV. Predictions based on the speculative relation (para. 5)

In Example 7.21, a key term topic sentence is used at each new step in the story. In each key term topic sentence, a key term from the previous paragraph is repeated and a new point is made about that key term. Thus, the reader can read sentences A and B of paragraph 1 and the first sentence of each of the remaining paragraphs (2–5) and see the overall story of this Discussion. Note that because Example 7.21 proceeds by a step-by-step technique, the outline has fewer subdivisions than does the outline of Example 7.20, which proceeds by an overview technique. Whichever technique you use in your Discussions, check that the outline of the overall story of the Discussion is apparent.

In a full-length Discussion, both the overview technique and the step-by-step technique can be used. For an example, see Exercise 7.1.

Topics That Do Not Fit Into the Story

In almost every Discussion, topics that do not fit into the story need to be included. For example, explanations of discrepancies and explanations of unexpected findings are often difficult to fit into the story. In these cases, the best you may be able to do is write a paragraph whose topic sentence does not have a transition or a key term that links it to the previous paragraph. An example of a paragraph that the authors could not fit into the story is paragraph 7 in Example 7.31 at the end of this chapter.

Another type of topic that does not fit into the story is a side issue that is relevant to a main topic. An example is sentences I–K in Example 7.20 above. These sentences add extra information (about how hilar stripping induces transient decreases in perfusion) that is not central to the story. If these sentences were omitted, the story would move more smoothly from paragraph 1 to paragraph 2. However, the author wanted to include this speculation since it makes a point that could save other workers unnecessary trial and error.

What is the best way to include this side issue? A separate paragraph is not defensible because the information does not contribute to the story announced in the section topic sentence ("perfusion and ventilation of transplanted lungs are decreased independently by the reimplantation response"). Also, if a separate paragraph were used, a reader reading the first sentence or two of every paragraph to see the story of the Discussion (sentences A, B, I, L) would get a step that in fact does not contribute to the story (sentence I). Sentences B and L are parallel ideas that support A; I interrupts this story. The solution is to use a subtopic sentence to introduce the new subtopic and to include the subtopic in the relevant paragraph. (In Example 7.20, sentences I–K are a subtopic included in paragraph 1; sentence I is the subtopic sentence.) Although the subtopic still interrupts the story, it is less noticeable and less disruptive than if it were in a separate paragraph.

Thus, the goal in dealing with topics that do not fit into the overall story of the Discussion is to preserve the chain of topic sentences at the beginning of each paragraph as best you can, because the chain of topic sentences tells the overall story.

How to End the Discussion: Make a Point

The Discussion should not simply stop. It should come to a definite, clear end.

Two standard ways to end the Discussion are to restate the answers to the questions, and to indicate the importance of the work by stating applications, implications, or speculations. These endings are explained and illustrated below.

A statement that further studies are needed is not a particularly strong ending. It is stronger to end by stating what knowledge you are contributing than by stating what remains to be studied. Some authors use statements about further studies to stake out territory for themselves ("We plan to study . . . " or "We are now doing experiments to determine . . . "). Such statements are inadvisable both because they are ungentlemanly and because unforeseen circumstances may prevent you from finishing the experiments.

Restating the Answers to the Questions

A straightforward way to end the Discussion is to restate the answers to the questions. This type of ending is also referred to as a *summary of conclusions*. It is particularly useful for Discussions in which the answers to the questions are given in successive paragraphs rather than all in the first paragraph.

The summary of conclusions should not contain detail and should include only conclusions that were presented earlier in the Discussion.

The summary of conclusions should be preceded by a signal such as "In summary, we have shown that . . . " or "In conclusion, this study shows that. . . ."

Example 7.22 Summary of Conclusions

In summary, we have shown that the biphasic inspiratory and expiratory airflow pattern of resting adult horses is brought about by the coordinated action of its respiratory pump muscles. Combined with a stiff chest wall, the resting neuromuscular strategy of the horse allows it to breathe around, rather than from, the relaxed volume of the respiratory system and thus to minimize the total elastic work of breathing.

In this example, the beginning of the first sentence ("In summary, we have shown that") signals the summary of conclusions. The rest of the paragraph states the conclusions. Note that the verbs that state the conclusions are in present tense ("is brought about," "allows").

Stating Applications, Implications, or Speculations That Indicate the Importance of the Work

Applications, implications, and speculations can be viewed as stages along a continuum: applications are the most certain, implications are less certain, and speculations are the least certain. Applications are uses to which answers can be put. Usually applications are fairly certain (see Examples 7.23 and 7.24 below). An implication is a logical step that follows from an answer. But whereas answers are solid because they are based on data, implications are tentative because they have no data to support them nor were any experiments done to obtain data for them. One type of implication is a clinical implication, for example, for treatment of patients (see Examples 7.25 and 7.28 below). Speculations are similar to implications, but speculations are even more tentative. Whereas an implication is a logical next step, a speculation is more of an imaginative leap. Nevertheless, reasonable speculation can be useful, for example, for suggesting relationships between ideas, and therefore should be included in a Discussion when warranted. For examples, see Examples 7.26, 7.27, and 7.29 below.

To use these indicators of importance as endings, first state the conclusion (or results) they are based on and, if necessary, remind the reader that it is a conclusion of your study. Then state the application, implication, or speculation, using a verb that indicates its degree of certainty. For greatest clarity, implications and speculations should be preceded by a signal. Signal implications by using the verb "suggest" or "imply." Signal speculations by using the verb "speculate."

Example 7.23   Application

Isolation of the genes for catabolism and the primary gene(s) for synthesis of L-3-*O*-methyl-*scyllo*-inosamine reported here provides a tool that <u>can be used</u> to analyze the mechanism by which the bacterial genes are involved in the synthesis of this compound in the nodule and to analyze the function of this compound in *Rhizobium*.

In this example, the subject of the sentence ("Isolation of the genes . . . ") is the conclusion, "reported here" reminds the reader that it is the conclusion, and the rest of the sentence gives two applications that indicate the importance of the conclusion. The verb used for the application indicates certainty: "can be used."

Example 7.24   Application

The availability of the purified cyclic GMP-dependent channel in a functional state <u>will</u> greatly <u>aid</u> the investigation of the molecular aspects of this protein and <u>lead</u> to a better understanding of how it functions and is modulated in the photoreceptor cell.

In this example, the subject of the sentence ("The availability of the purified cyclic GMP-dependent channel in a functional state") states the conclusion, but the conclusion is not identified as such. The rest of the sentence states the application. The verbs ("will aid . . . and lead") are certain.

Implications are usually stated after a summary of the conclusions, but sometimes implications are stated alone, as in Example 7.25.

Example 7.25   Implication

Our findings in dogs, together with findings from studies of human coronary arteries (2, 3, 21, 22, 31), <u>suggest</u> that H_1 blockers <u>may antagonize</u> histamine-mediated vasoconstriction and vasospasm in patients with atherosclerotic coronary artery disease and thus <u>may have</u> therapeutic value. Conversely, H_2 blockers <u>may permit</u> unopposed H_1-mediated vasoconstriction of epicardial arteries and <u>may</u> also <u>limit</u> vasodilation and thus <u>may not have</u> therapeutic value.

In this example, the findings the implications are based on are alluded to at the beginning of the first sentence. The implications are signaled by "suggest" and the verbs stating the implications indicate minimal certainty ("may antagonize," "may have," "may permit," "may limit," "may not have").

Example 7.26   Speculation

The chromosomal pattern encountered for the type IV genes leads us to <u>speculate</u> that <u>if</u> additional type IV collagen chains exist (49), the corresponding genes <u>will</u> also <u>be clustered</u> in the 13q33→q34 region. Interestingly, the B_1 and B_2 laminin genes, which are coordinately regulated with α1(IV) and α2(IV), have been shown to be tightly linked on mouse chromosome 1 (50). The physical proximity of these coding units <u>probably reflects</u> the mechanism of their genetic evolution and <u>may influence</u> their exclusive expression in basement membranes.

In this example, the subject of the first sentence ("The chromosomal pattern encountered for the type IV genes") is the conclusion, "encountered" reminds the reader that it is the conclusion, and "leads us to speculate that" signals the speculation, which is stated in the rest of the sentence. The verb used in the speculation ("will be clustered") indicates certainty, but it is tempered by the preceding "if." Two more speculations, based on a related conclusion reported by other authors (second sentence), are given in the last sentence. The verbs indicate moderate and minimal certainty ("probably reflects," "may influence").

Example 7.27 Speculation

The pulmonary venous waterfall we report here <u>could explain</u> why left atrial pulses were not faithfully transmitted to pulmonary arterial wedge catheters at low left atrial pressures. The presence of the pulmonary venous waterfall also <u>could account for</u> the inordinately high venous resistance to flow determined at low left atrial pressures (4, 12), the remarkable fall in this venous resistance when left atrial pressure increases slightly (5), and the constancy of the pressure drop through the pulmonary veins despite a threefold change in pulmonary venous flow (9).

In this example, "the pulmonary venous waterfall" is the conclusion and "we report here" reminds the reader that it is the conclusion. The rest of the sentence gives a speculative explanation of a finding from the author's study. The next sentence gives speculative explanations of findings from other studies. Although the verb "speculate" is not used, it is clear from the verbs indicating minimal certainty ("could explain," "could account for") that these statements are speculations.

These standard endings can also be used in combination. Usually a restatement of the answer(s) is given first and is followed by an application, an implication, or a speculation.

Example 7.28 Answer Plus Implication

<u>In summary, our results indicate that</u> expansion of plasma volume by 400 ml in untrained men increases stroke volume during exercise by 11% but that further expansion of plasma volume has no apparent hemodynamic benefit. These findings <u>imply</u> that in untrained men, the measurement of stroke volume during upright exercise when blood volume is normal <u>may not provide</u> an adequate measure of intrinsic myocardial function. It <u>appears</u> that about one-half of the difference in stroke volume normally observed between untrained and highly endurance-trained men during upright exercise is due to suboptimal blood volume in the untrained men.

In this example, the first sentence states the answer. The second sentence states a clinical implication of the findings. The third sentence quantifies the inadequacy mentioned in the second sentence. The implication is signaled by "These findings imply that," and the verbs used are cautious ("may not provide," "appears").

Example 7.29   Answer Plus Speculation

<u>In summary, we have shown that</u> the transforming activity of mutated *ras* is associated with two vertebrate cellular systems thought to be regulated by G proteins, namely phospholipases A_2/C and adenylate cyclase. In both cases the enzyme activity was reduced in cells expressing mutated *ras* at high levels. Since phospholipase and adenylate cyclase activities were also reduced in cells expressing c-*ras* at high levels, we <u>believe</u> that c-*ras* <u>may</u> normally <u>help</u> modulate systems that are regulated by G proteins and that *ras* transformation <u>may result</u> from a concerted aberration of guanine-nucleotide-regulated systems.

In this example, the first sentence summarizes the answers, the second sentence states supporting evidence, and the last sentence states two speculations. The speculations are signaled by "we believe that," and the verbs used are cautious ("may help," "may result").

As these examples show, restating the answers or indicating the importance of the work by stating applications, implications, or speculations gives the Discussion a sense of coming to a definite, clear end.

LENGTH

The Discussion section should be as long as necessary to state, support, explain, and defend the answer(s) to the question(s) fully and clearly and to discuss other important, directly relevant issues. However, in order not to obscure or overwhelm the message, the Discussion should be as short as possible. The more noise, the less message. To reduce noise and thus keep the Discussion short, do not use unnecessary words or add unnecessary detail, and do not include side issues.

DETAILS

Verb Tense

Use verb tenses to distinguish between answers to questions and results. The use of verb tenses is the same whether the answers and results are from your own study or from other studies.

For answers to questions and also for signals of answers, use present tense. Present tense indicates that a statement is considered permanently true. For example, "Our results *indicate* that alterations in glycosylation of IgE-binding factors expressed from a single cloned gene *result* in different biological activities of the factors." In this example, both the verb in the signal (*indicate*) and the verb in the answer (*result*) are in present tense.

For results use past tense. Past tense indicates action finished in the past. For example, "IgE-binding factors from carbohydrate-deficient cells *suppressed* an in vitro IgE response, whereas factors from untreated cells *potentiated* the IgE response."

The verb "found" is a special case. "Found" (past tense) is used to signal not only results but also answers, especially answers that are the same as results. For example, "found" signals a result in this sentence: "Only small regions of homology *were found*." However, "found" signals an answer in this sentence: "In this study, *we found that* the gene coding for the precursor of the human peptide hormones VIP and PHM-27 is 9 kb long and consists of seven exons." "Found" is appropriate for signaling answers because the action of finding was done in the past. In contrast, "show" and "indicate" (as in "This study shows" or "Our results indicate") are still true in the present. That is, the study still shows the answer and the results still indicate the answer. Therefore, present tense is appropriate for "shows" and "indicate." Finally, note that, like "found," "findings" is also used for both answers and results.

Precise Word Choice

Use verbs of the appropriate strength and degree of certainty for signals and statements of answers, applications, implications, and speculations.

To signal answers, implications, and speculations, use a verb that suits the strength of the statement you are signaling. "Prove" and "demonstrate" are very strong and are appropriate for signaling unequivocal answers to questions. "Show," "indicate," and "found" are not quite as strong and therefore are appropriate for signaling answers that are somewhat less certain, as is usually the case in the biomedical sciences. There is a big gap between these verbs and the verbs that express the next level of strength—"suggest" and "imply." "Suggest" and "imply" are fairly weak and therefore are appropriate for signaling implications. "Suggest" can also be used to signal speculations, but using "speculate" is clearer. Applications can be stated without a signal (see Examples 7.23 and 7.24 above).

The verbs used to state answers, applications, implications, and speculations can be weakened to the appropriate degree of uncertainty when necessary by adding a helping verb. For example, for answers that may not happen 100% of the time but are theoretically possible, add "can," as in, "This study in newborn goats demonstrates that continuous positive airway pressure (7.5 cm H_2O) *can impair* renal function in newborns." Some helping verbs, in order of decreasing degree of certainty, are as follows: "can" and "will" show a reasonable degree of certainty and are useful in answers ("can") and applications ("can," "will"); "should" and the adverb "probably" show less certainty and are useful for strong implications and speculations; "may," "might," "could," and the adverb "possibly" show the least certainty and are useful for weaker implications and speculations. An example of "could" used in a weak speculation is "We *suggest* that hypoventilation of the occluded lung *could* be the cause of the tendency to alveolar collapse."

Use of Others' Names

Generally it is unnecessary to use authors' names in the Discussion section of a scientific research paper. However, you may want to use names if a particular idea is linked with an author. For example, in Example 7.21 above, authors' names are used in paragraph 1 to identify those responsible for previous models of thick filament assembly. You may also want to use names to give credit to an author whose work stimulated your thought, as in paragraph 4 of Example 7.21. In contrast, when you are simply reporting others' results, names are not usually necessary, as in Example 7.21, paragraph 2, references 7 and 8. Similarly, when reporting results that agree or disagree with yours, it is often unnecessary to use authors' names (see Example 7.20, sentence G). When you do use names, remember that names do not make good transition words. Be careful to keep the story line going whether you use names or not.

Subtitles

Subtitles are not necessary in the Discussion. However, in long Discussions that have three or four sections, each dealing with a separate major topic, subtitles are sometimes used to signal the beginning of each section.

If you decide to use subtitles, keep in mind that subtitles are not a substitute for topic sentences. First write the Discussion from beginning to end, using paragraph topic sentences to indicate how each paragraph relates to the paragraph before it and section topic sentences to indicate how each section relates to the section before it. Then add brief subtitles before each section, as in Example 7.30.

Example 7.30 Subtitles

Discussion

Effects of α-Adrenoceptor Stimulation

The most important new conclusion of this study is that α-adrenoceptor stimulation by phenylephrine leads to an increase in the responsiveness of the myocardial contractile apparatus to Ca^{2+}. (etc.)

Effects of β-Adrenoceptor Stimulation

The results of our experiments on the inotropic effects of β-adrenoceptor stimulation by isoproterenol are not open to such unambiguous interpretation as are the results of the experiments with phenylephrine. (etc.)

Relation Between the Effects of α- and β-Adrenoceptor Stimulation

A significant difference between the inotropic effects of α- and β-adrenoceptor stimulation is that the maximum response to β-adrenoceptor stimulation appears to be determined by saturation of the contractile apparatus with Ca^{2+}, whereas the maximum response to α-adrenoceptor stimulation usually is not. (etc.)

In this example, the section topic sentence at the beginning of the first section states the answer to the first question. The section topic sentence at the beginning of the second major section states the relation of the second topic to the first topic and thus establishes a story line between the two topics. The section topic sentence at the beginning of the third section states a point showing the relation between the points of the first two sections. Thus, the point of each section is stated in the section topic sentences.

The topic of each section is also signaled visually by a subtitle. But note that the overall story of the Discussion is clear even if the subtitles are omitted. Thus, if topic sentences are well handled in the Discussion, subtitles are not necessary, but they do add a bonus—a signal for the eye. If topic sentences are not well handled, subtitles will not save the Discussion. Subtitles show what the major topics are, but if topic sentences are weak or missing, the reader will not know what the points are or what the overall story is, because points are conveyed by verbs, and subtitles have no verbs. So if you use subtitles in the Discussion, be sure to use them in addition to topic sentences, not in place of topic sentences.

SUMMARY OF GUIDELINES FOR DISCUSSIONS	

FUNCTIONS

Main function: to answer the questions posed in the Introduction.
Other important functions:
    To explain how the results support the answers.
    To explain how the answers fit in with existing knowledge.

CONTENT

State the answers to the questions.
    Answer each question exactly as you asked it (same key terms, same point of view, and, when appropriate, the same verb).
    Limit the answer to the appropriate population.
Support the answer.
    Use both your own results and others' results when relevant.
    Cite figures and tables when they would be helpful.
    Cite appropriate references for others' results.
Explain why the answer is reasonable or how the answer fits in with published ideas on the topic if necessary.
Defend your answer if necessary by presenting a pro-con argument.
Explain as best you can any results you got that do not support your answer.
Establish the newness of your answer if necessary.
Explain any discrepancies with published results.
Explain any unexpected findings.
State and explain any limitations of your methods and weaknesses in study design.
Explain the validity of any assumptions your methods are based on.
State the importance of the answer if necessary.

ORGANIZATION

The Discussion should have a beginning, a middle, and an end.
At the beginning of the Discussion, answer the questions and, if necessary, support, explain, and defend the answers.
    Precede the answer by
        A signal (necessary) (for example, "This study shows that . . . ").
        A restatement of the question (optional).
        Brief context (optional).
    State the species or the study population in the answer if the answer is limited to that species or population but in the signal if the answer is general.
    Use a transition or a topic sentence to link supporting results to the answer. A topic sentence ("Its presence has been demonstrated in two ways") is used in Example 7.2. Some possible transitions include
        "In our experiments," (Example 7.14).
        "Specifically," (Example 7.4).
        "The evidence is that" (Example 7.20).
        "Evidence that" (Example 7.1).
        "We found that" (Example 7.31) (but only if "In this study, we found that" is not used to signal the answer to the question).
In the middle of the Discussion, organize the topics in order of most to least important to the answer.
    Support, explain, and defend the answer first.

Then explain any of your results that do not support the answer, any discrepancies with others' results, unexpected findings, limitations of the methods, weaknesses in the study design, and the validity of assumptions.

State the importance of the answer last.

Group related paragraphs in one section, and organize paragraphs within each section from most to least important.

Tell a story on two levels: individual stories within each paragraph and an overall story throughout the Discussion, using either the overview technique or the step-by-step technique.

For the overview technique,

Use a section topic sentence at the beginning of each section and a transition topic sentence at the beginning of each paragraph.

Use stronger transitions in transition topic sentences for paragraphs farther from the section topic sentence. Repeating several key terms is stronger than repeating one or no key terms. Transition phrases and transition clauses are stronger than transition words.

For the step-by-step technique, use a key term topic sentence (repeating a key term from the previous paragraph) at the beginning of every paragraph.

Check that the outline of the overall story is apparent from reading the chain of topic sentences at the beginning of each paragraph.

For a point that does not fit into the story, either

Use an ordinary paragraph topic sentence without a transition or repetition of a key term and put the point in a separate paragraph, or

Use a subtopic sentence and include the point in another (relevant) paragraph.

At the end of the Discussion, conclude by making a point.

Restate the answers to the questions; precede the answers by a signal such as "In conclusion, this study shows that" or "In summary, our results indicate that."

If appropriate, indicate the importance of the work by stating

Applications of the answers.

Implications of the answers.

Speculations based on the answers.

LENGTH

Make the Discussion no longer than necessary to state, support, explain, and defend the answers to the questions and present any other necessary information.

DETAILS

Use present tense verbs for the answer and for signals of the answer.

Use strong verbs for conclusions and applications and weaker verbs for implications and speculations.

Use authors' names in the Discussion only if you have a particular reason for doing so.

If you use subtitles in the Discussion, use them in addition to, not instead of, topic sentences.

EXAMPLE OF A CLEARLY ORGANIZED DISCUSSION

Example 7.31 A Clearly Organized Discussion

Question: "To determine whether increasing heart rate rather than decreasing afterload, increasing preload, or increasing contractility is the most effective method of increasing cardiac output in young lambs."

Discussion

1 Contrary to our expectation, *this study shows that* **increasing contractility by infusing isoproterenol, not increasing heart rate by ventricular pacing, is the most effective method of increasing cardiac output in young lambs**. We found that increasing heart rate above baseline caused no significant change in cardiac output in the younger lambs (5–13 days) and only moderate increases in cardiac output in the older lambs (15–36 days). In contrast, increasing contractility caused substantially greater increases in cardiac output than increasing heart rate did.

2 **The reason for the unexpectedly small effect of increasing heart rate is uncertain. One possibility is that it was due to the pacing rate.** Although the baseline pacing rate we used, 200 beats/min, approximates the resting heart rate of 1- to 2-week-old lambs, it is faster than the resting heart rate of 170 beats/min of 3- to 4-week-old lambs. Therefore, one could argue that if the baseline pacing heart rate had been lower, larger increases in cardiac output could have been attained by increasing heart rate above baseline. However, our data show that the maximal percentage increase in cardiac output that would have been attained if 170 beats/min had been used as a baseline pacing rate would have been only 17.5% in the younger lambs and 21.0% in the older lambs. These increases are far less than those we found after increasing contractility (37% and 62%, respectively). Therefore, the small effect that increasing heart rate had on increasing cardiac output is probably not due to the pacing rate we used.

3 **Another possibility is that the method we used for controlling heart rate—ventricular pacing—may have caused smaller increases in cardiac output than would result from sequential atrioventricular pacing**. Indeed, it is well known that atrial systole plays an important role in determining effective ventricular stroke volume (9). However, it is unlikely that increases in cardiac output resulting from sequential atrioventricular pacing would have been greater than those resulting from increasing contractility by infusing isoproterenol because at the heart rate at which we were pacing, atrial contributions to cardiac output are minimal (unpublished observations; reference 6). Thus, heart rate appears to be less important than contractility for increasing cardiac output in young lambs. Nevertheless, heart rate is important for maintaining cardiac output, since we found that decreasing heart rate below baseline greatly decreased cardiac output.

4 **Of the other two methods of increasing cardiac output that we tested, neither decreasing afterload nor increasing preload while heart rate was fixed at 200 beats/min proved to be an effective method for causing large increases in cardiac output. Decreasing afterload** by infusing nitroprusside at a fixed heart rate did not cause significant increases in cardiac output in the younger lambs and caused only moderate increases in cardiac output in the older lambs. The reason for this minimal effect on cardiac output may relate to the fact that nitroprusside not only decreases afterload but also decreases preload by venodilation. Thus, if the initial preload is not optimal for the afterload, decreasing preload will decrease cardiac output. As a result, the increase in cardiac output induced by decreasing afterload will be counteracted by the decrease in cardiac output induced by decreasing a suboptimal preload. This mismatch between afterload and preload (10), which has been described for failing hearts (10, 11), may also be occurring in the hearts of our lambs. If so, this mismatch may be the reason that decreasing afterload by infusing nitroprusside in young lambs does not cause large increases in cardiac output within the range of preloads seen in our lambs.

5   The last method of increasing cardiac output that we tested, increasing preload by infusing blood or 0.9% NaCl, was not only minimally effective in increasing cardiac output but also yielded a smaller percentage increase in cardiac output than that previously reported after infusion of 0.9% NaCl in lambs of similar ages (1). The reasons for the smaller percentage increase are partly that we infused smaller volumes and partly that the baseline preloads were somewhat higher in our lambs because of ventricular pacing. Since the preloads of the lambs in our study were higher than normal, the percentage increase attainable by increasing preload was less. It is possible, therefore, that larger increases in cardiac output are attainable by infusing larger amounts of fluid into young lambs that have normal atrioventricular node conduction.

6   Another reason for our smaller percentage increases in cardiac output after increasing preload could be that our indicator of preload was inaccurate. The indicator we used, mean left atrial pressure, may not be a sensitive indicator of preload in the presence of atrioventricular blockade. To obtain a more accurate assessment of preload we measured left ventricular end-diastolic pressure in two lambs. However, left ventricular end-diastolic pressure was difficult to interpret because of wide variations in pressure at the same heart rate. These variations resulted either from alterations in the temporal relationship between atrial and ventricular contractions or from movement of the ventricular septum into the left ventricle during right ventricular pacing. Therefore, we used mean left atrial pressure to measure preload. We believe that although mean left atrial pressure may not reflect rapid variations in preload in the presence of atrioventricular blockade, it accurately measures general preload state and changes in preload state.

7   In contrast to previous reports, we found that isoproterenol did not consistently have hypotensive effects. Mean aortic pressure decreased in the younger lambs during isoproterenol infusion (Fig. 4A), as it did in previous studies (11–13). However, mean aortic pressure increased in the older lambs, and systolic aortic pressure increased in both groups of lambs during isoproterenol infusion. These increases are in contrast to previous reports of decreases in mean and systolic aortic pressures during isoproterenol infusion (12, 14). Since the major difference between our study and these other studies was that the heart rate was fixed in our lambs, it is possible that some of the hypotensive effects of isoproterenol are due to its strong effects on heart rate.

8   *In summary, this study shows that* increasing contractility, and not increasing heart rate by ventricular pacing, is the most effective method of increasing cardiac output in young lambs. Although the increase in cardiac output in response to increasing contractility is less in younger than in older lambs, it is still greater than that attainable by changes in heart rate, afterload, or preload.

This Discussion follows the guidelines in the Summary of Guidelines for Discussions listed above.

Functions

The answer to the question is stated in paragraph 1.

Another important function of the Discussion is also fulfilled: paragraphs 2–4 speculate about why the authors got the results they got and thus explain how the results support the answer.

Content

The answer to the question is stated.

Both the negative answer and the positive answer (para. 1, sentence 1) use the same key terms, the same verb, and the same point of view as the question.

The answer is limited to the appropriate population (young lambs).

The answer is supported by the authors' results (para. 1, sentences 2 and 3) and data (para. 2, second-to-last sentence).

The answer is explained. In fact, half of the Discussion is an explanation of the answer (paras. 2–4).

The Discussion also includes explanations of two discrepancies. Since the discrepancies involve minor findings, the explanations are appropriately late in the Discussion (paras. 5 and 6; para. 7).

A limitation of the method is also explained (para. 6). This explanation is woven into the explanation of a discrepancy.

Organization

The Discussion has a beginning (para. 1), a middle (paras. 2–7), and an end (para. 8).

At the beginning, the answer is stated and supported.

The answer is preceded by a signal ("this study shows that").

The species is stated in the answer, since the question was about that species (young lambs).

The results are linked to the answer by a transition phrase ("We found that").

In the middle of the Discussion, the topics are arranged from most to least important. Paragraphs 2–4 explain the answer; paragraphs 5–7 explain discrepancies with previous findings. The explanations of the answer are also organized from most to least important. First is the explanation of the answer the authors expected but did not get (paras. 2 and 3). Second is the explanation of another negative answer (para. 4). Similarly, the explanations of the discrepancies are organized from most to least important: first a discrepancy for a result directly related to the answer (paras. 5 and 6), then a discrepancy for a result less directly related to the answer (para. 7).

The Discussion tells a story on two levels: within each paragraph and throughout the Discussion (overall story). The overall story proceeds by the overview technique.

Paragraph 2 begins with a section topic sentence for paragraphs 2 and 3 and then has a paragraph topic sentence that includes a transition word ("one possibility"). Note that the section topic sentence is a key term topic sentence; it repeats "increasing heart rate" from the topic sentence of paragraph 1. In addition, "unexpectedly" in the section topic sentence reminds us of "contrary to our expectation" in the topic sentence of paragraph 1, and "small effect" summarizes the point in the second sentence of paragraph 1. All these repetitions ensure that the overall story runs smoothly from paragraph 1 to paragraph 2.

Paragraph 3 begins with a transition word topic sentence similar to the transition word topic sentence of paragraph 2 ("another possibility").

Paragraph 4 begins with a transition phrase topic sentence that introduces the last topic of the section. The transition phrase is "Of the other two methods of increasing cardiac output that we tested." This transition phrase indirectly summarizes the two preceding paragraphs by using "the other two methods" to indicate that the first two methods have already been discussed. The second sentence of paragraph 4 uses a key term from the transition phrase topic sentence of paragraph 4 to introduce the topic of the paragraph ("Decreasing afterload").

Paragraph 5 begins with a transition clause topic sentence that changes the topic and is a section topic sentence for paragraphs 5 and 6. The transition clause restates the point (answer) for the fourth method tested ("was minimally effective"); the topic sentence then makes another point about this method (that it yielded a smaller percentage increase than previously reported). Thus, this strong transition topic sentence is used at a major junction of the Discussion: the end of the explanation of the answers to the questions and the beginning of an explanation of a discrepancy. The second sentence of paragraph 5 both introduces a new key term ("reasons") and repeats a key term ("smaller percentage increase") from the first sentence of paragraph 5 to state the topic of the paragraph ("The reasons for the smaller percentage increase are partly that . . . ").

Paragraph 6 uses a transition word topic sentence to continue the story of the explanation of the discrepancy begun in paragraph 5. The topic sentence repeats more key terms than the topic sentence of paragraph 5 does ("Another reason for our smaller percentage increases *in cardiac output* . . . ").

Paragraph 7 does not fit into the story. It explains another discrepancy. The topic sentence begins with a transition phrase but does not relate to the previous paragraphs.

The end of the Discussion makes a point by restating the answer to the question. The answer is preceded by a signal ("In summary, this study shows that").

The outline of the overall story (see below) is apparent from reading the topic sentences of paragraphs 1–7 (boldfaced) and the last paragraph. (Check this by reading those sentences.)

Length

The Discussion is no longer than necessary: it states, supports, and explains the answer and explains two discrepancies.

Details

Both the signal of the answer and the answer in paragraph 1 use present-tense verbs ("shows" and "is").

The verb in the answer is strong ("is").

Authors' names are not used; references are identified by number only.

OUTLINE

I. Answer to the question plus supporting evidence (para. 1)

II. Explanation of the answer (paras. 2–4)
   A. Speculative explanation for the surprising negative answer (paras. 2 and 3)
      1. One possible but unlikely explanation (rate of pacing) (para. 2)
      2. Another possible but unlikely explanation (method of pacing) (para. 3)
   B. Explanation of another negative answer (the effect of decreasing afterload possibly counteracted by the effect of decreasing preload) (para. 4)

III. Explanations of discrepancies with previous findings (paras. 5–7)
   A. Reasons for a smaller percentage increase in cardiac output than previously reported after increasing preload by infusing blood or 0.9% NaCl (paras. 5 and 6)
      1. Smaller volumes infused (yes) (para. 5)
      2. Higher preload (yes) (para. 5)
      3. Inadequate indicator of preload (no) (para. 6)
   B. Reason for inconsistent hypotensive effects of isoproterenol (para. 7)

IV. Summary of conclusions (para. 8)

Finding the Forest Among the Trees

In this Discussion, the organization and the story line are clear. However, they did not start out that way. In an early draft, the trees were there but none of the forest. That is, the topic sentences that tell the story (boldfaced) were missing. In addition, the details in paragraphs 1 and 2 were run together, which blurred the story line further. Finally, a paragraph was included that had no clear relation to the question and interrupted the story of the factors that affect cardiac output; this paragraph was omitted in the final draft. The version we have here, which may seem embarrassingly obvious, in fact emerged only after a careful process of examining every paragraph and asking "What is the point?" and then writing that point in a topic sentence at the beginning of the paragraph. Thus, the story (forest) in this Discussion is clear because the answer is stated at the beginning and because transition topic sentences or transitions are used at the beginning of every paragraph to link each paragraph (except para. 7) to the paragraph before it and thus guide the reader through the story.

■ *EXERCISE 7.1: OVERALL STORY IN A COMPLEX DISCUSSION*

Below is the beginning of a long, complex Discussion from a paper entitled, "Power Spectral Analysis of Inspiratory Nerve Activity in the Decerebrate Cat." This Discussion does not give the answer to the question at the beginning. Instead it assesses an unexpected finding that turned out to be more important. Although this Discussion is long and complex, you should be able to follow the overall story.

1. *Read the entire Discussion once rapidly to get an overview. Do not get lost in technical details or in the individual stories within each paragraph. Concentrate on the overall story as revealed by the topic sentences.*

2. *Read the first sentence of every paragraph. Do you get the essence of the story?* _____

3. *List the letters of all topic sentences in this Discussion and identify each one as a section topic sentence, paragraph topic sentence, or subtopic sentence; also identify all transition word topic sentences, transition phrase topic sentences, transition clause topic sentences, and key term topic sentences.*

4. *How does the story proceed—by the overview technique?* _____

   by the step-by-step technique? _____

5. *Based on the chain of topic sentences you identified, outline the topics and subtopics that compose the overall story of this Discussion (as done after Examples 7.20, 7.21, and 7.31).*

6. *Are you familiar with this field of research?* _____

7. *Was it difficult for you to figure out the overall story?* _____

Discussion

1 *A*The appearance of a second peak in the power spectral densities of the whole nerve signal was a surprise. *B*There are three reasons why the second peak had not been noted before. *C*One reason is the disadvantages of the techniques previously used to detect frequencies—detection by eye and detection by time autocorrelation. *D*The detection of a single frequency in a noisy signal by eye (9, 27, 29) is a difficult and subjective procedure. *E*The detection of more than one frequency in a noisy signal is much more difficult; hence, there is a bias towards identifying only one. *F*Although the technique of time autocorrelation (7) has the advantage of canceling random noise and clarifying the signal by summing and averaging, a disadvantage is that multiple frequencies interfere with each other, making the autocorrelation appear noisy. *G*In addition, the significance of amplitude variations in the autocorrelogram is difficult to interpret unless the correlation function is transformed to the correlation coefficient by dividing by the correlation function at zero lag time (3), although this has not commonly been done. *H*Furthermore, in the auto-correlation study, the lower peaks were computed over an interval of 32 ms. *I*This short time interval has only about 1.72 cycles of the 55 Hz signal and about 1.16 cycles of the 37 Hz signal and therefore provides no clear indication of their presence. *J*Thus, detection by eye or by autocorrelation would tend to identify a signal as having a single periodic component or none at all.

2 *K*Another reason for not noticing the second peak is that experimental conditions may mask low peaks. *L*Raising the end-tidal CO_2 increased the amplitude of the 88 Hz oscillation well above the random noise, making it detectable by eye (9, 29) and by autocorrelation (7), but a strong high-frequency oscillation at 88 Hz could have masked the 37 Hz oscillation in the phrenic nerve activity and the 55 Hz oscillation in the recurrent laryngeal nerve activity.

3 *M*Finally, anesthetics can eliminate the peaks. *N*In studies by eye or by autocorrelation, barbiturates reduced or eliminated the high-frequency oscillations (7). *O*Similarly, in our experiments, ketamine reduced or eliminated the spectral peak at 88 Hz, though it increased the amplitude of lower frequency spectral peaks in the phrenic and recurrent laryngeal nerves. *P*Chloralose-urethane tended to flatten the spectra of both nerves. *Q*Anesthetics might cause these changes in two ways. *R*First, if the spectral peaks in the nerve activity are due to synchronous drives from specific central pattern generators or from specific neuronal groups such as the dorsal and ventral respiratory groups, an anesthetic might excite one group and depress another, perhaps increasing the amplitude of a low-frequency peak and decreasing that of a high-frequency peak. *S*Or an anesthetic might act on the pathways between the source of the synchronous drive and the motoneuron by interfering with synaptic transmission or cell thresholds and adding random noise to the signal in the nerve.

4 *T*By avoiding these problems we were able to discover the second peak. *U*We avoided the problems associated with anesthesia by recording nerve signals from decerebrate cats. *V*We overcame the technical difficulties and detected a second peak in each nerve by using power spectral analysis. *W*This technique has two advantages over previous methods. *X*First, it provides a simple means for detecting multiple frequencies because the power in the signal is plotted as a function of frequency, not as a function of time. *Y*Second, it allows a statistical test for the flatness of the power spectral density function, an objective method for detecting significant peaks.

5 ***Z***When we found two peaks in the power spectral densities of the phrenic and recurrent laryngeal nerves, one of the first hypotheses we considered to interpret the second peak was based on the notion that the oscillations are dependent on each other. ***AA***Specifically, we hypothesized that a central respiratory pattern generator with an inherent rhythm of 88 Hz was driving a pool of upper motoneurons in the dorsal respiratory group, which were in turn driving the phrenic motoneurons in the spinal cord and the recurrent laryngeal motoneurons in the ventral respiratory group. ***BB***Since Merrill (18) had concluded that the dorsal group projected to the ventral group but the ventral group did not project to the dorsal group, we reasoned that the synchronies at 55 Hz and 37 Hz must originate downstream from the dorsal respiratory group, in the laryngeal motoneuron pool and in the phrenic motoneuron pool, respectively. ***CC***We postulated that interconnections within the pool of phrenic motoneurons accounted for the synchrony on the phrenic nerve at 37 Hz. ***DD***Similarly, we postulated that interconnections within the pool of motoneurons in the rostral portion of the nucleus ambiguus and the caudal portion of the retrofacial nucleus projecting to the intrinsic muscles of the larynx accounted for the synchrony on the recurrent laryngeal nerve at 55 Hz.

6 ***EE***The power spectral densities of single fibers contradicted this hypothesis. ***FF***Although 68% of the recurrent laryngeal fibers had power spectral densities similar to that of the recurrent laryngeal nerve, 26% had power spectral densities with a lower peak matching that of the phrenic nerve. ***GG***Because the cell bodies of the recurrent laryngeal motoneurons are in the brain stem and the cell bodies of the phrenic motoneurons are in the spinal cord and there are no known projections from the phrenic motoneurons to the laryngeal motoneurons, this finding implied that the source of the synchrony at 37 Hz cannot be the phrenic motor nucleus, but is probably in the brain stem and projects to phrenic motoneurons and to some laryngeal motoneurons. ***HH***Similarly, a minority of the phrenic fibers (21%) had a lower peak in their power spectral densities, matching the lower peak of the recurrent laryngeal nerve. ***II***This finding implied that the source of the synchrony at 55 Hz projects from the brain stem to laryngeal motoneurons and to some phrenic motoneurons.

7 *JJ*Since it appears that the sources of the 88 Hz, 55 Hz, and 37 Hz oscillations in the inspiratory activity on the respiratory nerves are in the brain stem, the next hypothesis that we considered was based on the notion that the oscillations are independent. *KK*Whether the oscillations are indeed independent cannot be answered until the source of each oscillation has been identified, that is, until one or more central respiratory pattern generators have been located anatomically, identified physiologically, and associated with the specific oscillations. *LL*Lacking this direct evidence, we suspect that the oscillations are independent, for two reasons. *MM*First, they are not simple multiples of one another. *NN*If the primary signal were at 88 Hz and neurons being driven by it could not follow at 88 Hz but acted as frequency dividers, the resulting frequencies would be rational fractions of 88 Hz, that is, 44 Hz, 29.3 Hz, 22 Hz, and so on. *OO*Second, the amplitudes at each frequency are not necessarily proportional at any given time but can vary independently. *PP*For example, in the power spectral density of the recurrent laryngeal nerve in Figure 3, the peak at 88 Hz is maximal at 0.8 s but the peak at 55 Hz is maximal at 1.6 s.

8 *QQ*If the sources for each oscillation frequency are independent, how can the independence be explained? *RR*We propose that in the brain stem of the cat there are two central respiratory pattern generators, each characterized by specific spectral lines in the respiratory motor outputs. *SS*We further propose that, as previously described by Mitchell (19, 20), an evolutionarily younger pattern generator, associated with the dorsal respiratory group and the diaphragm, dominates a second and evolutionarily older pattern generator, associated with the ventral respiratory group in the nucleus ambiguus and the branchiomeric muscles.

9 *TT*Based on this explanation, the hypothesis we developed to interpret the second peak is as follows. *UU*The spectral peak at 88 Hz is the signature of the younger pattern generator, located in the vicinity of the dorsal respiratory group. *VV*It dominates and drives the second, older pattern generator, which has its own characteristic frequency of 55 Hz. *WW*The drives from each pattern generator are distributed with unequal weights to respiratory motoneurons. *XX*The mixing of the 88 Hz and the 55 Hz drives, coupled with the threshold nonlinearity, produces a beat frequency of about 37 Hz evident in the power spectral densities of some single fibers in each nerve.

etc.

■ EXERCISE 7.2: CONTENT AND ORGANIZATION IN A DISCUSSION

1. *After reading this Discussion once, write the topic of each paragraph in the margin, making sure to identify the answers to the two questions.*

2. <u>*Rewrite*</u> *this Discussion.*
   a. *Omit unnecessary information.*
   b. *Tell a story that has a strong beginning, a clear middle, and a brief end.*
   c. *State the answers to the questions. Answer the questions exactly as they were asked; that is, use the same key terms, the same or similar verbs in present tense, and the same point of view; signal the answers.*
   d. *Support the answers with results. Organize to emphasize the most important results.*
   e. *Use a topic sentence at the beginning of every paragraph. In the topic sentences, try to relate each paragraph to the previous paragraph, creating an overall story. Paragraphs 6 and 7 have no topic sentence. Try to write topic sentences for these paragraphs.*
   f. *Write a brief, relevant conclusion.*

The Introduction of this paper is given below. Note the two questions.

RETROGRADE CEREBRAL BLOOD FLOW IN PRETERM INFANTS WITH A LARGE SHUNT THROUGH A PATENT DUCTUS ARTERIOSUS

Introduction

Preterm infants who have a large shunt through a patent ductus arteriosus have retrograde flow of blood from the descending aorta through the ductus arteriosus into the pulmonary circulation during diastole. This retrograde blood flow may impair circulation to the bowel and cause necrotizing enterocolitis (4, 5). Recently, a similar but less severe finding—decreased flow velocity—was demonstrated in the anterior cerebral arteries of infants who have a large ductal shunt (6). If retrograde flow also occurs in the cerebral arteries of these infants, cerebral ischemia or intraventricular hemorrhage could result.
Question 1
Question 2
<u>In order to determine if retrograde diastolic blood flow can occur in the cerebral arteries of preterm infants who have a large shunt through a patent ductus arteriosus</u> and <u>to relate alterations in cerebral blood flow to alterations in aortic blood flow</u>, we examined the cerebral arteries and the aorta of preterm infants with a patent ductus arteriosus using a range-gated, pulsed-Doppler ultrasound system.

Discussion

1 *A*Patients with a large shunt through a PDA have retrograde flow of blood from the descending aorta through the ductus arteriosus into the pulmonary circulation during diastole. *B*This retrograde diastolic flow pattern was demonstrated on electromagnetic flowmeter curves obtained by Spencer and Denison (9) in 1963 from the descending thoracic aorta of a child at surgery for a PDA and by Rudolph and colleagues (10) in 1964 in dogs in which a prosthetic aortopulmonary shunt had been placed. *C*Subsequently, Cassels (11) recorded numerous electromagnetic flowmeter curves from patients during surgery for a PDA and showed that marked retrograde diastolic flow in the descending thoracic aorta occurred only in patients with a large left-to-right shunt. *D*The angiographic studies of Spach and co-workers (5) showed that most of the diastolic left-to-right shunt through the PDA is from the descending aorta and may result in a steal of blood during diastole from the abdominal organs. *E*These investigators suggested that diastolic steal might have a relationship to the development of necrotizing enterocolitis in infants with a large PDA.

2   *F*Several investigators have used the noninvasive technique of Doppler ultrasonography to examine patients with a PDA (12–14). *G*Using continuous-wave Doppler ultrasonography, Serwer and colleagues (4) showed retrograde diastolic flow in the descending aorta in infants with a large shunt through a PDA. *H*Retrograde diastolic flow disappeared after ductal ligation.

3   *I*Recently, Perlman and colleagues (6) used a continuous-wave velocitometer to record velocity-time profiles in the anterior cerebral arteries of preterm infants with a PDA. *J*These investigators showed that there was a marked decrease in diastolic flow velocity in the cerebral arteries in infants with a large shunt through a PDA. *K*In addition, the decrease in diastolic flow velocity seemed to parallel decreases in the diastolic blood pressure. *L*These findings suggest that changes in cerebral blood flow reflect changes in aortic blood flow.

4   *M*There are important differences between our study and the study of Perlman and associates (6). *N*In addition to decreased diastolic flow, we observed absent and retrograde diastolic flow in the cerebral arteries of infants with a large shunt through a PDA. *O*There are several factors that might explain the more severe alterations in cerebral blood flow observed in our infants. *P*First, the infants in our series may have had a larger left-to-right ductal shunt and, therefore, greater amounts of diastolic steal from the cerebral arteries than the infants in Perlman's series. *Q*Second, whereas Perlman used a continuous-wave Doppler velocitometer, we recorded the cerebral artery Doppler signals with a range-gated pulsed-Doppler system, which allowed us to examine the signals arising only from the vessel within the sample volume. *R*The velocity-time profile obtained with the continuous-wave Doppler system may contain contributions from several vessels. *S*Also, most continuous-wave

Doppler systems use a zero-crossing detector to convert the spectrum of Doppler frequency shifts to an analog signal. *T*The zero-crossing detector method of analysis has limitations, which include loss of low-frequency signals, loss of signals during rapid changes in the direction of blood flow, and analysis of noise on the zero-amplitude line as a frequency (15, 16).

5   *U*Changes in the cerebral blood flow patterns closely paralleled changes in aortic blood flow patterns in the infants in our study. *V*All control infants and all infants with a small shunt through the PDA had significant forward flow in the cerebral arteries throughout diastole and no retrograde diastolic flow in the descending aorta. *W*All infants with a large ductal shunt had retrograde diastolic flow in the descending aorta and markedly decreased or retrograde diastolic flow in the cerebral arteries. *X*After closure of the PDA, all of these infants had significant forward diastolic flow in the cerebral arteries and no evidence of retrograde diastolic flow in the descending aorta. *Y*These findings support the observation that cerebral blood flow is directly related to aortic blood flow in sick preterm infants (6, 17).

6   *Z*In the presence of a large ductal shunt, the low resistance pulmonary vascular bed communicates with the higher resistance systemic vascular bed. *AA*This results in a steal of blood from the aorta during diastole and a concomitant decrease in diastolic blood pressure (5). *BB*As the diastolic blood pressure falls, diastolic flow in the cerebral arteries decreases and eventually reverses, resulting in diastolic steal from the cerebral circulation. *CC*The failure of the cerebral circulation to decrease resistance and maintain diastolic forward flow is probably due to maximum vasodilation or impaired autoregulation, which are believed to occur in sick preterm infants (6, 17, 28).

7   *DD*The forward diastolic flow in the transverse aorta proximal to the ductus arteriosus disappeared after PDA closure. *EE*We believe that this forward diastolic flow reflects diastolic flow from the carotid and subclavian arteries toward the PDA. *FF*Electromagnetic flowmeter curves recorded by Cassels (11) and by Rudolph et al. (10) and angiographic studies by Spach et al. (5) indicate that forward flow does occur during diastole in the aortic arch proximal to a large aortopulmonary shunt. *GG*In Doppler tracings taken from the ascending aorta just above the aortic valve, we were unable to show any differences between control infants and infants with a large PDA. *HH*Thus, if diastolic steal also occurs from the coronary arteries toward the pulmonary artery, the volume of blood flow was too small to be detected by our technique.

8 *II*In conclusion, we found decreased, absent, and retrograde blood flow in the cerebral arteries during diastole in preterm infants with a large shunt through a PDA. *JJ*Our cerebral Doppler tracings suggest that a large ductal shunt leads to diastolic steal of blood from the cerebral circulation and to cerebral ischemia. *KK*Recent studies have shown a direct correlation between cerebral ischemia and brain cell structural damage and necrosis (19, 20). *LL*Although it has been suggested that the incidence of intraventricular hemorrhage is increased in preterm infants with a PDA, it remains to be seen if cerebral ischemia is an important factor in this relationship. *MM*In this regard, further studies are necessary to determine the effect on cerebral blood flow of such common medical interventions as fluid restriction. *NN*Also, wide fluctuations in cerebral blood flow patterns in infants with a large ductal shunt may predispose these infants to hemorrhagic brain injury. *OO*Further studies are also necessary to determine if there is a difference in cerebral blood flow after abrupt closure of the ductus arteriosus by surgical ligation or more gradual closure of the ductus arteriosus with indomethacin.

9 *PP*Range-gated pulsed Doppler echocardiography is a safe, noninvasive method for assessing the patency of the ductus arteriosus as well as the alterations in cerebral and systemic blood flow that accompany this abnormality. *QQ*This study shows that a large shunt through a PDA results in significant diastolic steal of blood from the cerebral arteries as well as from the descending aorta. *RR*This altered perfusion may predispose infants with a large ductal shunt to systemic complications such as necrotizing enterocolitis and to cerebral complications such as ischemia or hemorrhagic brain injury.

SUPPORTING INFORMATION

So far we have looked only at the written text of a biomedical journal article. We turn now to two types of crucial supporting information— first figures and tables, which illustrate and provide evidence for statements in the text, and then references, which direct readers to published works that support statements in the text.

FIGURES AND TABLES

In Section II, The Text of the Biomedical Research Paper, we saw how to write each section of the text to tell a clear story. However, many readers do not read the text, or read only part of it. Instead these readers look at the figures and tables. Therefore it is important that the figures and tables are clear and tell the story of the paper.

Clear figures and tables result from careful design and from informative legends for figures and informative titles and footnotes for tables. Careful design is important because figures and tables are visual means of conveying information and therefore should have strong visual impact. Informative legends, titles, and footnotes are important to ensure that the topic of each figure and table is clear.

Figures and tables that tell the story of the paper result from designing the figures and tables to form a clear sequence that relates clearly to the text.

Chapter 8 presents guidelines for designing clear figures and tables, for writing informative legends for figures and informative titles and footnotes for tables, and for designing figures and tables to tell the story of the paper.

FIGURES

In scientific research papers, most figures are used in the Methods and Results sections, though figures can also be used in the Introduction and the Discussion. In Methods, the main use of figures is to clarify or amplify the methods. For example, figures can be used to show apparatus or anatomic relations. In Results, the main use of figures is to present evidence that supports the results. Figures present either primary evidence (for example, electron micrographs) or numerical data (in graphs).

Drawings and Diagrams

Drawings illustrate anatomy, apparatus, and other concrete things. Diagrams illustrate concepts such as flow systems. Drawings and diagrams can be either realistic or schematic (Fig. 1).

For animals and apparatus, drawings are preferable to photographs, because drawings can eliminate unnecessary detail and emphasize important features (Fig. 2).

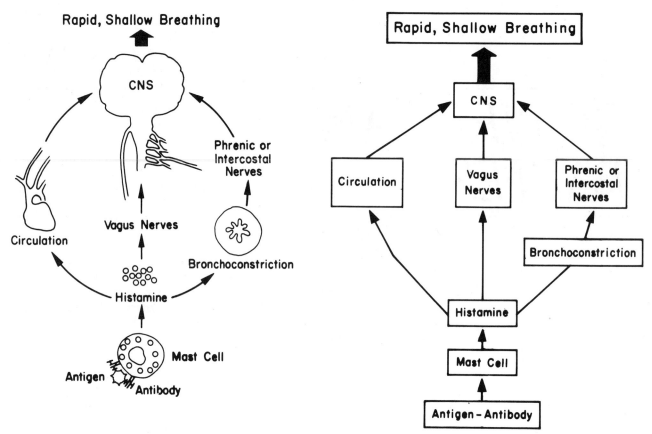

Figure 1. A diagram drawn both realistically (left) and schematically (right). The schematic diagram is simpler, but the realistic diagram may have more impact for some readers. The drawing is black on white, and the labels are uppercase and lowercase letters in a vertical, uncrowded, sans serif typeface of medium weight.

Drawings and diagrams should be black on white and should be kept simple. Labels should be large enough to be visible but not overwhelming. The letters used for labels should be uppercase and lowercase in a vertical, uncrowded, sans serif typeface of medium weight (Fig. 1).

Primary Evidence

Primary evidence includes photographs of patients and tissues, radiographs, micrographs, and experimental records (for example, gel electrophoretograms, chromatograms, spectrophotometer curves, polygraph recordings).

Show primary evidence when that is the type of data you have (for example, electron micrographs, gel electrophoretograms). Also show primary evidence to indicate the quality of your data when appropriate. For example, for a study of various pressures, in addition to presenting summarized data in graphs, also show a representative polygraph recording. Select your best quality recording for publication.

Some types of primary evidence (for example, photographs of patients, radiographs, micrographs, electrophoretograms) are reproduced as halftone figures. That is, they have gray tones as well as black and white (Figs. 3–5). For halftone figures, make the photograph sharp and clear.

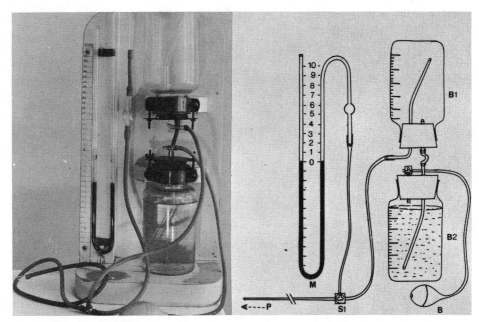

Figure 2. Photograph (left) and drawing (right) of an apparatus for measuring intrapleural pressure. The drawing shows the apparatus more clearly and simply than the photograph does.

Photographs of Patients

Use photographs of patients only if the patient gave written, informed consent before the photograph was taken. Cover facial features whenever possible to prevent identification of the patient. If you need to refer to patients, use A, B, etc., not the patient's initials.

Micrographs

Clarity. Make glossy prints of micrographs and ensure that the prints have sufficient contrast to make the features of interest clear.

Size. Make the micrograph large enough to show the important features clearly (Figs. 3, 4). The important features should nearly fill the space. The micrograph should be just enough larger than the features of interest to give a sense of where they are in their context.

To obtain micrographs of optimal size, decide before printing the negative what dimensions you need so that the features of interest will nearly fill the photograph and the photograph will fill the column or page of the journal. Then print the photograph the appropriate size and crop (trim) the photograph to fit the column or page. Submit photographs of micrographs the size they will appear in the journal, not larger.

Labeling. Labels used on micrographs include arrows and arrowheads, letters and numbers, and symbols such as *.

The amount of labeling needed depends on the audience. More labels are needed for a general audience (for example, for micrographs in general journals or in, say, physiology journals). Fewer labels are needed for a specialty audience.

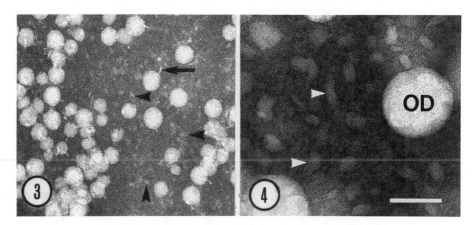

Figures 3 and 4. Well-prepared electron micrographs. Figure 3 shows negatively stained low-density lipoprotein treated with sodium decyl sulfate. The arrow points to one of the disc-like structures and the arrowheads point to tiny particles. Figure 4 shows the same lipoproteins after elastase digestion. The arrowheads point to irregularly shaped structures. OD identifies an oil droplet. The scale bar in the lower right corner represents 75 nm. In these micrographs, both the large, obvious structures and the small, subtle features are clearly visible.

Since labels cover up and detract from the data on the micrograph, make labels brief and few and just big enough to be readily visible (Figs. 3, 4). Define the labels in the figure legend.

To show magnification, a scale bar can be placed on the micrograph, in the lower right corner (Fig. 4). The scale bar should be a thin, horizontal line without cross bars at the end so that the distance is clear. (Cross bars create the ambiguity of inner distance versus outer distance.) In the figure legend, identify the distance that the bar represents by writing, for example, "Scale bar = 75 nm." For specialty audiences, magnification can be indicated by a number (for example, "× 32,000") in the legend rather than by a bar on the micrograph.

Plates. Micrographs being discussed together in the text can be grouped into plates. Group micrographs to allow comparisons and to avoid wasting space. The best arrangements are across the top or bottom of a page, down a column, or filling a page. Make all the micrographs in a plate the same length or width, or both, so that there are no rectangles of white space between photographs. When mounting micrographs in plates, leave uniform, thin (1–2 mm) white lines between micrographs (Figs. 3, 4). The reasons for avoiding large white spaces are that they pull the eye away from the micrographs and distract the eye from the gray tones of the micrographs.

Mount micrographs by gluing them onto white bond paper or board and hot pressing them. Do not use tape to mount micrographs.

If the magnification is the same in all micrographs, one scale bar is sufficient (as in Figs. 3, 4).

Numbering. It is conventional to give each micrograph a separate number, even when several micrographs are grouped into a plate. Place the number in the lower left corner. [In contrast, when graphs are grouped into composite figures, the whole composite is given a single number and the parts are identified by capital letters or brief labels (see Fig. 12 below)].

Numbers should be the same style on all micrographs (Figs. 3, 4), not some white and others black. The simplest and clearest numbering method is to put a black number inside a white circle outlined by a black line. This number will show up against all backgrounds—black, white, and gray.

Gel Electrophoretograms

Gel electrophoretograms are halftone figures. Make the photograph of the gels sharp and clear (Fig. 5).

Identify material in each gel by adding capital letters or labels along the top or bottom of the photograph (Fig. 5). Identify important fractions by adding labels along the side. Use leader lines to join labels to their fractions. Labels and letters should not overwhelm the data.

Polygraph Recordings

Polygraph recordings are made as black lines on a grid. If the grid lines are not needed, they can be eliminated by filter photography. To be able to eliminate grid lines, use recording ink that differs in color from the printed grid lines on the recording paper.

After removing grid lines, add vertical scales and either horizontal scales or horizontal scale markers (for example, temperature in °C, time in minutes) (Fig. 6). Check that the scales and scale markers you add are perfectly accurate.

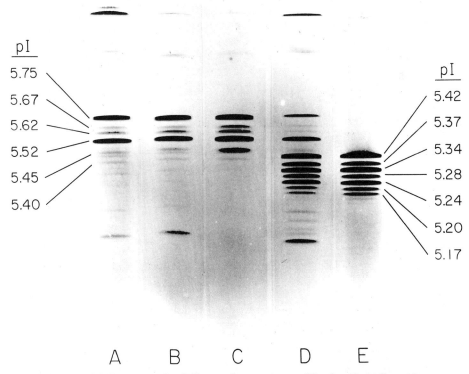

Figure 5. Well-prepared gel electrophoretograms. The fractions (here, isoelectric points, pI) are sharp and clear. Each gel is identified by a capital letter along the bottom of the photograph. Important fractions are identified by labels along the sides. Leader lines join each label to the appropriate fraction. The labels do not overwhelm the data.

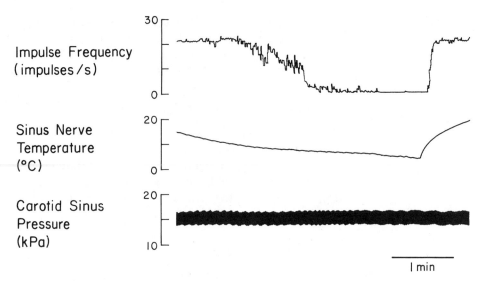

Figure 6. Well-prepared polygraph recordings. Grid lines have been elim- inated, and vertical scales and a horizontal time marker have been added. Y-axis labels are aligned along the left and do not protrude into the column of scale numbers. The labels do not overwhelm the data.

Label each axis with the name of the variable followed by the unit of measurement in parentheses (Fig. 6). Use uppercase and lowercase letters for the name of the variable; use International System abbreviations for units of measurement. Label each scale marker with the unit it represents.

Horizontally oriented axis labels should align on the left and should not protrude into the column of scale numbers (Fig. 6). Scale numbers should be slightly smaller than the capital letters in the axis labels. Scale numbers and axes should be thinner than letters in labels. Labels should not overwhelm the data.

Graphs

Use the appropriate type of graph to display the type of data you have. Some commonly used types of graphs are described below.

Line Graphs

A line graph is a two-axis graph on which curves, data points, or both show the relation between two variables such as weight, volume, pressure, time, concentration. Conventionally, the independent variable is on the X axis, and the dependent variable is on the Y axis. If the scale of an axis is linear, it must look linear: tick marks must be spaced at equal distances and scale numbers must be placed at equal intervals, starting where the axes meet (Fig. 7).

Scattergrams

A scattergram is a two-axis graph that plots individual data points and fits a mathematical function to the points to show how strongly two variables are correlated. For example, a straight regression line shows a linear correlation (Fig. 8).

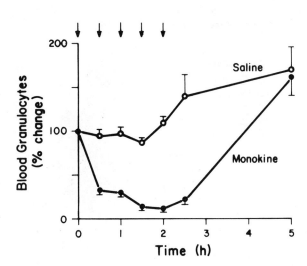

Figure 7. A line graph. The scales on both axes are linear, as indicated by equally spaced tick marks and equally spaced scale numbers. Curves are identified by individual labels. Arrows indicate the times when saline or monokine was injected.

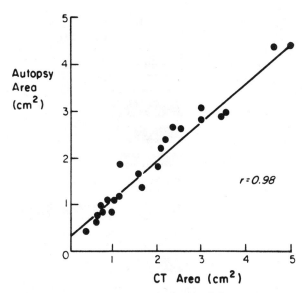

Figure 8. A scattergram. Individual data points are plotted, a regression line shows a linear correlation, and the correlation coefficient (r) indicates that the correlation is strong.

Bar Graphs

A bar graph is a one-axis graph that compares amounts or frequencies for classes of a discontinuous variable (for example, types of bacteria) or a "relative-scale variable" (for example, responses graded from least to most). A bar graph may be horizontal (Fig. 9) or vertical (Fig. 10). In a bar graph, the axis must include zero to avoid falsifying the differences between bars. Bars should all be the same width, and bars should be as wide as or wider than the spaces between them. The exact amount of space depends on the number and width of the bars. No tick marks should appear along the baseline, and the baseline need not be drawn; the baseline is not an axis.

Individual-Value Bar Graphs

An individual-value bar graph is a variation on vertical bar graphs in which individual data points are shown either in addition to the mean (Fig. 11) or instead of the mean (Fig. 12). For paired data, lines can be drawn to show the direction of change (Fig. 12). When more than one data point occurs at one amount, the data points are arranged horizontally (Fig. 11).

Histograms

A histogram is a two-axis graph that shows a single frequency distribution by means of a series of contiguous rectangles (Fig. 13). The rectangles should be of equal widths so that the height, and not just the area, of each rectangle represents the frequency of its class. The area of the histogram represents the distribution. The outlines of individual rectangles may be drawn, as in Fig. 13, or omitted, to emphasize the shape of the distribution.

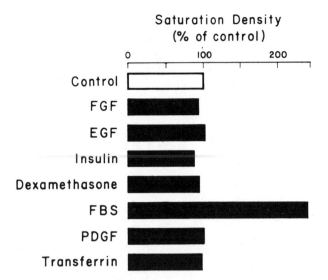

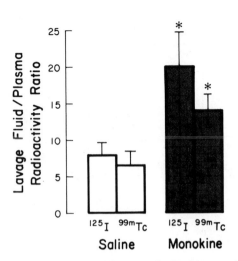

Figure 9. A horizontal bar graph. The axis includes zero, the baseline is not drawn, bars are all the same width, and bars are wider than the spaces between them.

Figure 10. A vertical bar graph. Ratios are shown for two variables (^{125}I, ^{99m}Tc), each under two conditions (saline, monoline). The variables and the conditions are identified in the labels under the bars.

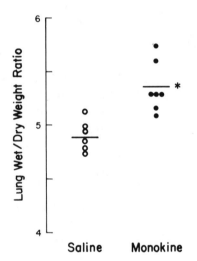

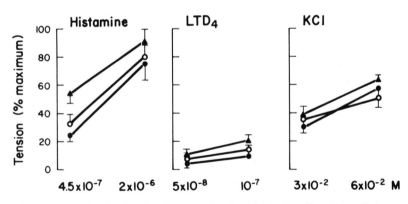

Figure 11. An individual-value bar graph. Data points show the individual values. Means are shown by horizontal lines. The asterisk (*) indicates a statistically significant difference between the means. Note that when more than one data point occurs at one amount, the data points are arranged horizontally.

Figure 12. Individual-value bar graphs in which the direction of change is shown by lines connecting the data points. In this composite figure, each part of the composite is identified by a brief label in the upper right corner of the graph. The letters in these labels are the largest letters on the figure.

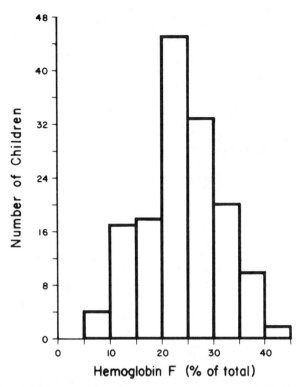

Figure 13. A histogram showing a single frequency distribution. All rectangles are the same width, so the height of each rectangle shows the frequency for its class. The area of the histogram represents the frequency distribution.

Frequency Polygons

A frequency polygon is a two-axis graph that uses data points joined by lines to show two or more overlapping frequency distributions (Fig. 14) or a single distribution. Data points are plotted at the midpoint of each class, and the

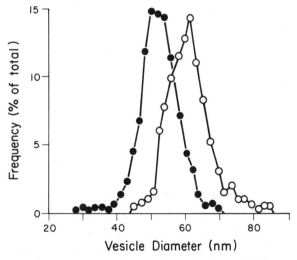

Figure 14. Two frequency polygons showing two overlapping frequency distributions.

lines joining the data points are extended to the baseline to complete the distribution.

For further details about these types of figures, see *Illustrating Science: Standards for Publication*, Chapter 4, Graphs and Maps. For further details about these and other kinds of figures, see Briscoe, *A Researcher's Guide to Scientific and Medical Illustrations*.

General Guidelines for Figures

Readability

Make each figure easy to read. The lettering should be large enough to be legible after the graph is reduced to fit the width of the journal's column. Check legibility by reducing the figure to publication size on a photocopier. The smallest letter in a published graph should be at least 1.5 mm high. Symbols should be large enough to be seen easily. The shapes should be easy to distinguish. (The easiest data point symbols to distinguish are ● and ○.) The graph should be uncluttered. For example, if there is no room for curve labels or a key on the face of the graph, define the curves in the figure legend.

Emphasis

Make each figure emphasize the important information (the data) by using different line weights. For example, in line graphs, curves should be the darkest lines, letters in axis labels should be less dark, and axes, tick marks, error bars, keys, and curve labels should be least dark, as in Fig. 7.

Point

Ensure that each figure makes a clear point. For example, a decrease should look like a decrease. In Fig. 7, the point that monokine injection decreased the numbers of circulating granulocytes in rabbits for 2.5 hours is clear.

Figure Legends

A figure legend is a descriptive statement that is printed below or next to a figure in a published article. A legend is needed so that the figure will be intelligible without reference to the text.

A figure legend typically has four parts: a brief title; experimental details; definitions of symbols, line or bar patterns, and abbreviations not defined earlier in the legend; and, for graphs, statistical information.

Some journals do not follow this format. For example, some journals request only a title. Other journals request complete experimental details in the legend and none in the Methods section of the paper. When the journal gives explicit instructions, follow them.

The Title

The title is the first item in the figure legend; it does not appear on the figure itself. The title is a phrase (not a sentence); that is, the title does not contain a verb. The title identifies the specific topic of the figure. The title should be brief. It should not contain abbreviations. The details included in the title depend on the type of figure.

Titles for Drawings, Diagrams, and Primary Evidence. For drawings, diagrams, and primary evidence, the title should identify the type of figure shown, if necessary, and the specific apparatus, concept, or biological specimen shown, as in Examples 8.1 and 8.2.

Example 8.1 Title for a Drawing

Fig. 1. Apparatus used for measuring intrapleural pressure.

In this title for a drawing, only the specific apparatus shown is identified.

Example 8.2 Title for a Diagram

Fig. 1. Schematic diagram of the relationship of the return cycle during resetting of ventricular tachycardia to the absence or presence of electrocardiographic fusion.

In this title, "schematic diagram" identifies the type of figure shown and the remaining words identify the concept shown.

The specific feature of interest may also be included in the title, as in Example 8.3.

Example 8.3 Title for Primary Evidence

Fig. 1. Bright-field light micrograph of a segment of a bacterial filament showing intracellular sulfur inclusions.

In this title, "bright-field light micrograph" identifies the type of figure shown and the remaining words identify the biological specimen shown (a segment of a bacterial filament) and an important feature (intracellular sulfur inclusions).

Titles for Graphs. For a graph that depicts the results of an experiment in which a manipulation was made and a variable was measured or observed, the standard title is

Effect of X on Y in Z,

where X is the independent variable (cause), Y is the dependent variable (effect), and Z is the species or material studied, or both (Example 8.4). The species is usually omitted for humans (as in Example 8.14 below) unless the data are for a specific subpopulation.

Example 8.4 Title for a Bar Graph

X

Fig. 1.   Effect of <u>increasing concentrations of doxorubicin</u> on <u>release of</u>

Y   Z

<u>histamine and lactate dehydrogenase</u> from <u>dog mastocytoma cells</u>.

Alternatively, the dependent variable can come first in the standard title. In this case, the title is in a form such as

Y in response to X in Z

Y during X in Z.

Example 8.5   Title for a Line Graph

$$Y$$

Fig. 1. <u>Release of ^{14}C-labeled lipid and lactate dehydrogenase</u> in response to

$$X \qquad\qquad\qquad\qquad\qquad\qquad\qquad Z$$

<u>increasing concentrations of the ionophore A23187</u> in <u>alveolar type II cells
from rats.</u>

Example 8.6   Title for a Line Graph

$$X \qquad\qquad\qquad\qquad\qquad\qquad\qquad\qquad\qquad\qquad\qquad\qquad Y$$

Fig. 1. <u>Mean arterial pressure</u> before, during, and after <u>stimulation of the</u>

$$Z$$

<u>carotid nerve</u> in <u>young and old piglets.</u>

For graphs of data from experiments that have no independent variable,
the title states the dependent variable (Y) and the species or material, or both
(Z). The form is

Y in Z.

Example 8.7   Title for a Histogram

$$Y \qquad\qquad\qquad\qquad\qquad\qquad\qquad\qquad\qquad Z$$

Fig. 1. <u>Distribution of resting membrane potential (E_{m})</u> in <u>bovine trachealis muscle.</u>

Sometimes the type of figure shown is also stated in the title of a graph,
usually for histograms and frequency polygons, which show frequency distributions (Example 8.7: "Distribution"), and also for special types of graphs, such
as Scatchard plots (see Example 8.11 below).

Titles That State a Point.   The standard title states only the *topic* of the
graph. However, the title can also state the *point* the graph is making when
there is a single, clear point. For example, it is generally more useful to write

Fig. 1. Inhibition of Y by X in Z,

which states the point (inhibition), than to write

Fig. 1. Effect of X on Y in Z,

which states only the topic (effect).

Example 8.8   Title That States a Point

Fig. 1. <u>Inhibition</u> of antiviral response in MDA-MB-231 (human breast car-
cinoma) cells by oxyphenbutazone.

Example 8.9   Title That States a Point

Fig. 1. <u>Elevation</u> of acute-phase reactants after a single 3-hour exposure to
ultraviolet radiation.

Overloaded Titles.   Do not overload the title with details. Instead give
details in the rest of the legend.

Example 8.10 Overloaded title

Fig. 1. Mean resting tension of left ventricular papillary muscles (grams per mm^2 of muscle cross-sectional area) from starved rats (●——●) ($n = 8$) and their controls (○——○) ($n = 6$), and from streptozotocin-treated rats (▲——▲) ($n = 16$) and their controls (△——△) ($n = 18$) plotted against muscle length over the range from 84 to 102% of L$_{max}$.

Revision

Fig. 1.*A* Mean resting tension of left ventricular papillary muscles at various muscle lengths in rats. *B* Resting tension was measured as g/mm^2 of muscle cross-sectional area. *C* ●, 8 starved rats; ○, their 6 controls; ▲, 16 streptozotocin-treated rats; △, their 18 controls.

In the revision, the title (A) contains only the important details: mean resting tension is the dependent variable, left ventricular papillary muscles is the material, muscle length is the independent variable, and rats is the species. The experimental details, which expand the Y-axis label [Resting Tension (g/mm^2)], are in a separate sentence (B). "Over the range from 84 to 102% of L$_{max}$" is omitted because it is obvious from the X axis. Symbols are defined at the end of the legend (C). Only one symbol is used for each definition, not two symbols connected by a line.

Abbreviations in Titles. Avoid using abbreviations in the title so that the reader does not have to search through the text of the paper to find the meaning.

Titles for Composites. For composite figures, such as Figs. 1, 2, and 12 above, provide a title for the entire figure and also identify each individual part. The title should indicate the common topic illustrated in all the parts of the composite so that the reader understands why they are grouped together. The parts can be identified either within the title (Example 8.11) or in separate subtitles (Example 8.12). Subtitles, like titles, are phrases, not sentences.

Example 8.11 Parts of a Composite Figure Identified in the Title

Fig. 1. Representative Scatchard plots of the dose-response of [^{125}I] T$_3$-binding to lung nuclei from (A) adult and (B) 28-day-old fetal rabbits.

In this example, the parts of the composite are identified by the words "(A) adult" and "(B) 28-day-old" in the title. The rest of the title identifies the topic shown in both graphs.

Example 8.12 Parts of a Composite Figure Identified in Subtitles

Fig. 1. Representative coronary angiograms in a patient with organic stable obstruction without thrombus. Insets show the electrocardiogram (lead V$_4$) obtained during each angiographic assessment. A. The initial appearance of the left coronary arteries during chest pain. Note the eccentric segmental narrowing (arrow) in the proximal left anterior descending coronary artery and the delayed distal filling. B. The unchanged appearance of the coronary arteries after a 60-min infusion of urokinase (960,000 U). C. The unchanged appearance of the coronary arteries 4 weeks after the initial angiograms.

In this example, the title states the topic shown in all three parts of the composite, and the topic of each part is identified by a separate subtitle (underlined). Note that subtitles B and C make a point: "unchanged appearance."

Experimental Details

Give just enough experimental details to permit the reader to understand the figure. If no experimental details are needed, do not give any. In legends for graphs, do not simply repeat the information in the axis labels. Write experimental details in sentences.

Example 8.13   Experimental Details in a Sentence After the Title

Fig. 1. Nuclear T_3-binding capacity in rabbit lung during prenatal and postnatal development. <u>Dose-response experiments were done with isolated nuclei (50–120 μg of DNA) under optimal conditions, data were analyzed by Scatchard analysis, and results were corrected for released receptor</u>.

Statements such as "For details, see Methods" are unnecessary.

Definitions

Symbols, line or bar patterns, and abbreviations that are not defined in the figure or earlier in the legend should be defined after experimental details are given (see C in the revision of Example 8.10 above). Definitions can be written as phrases (as in the revision of Example 8.10) or as sentences.

For definitions of symbols or line patterns, draw the symbol or line pattern in the legend. For example, "O, control" (rather than "open circles, control," which is not visually effective). Only one symbol is needed, not two symbols connected by a line (see the revision of Example 8.10). For bar patterns, be careful that the patterns in the legend match the patterns in the graph. For example, if the bar pattern is ◧, the pattern in the legend must be ◧, not ▨.

If the same symbols, line or bar patterns, or abbreviations are used in more than one figure, define them in the legend for the first relevant figure only. In succeeding legends, refer the reader to that legend.

Example 8.14   Avoiding Repetition of Definitions

Fig. 3. Autoregulation of coronary blood flow during balloon pumping. Abbreviations as in Fig. 1.

Statistical Information

The explanation of statistical information in graphs should include the following details: whether the data points or bars represent individual or mean values; whether error bars represent standard deviations (SD), standard errors of the mean (SEM), confidence intervals (CI), or ranges; and the sample size (n).

Example 8.15   Statistical Details for Summarized Data

Fig. 1. Nuclear T_3-binding capacity in rabbit lung during prenatal and postnatal development. Dose-response experiments were done with isolated nuclei (50–120 μg of DNA) under optimal conditions, data were analyzed by Scatchard analysis, and results were corrected for released receptor. <u>Values are means ± SD for 8 samples, except 28-day-old prenatal = 34 samples.</u>

Avoid writing "$n = 12$." It is much clearer to be specific—for example, "12 samples," "12 measurements," "12 dogs." What does "$n = 12$" mean in this example? "Fig. 1. Results of glucose absorption in milligrams (means ± SD) obtained by the segmental-perfusion technique ($n = 12$)." Twelve patients? Twelve samples from one patient? Twelve samples from four patients?

For data in bar graphs that have been analyzed by a statistical test, state which values were compared by statistical analysis and the significance value (for example, the P value). It is not necessary to name the statistical test used. Two ways to state which values were compared and to identify the P value are shown in Examples 8.16 and 8.17.

Example 8.16   Statistically Significant Differences

Fig. 2. Effect of dopamine on the major determinants of left-ventricular circumferential end-systolic wall stress. *, ** significantly different from control, *$P < 0.05$, **$P < 0.01$.

In this legend, the title is followed by an explanation of the statistical analysis. First the values being compared are stated ("significantly different from control") and then the P values are identified.

Example 8.17   Statistically Significant Differences

Fig. 2. Effect of dopamine on the major determinants of left-ventricular circumferential end-systolic wall stress. *$P < 0.05$, **$P < 0.01$ vs. control.

In this legend, P values are given first and then the values being compared are identified by "vs. control."

Other Information

In addition to these standard parts of a figure legend, a legend may also include other information, such as statements pointing out an unusual or an interesting feature.

Example 8.18   Unusual Feature

Fig. 6. Effects of hyperthermia (43°C) on immune cytolysis by cytotoxic lymphocytes and on survival of P815 mastocytoma cells. <u>The curves were plotted from the data in Figs. 3 and 5.</u>

In this legend, the last sentence calls the reader's attention to the relationship between this figure and previous figures.

Example 8.19   Interesting Feature

Fig. 1. End-diastolic angiographic appearance of (A) the right ventricle in the dog placed in the right lateral decubitus position (35-mm frame) and (B) the left ventricle of the same dog. <u>Note how the anterior border of the left ventricular cavity approaches the anterior border of the heart, which has been retouched for clarity.</u>

In this legend, the last sentence points out a feature of particular interest and also calls the reader's attention to the retouching of the photograph. Note that when describing what the figure shows, you use present tense ("approaches the anterior border").

Indicating Results

Results as such are not normally given in figure legends, since that would repeat the Results section. However, results can be indicated. To indicate results in graphs, include the point the graph makes (that is, the result shown by the graph) in the title (as in Examples 8.8 and 8.9 above: "Inhibition of antiviral response . . . ," "Elevation of acute-phase reactants . . ."). To indicate results in figures showing primary evidence, point out a feature in the figure by writing "Note . . ." (as in Examples 8.12 and 8.19 above) or ". . . showing . . ." (as in Example 8.3 above).

Republishing Figures

To republish a figure that has already been published, first obtain permission from the copyright holder (usually the publisher); this is a legal requirement. Also obtain permission from the author (unless you are the author); this is common courtesy. Standard permission forms are available from your publisher.

In your paper, give full credit to the source and the publisher by citing the reference in the figure legend and stating that you have permission to republish the figure. Two possible ways of giving credit are shown in Examples 8.20 and 8.21. If the copyright holder specifies another way, use it. Credit is always given as the last item in the figure legend. The complete reference is included in the list of references at the end of the text.

Example 8.20   Credit Line for a Republished Figure

From Fraser et al. (1975), with permission.

Example 8.21   Credit Line for a Republished Figure

From ref. 7, with permission from the American Review of Respiratory Disease.

You must obtain permission whether you use *all* of the originally published figure, use *part* of the originally published figure, or use a *modified version* of the originally published figure. For modified versions, one possible credit line is illustrated in Example 8.22.

Example 8.22   Credit Line for a Modified Figure

Redrawn from Fraser et al. (1975); reproduced with permission.

TABLES

In scientific research papers, tables are commonly used for two purposes: to present background information related to methods (for example, the characteristics of patients in a study, Table 1) and to present data that support results (Tables 2–5). Tables that present data, in turn, have two purposes: to present individual data for all the subjects, animals, or specimens studied or to make a point. Tables that present individual data can get rather large. However, their advantage is that other workers, analyzing the data for other purposes or comparing the table with other similar tables, might see trends or relationships the author did not notice.

All tables, whatever their purpose, have the same parts and are arranged in the same way. Since tables are a visual medium, it is important to arrange tables clearly, for maximal visual impact, so that the reader can find the specific data or see the point easily.

Tables have four main parts: the title, column headings, the body, and footnotes.

The Title

The title of a table, like the title of a figure, is a phrase, not a sentence, that states the topic or the point of the table. The title should be brief. The details included in a title depend on the type of table.

For tables that give background information, the title should state the topic of the information listed in the body of the table (that is, the variables) and also the species or population, the material described, or both. The form is

Y in Z   or   Y of Z.

For example, in the title of Table 1, "Clinical Characteristics of the Infants," "clinical characteristics" is the topic (Y) and "the infants" (that is, the infants in the study) is the population described (Z). In the title "Phospholipid Composition of Cardiac Lymph from Normal Dogs," "phospholipid composition" is the topic (Y), "normal dogs" is the species (Z), and "cardiac lymph" is the material described (Z).

For tables that present data from experiments that have only dependent variables, similar titles are appropriate. For example, in the title "Dimensions of Cell Bodies in the Tracheal Ganglia of Ferrets," "dimensions" is the topic (dependent variable) (Y), "ferrets" is the species (Z), and "cell bodies in the tracheal ganglia" is the material described (Z).

For tables that present data from experiments that have both independent and dependent variables, the title should state the independent variable(s) (X), the dependent variable(s) (Y), and the species or population, the material described, or both (Z). It is not necessary to mention the controls in the title. Two standard forms for these titles are

Effect of X on Y in Z

Y during X in Z.

For example, in the title "Effects of Methacholine on Electrical Properties and Ion Fluxes in Tracheal Epithelium From Cats and Ferrets," "methacholine" is the independent variable, "electrical properties and ion fluxes" are the dependent variables, "tracheal epithelium" is the material, and "cats and ferrets" are the species. (See also the title for Table 2.) In the title "Plasma Variables Before and After Protein Loss in Lambs," "plasma variables" are the dependent variables, "before and after" is used instead of "during," "protein loss" is the independent variable, and "lambs" is the species. (See also Table 3.)

Even better than stating the topic in the title of the table is stating the point. When the title states the point, the reader knows exactly what to look for in the table. For example, in the title "Increase in Helicity of Abortifacient

TABLE I
CLINICAL CHARACTERISTICS OF THE INFANTS

Infant	Sex	Birth Weight (g)	Gestational Age (wk)	Age at Study (wk)	Post-conceptual Age (wk)	Diagnosis
1	F	1,080	30	7	37	Mild RDS,[a] apnea
2	F	1,710	34	5½	39½	RDS, apnea
3	F	1,980	35	7	42	Severe RDS, ventilator, aborted SIDS[b]
4	M	2,240	37	2½	39½	Aborted SIDS
5	F	2,330	37	14	51	Aborted SIDS[c]
6	M	2,520	32	4	36	Severe RDS, apnea
7	F	2,810	40	7	47	Aborted SIDS
8	F	3,300	37	5	42	Severe RDS, ventilator, aborted SIDS

[a]RDS = respiratory distress syndrome.
[b]SIDS = sudden infant death syndrome.
[c]History from parents only.

Table 1 gives background information related to methods—clinical characteristics of the infants in the study. In this table, the terms in the title correlate with the terms in the column headings: "infants" in the title is the same as "infant" in the first column heading, and "clinical characteristics" in the title is a category term for all the other terms in the column headings. Three horizontal lines are drawn: one above the column headings, one below the column headings, and one below the data.

Proteins in the Presence of Sodium Dodecyl Sulfate," "increase in helicity" is the point.

To keep titles brief, use a category term instead of listing all the dependent variables. For example, in Table 3, "hemodynamic variables" is the category term for all the dependent variables in the table.

To ensure that the title relates clearly to the table, use the same terms in the title as in the column headings, or use a category term in the title instead of two or more column headings. For example, in Table 1, "infants" in the title corresponds with "infant" in the first column heading, and "clinical characteristics" is a category term for the remaining column headings (sex, birth weight, gestational age, age at study, postconceptual age, diagnosis).

Column Headings

Column headings consist of headings that identify the items listed in the columns below them, subheadings as necessary, and units of measurement as necessary. Column headings should be brief.

Headings

There are two main groups of headings, corresponding to the two main groups of information in the body of the table: the items for which data are given, in one or more columns on the left side of the table, and the data, in one or more columns on the right. In tables for experiments that have both independent and dependent variables, the independent variable(s) are in the column(s) on the left and the dependent variable(s) are in the column(s) on the right, as in Tables 2–5. For example, in Table 3, the column labeled "Ventilatory condition" is the independent variable and the remaining columns are the dependent variables. In Table 4, the columns labeled "Incubation conditions" and "Sample" describe the independent variable and the remaining columns are the dependent variable.

Each type of information should have its own vertical column, and each column should have its own heading. Do not combine two types of information in one column. For example, under a column headed "Drug," only the names of the drugs should appear, not both the drugs and the doses.

Do not omit the heading that states the name of the first column on the left. For example, in Table 3, the first column on the left (the independent variable) needs a heading ("Ventilation condition") just as the other columns (the dependent variables) do.

Do not omit the column heading that states the name of the dependent variable (for example, "Recovery (%)" in Table 5), even in simple tables that have only one dependent variable that is named in the title. It is clearest for

TABLE 2. Effect of hormones on saturation of phosphatidylcholine in explants of human fetal lungs, assessed by two methods

Hormone	Number of explants	Saturated phosphatidylcholine (% of total phosphatidylcholine)		a/b
		a) By Pi	b) By cpm	
Control	8	27.4 ± 2.3	17.8 ± 2.3	1.57 ± 0.17
T_3	6	30.4 ± 5.4	20.2 ± 4.7	1.44 ± 0.22
Dexamethasone	9	$33.8 \pm 3.9*$	$28.9 \pm 2.7*$	$1.17 \pm 0.09*$
T_3 + dexamethasone	8	$32.6 \pm 3.7*$	$27.6 \pm 0.6*$	$1.19 \pm 0.11*$

Explants (19–23 weeks of gestation) were exposed to 2 nM T_3, 10 nM dexamethasone, or both for 6 days. Phosphatidylcholine was isolated by thin-layer chromatography and was treated with OsO_4. Saturated phosphatidycholine and unsaturated phosphatidylcholine were separated by thin-layer chromatography and were quantitated by Pi assay or by counts per minute [^{3}H]choline incorporated. Values are the mean $\pm$ SD.

$*P < 0.01$ vs. control.

Table 2 presents data that make two points: that dexamethasone, alone or with T_3, increased the saturation of phosphatidylcholine in explants of human fetal lungs and that the values determined by Pi assay were greater than the values determined by incorporation of [^{3}H]choline. In this table, the title is in the form "Effect of X on Y in Z." The independent variable is in the first column on the left, the dependent variables are in the last three columns on the right, and the sample size (number of explants) is given between the independent and dependent variables. Subheadings ("By Pi," "By cpm") are used to divide a column heading into two categories. Control data are given first (top row). Trends read down the columns. Comparisons are made both between columns and between rows. Footnotes that apply to the entire table are in one paragraph and are not identified by a symbol. The footnote explaining statistically significant differences is in a separate paragraph and is identified by a symbol. This footnote states not only the P value but also what values are being compared.

the reader if the dependent variable is named both in the title and in the column headings. For example, in a table titled "Effects of Enzymes on Antibody Reactivity," the column headings should not be merely "Enzyme," "4E4," "3F11," "4D4," "4D8." The last four headings, which are names of antibodies, should be subheadings under "Antibody Reactivity (% of control)," because the data in the columns are antibody reactivity, not types of antibodies.

Subheadings

When necessary, subheadings can be used to subdivide a heading into two or more categories. For example, in the column heading

Cyclic GMP Concn (fmol/mg wet wt)

Left Atrium   Right Atrium

the dependent variable and the unit of measurement are in the main heading and two sites in which this variable was measured are in the subheadings. (See also Tables 2, 4, and 5.)

Note that column headings and subheadings are singular, not plural (for example, "Recovery," not "Recoveries").

Units of Measurement

Units of measurement are given (usually in parentheses) after or below the name of the variable in the column heading. Repeating the unit of measurement after each value is inefficient. For example, in Table 4, the second column is appropriately

Incubation Time (min)   *not*   Incubation Time

30   30 min
90   90 min

Use International System (SI) abbreviations for units of measurement.

Try to choose units of measurement that eliminate unnecessary zeros. For example, if the unit is grams and the values in the column are 120,000, 98,000, etc., change the unit to kilograms and report the values as 120, 98, etc. Make the same change in the text.

Avoid using multipliers in the column headings (for example, "$\times 10^3$") as a way of eliminating unnecessary zeros, because multipliers are confusing.

The Body of the Table

The body of the table contains the listing of individual items for which data are given (columns on the left) and the corresponding data (columns on the right).

The Columns on the Left

Just as the column headings identify the information in the columns below them, so the items listed in the column(s) on the left identify the information in each row. The items in the columns on the left (usually the independent variable) should be listed in a logical order according to the experimental design. For example, in Table 5, the media are listed in order of decreasing ionic strength. In Table 2, the hormones are listed in increasing order: control (no hormone), each hormone, both hormones.

The control, if any, is conventionally the first item in the list of independent variables. Thus, control data are given in the top row of the table (Table 2). In Table 3, control data are given in the top row in each group (Normoxic, Hypoxic).

When the independent variable in the column on the left contains two or three groups, one clear way to show the groups is to place the group name at the far left of the table and indent the items in the first column under them, as in Table 3 (the two groups of independent variables are Normoxic and Hypoxic). Another possibility is to place group names at the center of the table rather than at the far left (see Table 4 in Woodford, Chap. 10, Design of Tables and Figures).

If the sample sizes (*n*) are different, they can be given in the body of the table. Sample size is conventionally placed between the independent and the dependent variables (Table 2).

The Columns on the Right

Presentation of Data.   In the columns on the right, the data are usually presented in numbers, but data may also be in words (see Table 1, last column), letters (Table 1, second column), or symbols such as +.

Arrangement of Data.   Arrange the columns and rows of data to reveal trends or to permit easy comparison. Trends can be read either down a column (Tables 3, 5) or across a row (Table 4). Comparisons can be made between adjacent columns (Table 2) or between adjacent rows (Table 3, top two rows; Table 4). Comparison across intervening columns or rows is more difficult (Table 2, all four rows; Table 3, bottom four rows).

Placement of SDs.   A problem arises when data are presented as mean and standard deviation (SD) or mean and standard error of the mean (SEM), confidence intervals (CI), or ranges. If the SDs are placed to the right of the means, it is difficult to read across the rows or to compare two adjacent columns. If the SDs are placed below the means, it is difficult to read down the columns or to compare two adjacent rows. To decide where to place the SDs, consider whether you want readers to read across the rows (if so, place SDs below the means, as in Table 3A) or to read down the columns (if so, place SDs to the right of the means, as in Table 3). If readers need to read both across and down, try both placements of the SDs and see which you prefer. Another point to consider is that placing the SDs below the means can help keep the table from getting too wide. Finally, a trick for helping the reader skip over the SDs is to place the SDs in parentheses (as in Table 3A) instead of using ±.

Number of Decimal Places.   Use the fewest decimal places necessary to convey the precision of the measurement. Have the same number of decimal places in all values for one variable (Tables 2–5). Have the same number of decimal places in the SD as in the mean (Tables 2, 3).

Alignment of Data.   In each column, the data should align on the decimal point, whether or not a decimal point is present (Tables 4, 5). For data that are given as mean ± SD or mean ± SEM, the data should also align on the ± (Tables 2, 3). In Tables 2–5, because the independent variable is on the left

Table 3. *Hemodynamic variables in newborn lambs during various conditions of ventilation with normoxic and hypoxic gases*

Ventilation condition	Mean pulmonary arterial pressure (mmHg)	Pulmonary vascular resistance (mmHg/liter/min/kg)	Mean systemic arterial pressure (mmHg)	Heart rate (beats/min)	Cardiac output (liter/min/kg)
Normoxic					
Control	22.3 ± 4.4	52.7 ± 14.4	74.1 ± 11.2	206.3 ± 43.9	0.38 ± 0.08
Respiratory alkalosis	18.6 ± 4.2*	48.1 ± 13.2	75.0 ± 13.6	217.0 ± 44.0	0.34 ± 0.06
Hypoxic					
Control	40.1 ± 7.6	111.7 ± 86.6	87.8 ± 13.3	241.1 ± 45.7	0.39 ± 0.12
Respiratory alkalosis	26.7 ± 5.9†	76.9 ± 51.1†	76.7 ± 8.5†	260.2 ± 39.1	0.33 ± 0.10
Metabolic alkalosis	26.8 ± 4.7†	74.8 ± 39.1†	75.3 ± 12.8†	245.0 ± 50.8	0.37 ± 0.14
Hypocapnia	43.7 ± 7.1†	172.1 ± 78.3†	87.1 ± 7.0	239.4 ± 31.7	0.24 ± 0.08†

Data are means ± SD for 8 normoxic and 9 hypoxic lambs.
*$P < 0.05$ vs. normoxic control.
†$P < 0.05$ vs. hypoxic control.

Table 3 presents data that make the points that both respiratory and metabolic alkalosis reduced hypoxia-induced pulmonary vasoconstriction but that hypocapnia increased it, as indicated by changes in mean pulmonary arterial pressure and pulmonary vascular resistance. The points could be stated in the title: "Reduction of hypoxia-induced pulmonary vasoconstriction by respiratory and metabolic alkalosis but not by hypocapnia in newborn lambs." As written, the title states only the topic of the table, in a modification of the form "Y during X in Z"—"Y in Z during X." In the table, the independent variable is in the first column on the left and the dependent variables are in the remaining columns. Column headings are written out rather than being abbreviated, to avoid excessive footnotes. Note that every column, including the first column, has a heading. The independent variable is divided into two groups: normoxic and hypoxic. To identify the groups visually, the names of the groups are at the far left of the first column and the ventilation conditions are indented under the group names. Data are aligned on the decimal point and on the ±, thus making values easy to compare. Trends run down each column, so SDs are placed to the right of means. The same number of decimal places is used in all values for each variable, and the same number of decimal places is used in the SDs as in the means. The sample size (*n*) is stated in the footnote that identifies the data as means ± SD.

and the dependent variables are on the right, the values in each column align neatly on the decimal point, thus making differences between numbers easy to see.

Arranging Wide Tables. Sometimes a table that has a great many dependent variables would be too wide for the page of the journal if the dependent variables were listed across the top. One solution is to put the SDs, SEMs, confidence intervals, or ranges below the means (as in Table 3A), but this solution may not save enough space. Another solution is to switch the independent and dependent variables, thus listing the dependent variables down the first col-

Table 3A. *Hemodynamic variables in newborn lambs during various conditions of ventilation with normoxic and hypoxic gases*

Ventilation condition	Mean pulmonary arterial pressure (mmHg)	Pulmonary vascular resistance (mmHg/ liter/min/kg)	Mean systemic arterial pressure (mmHg)	Heart rate (beats/min)	Cardiac output (liter/min/kg)
Normoxic					
Control	22.3 (4.4)	52.7 (14.4)	74.1 (11.2)	206.3 (43.9)	0.38 (0.08)
Respiratory alkalosis	18.6* (4.2)	48.1 (13.2)	75.0 (13.6)	217.0 (44.0)	0.34 (0.06)
Hypoxic					
Control	40.1 (7.6)	111.7 (86.6)	87.8 (13.3)	241.1 (45.7)	0.39 (0.12)
Respiratory alkalosis	26.7† (5.9)	76.9† (51.1)	76.7† (8.5)	260.2 (39.1)	0.33 (0.10)
Metabolic alkalosis	26.8† (4.7)	74.8† (39.1)	75.3† (12.8)	245.0 (50.8)	0.37 (0.14)
Hypocapnia	43.7† (7.1)	172.1† (78.3)	87.1 (7.0)	239.4 (31.7)	0.24† (0.08)

Data are means and (SD) for 8 normoxic and 9 hypoxic lambs.
*$P < 0.05$ vs. normoxic control.
†$P < 0.05$ vs. hypoxic control.

Table 3A illustrates how to save space in a table and simultaneously permit easier reading across the rows by placing SDs in parentheses below the means rather than to the right of the means. (In this particular table, however, since we need to read down the columns to see the trends, putting the SDs to the right of the means, as in Table 3, is clearer.) Note that placing SDs in parentheses makes them easier to skip over.

umn on the left and the independent variables across the top (Table 6). In this case, aligning the numbers on the decimal point would give the columns jagged edges. Therefore, for a neater appearance, the numbers are usually centered on the $\pm$ and the alignment on the decimal point is ignored. However, this neatness can be deceptive. For example, in Table 6, at first glance, the numbers in the column 50.7, 56.7, 2730 look about the same size, but in fact the third number is two orders of magnitude larger than the other two. Other solutions for a table that is too wide for the page are to print a wide table across two pages, if the journal will do this, or to rotate the table 90 degrees to run the length of the journal's page, but this last solution is inconvenient for the reader and should be avoided.

Indicating Significant Differences. To indicate statistically significant differences between data, it is clearest to use symbols, such as asterisks (*), after the values that are different, and then to define the symbols in a footnote (for example, "*$P = 0.02$ vs. control") (Tables 2, 3). (Symbols indicating significant differences are not placed after control values or halfway between two values.) Putting P values in a separate column is less effective visually (Table 6A),

Table IV. Recovery of [¹⁴C]PC and [¹⁴C]LPC Standards Incubated with Cardiac Lymph from Dogs

Incubation conditions			% of total applied dpm recovered from TLC plate		
			LPC region	PC region	FA region
Temperature	Time	Sample			
°C	min		%	%	%
4	30	[¹⁴C]PC + buffer	1	98	1
		[¹⁴C]PC + lymph	1	97	1
		[¹⁴C]LPC + buffer	99	ND	ND
		[¹⁴C]LPC + lymph	99	ND	ND
37	90	[¹⁴C]PC + buffer	1	97	1
		[¹⁴C]PC + lymph	2	94	2
		[¹⁴C]LPC + buffer	80	1	19
		[¹⁴C]LPC + lymph	96	1	2

Disintegrations per minute (dpm) were obtained from measured counts per minute after correction for quenching using a ¹⁴C label as an internal standard. Values are means of three experiments. TLC, thin-layer chromatography; LPC, lysophosphatidylcholine; PC, phosphatidylcholine; FA, fatty acid; ND, not detectable.

Table 4 presents data that make the points that there was virtually no hydrolysis of lysophosphatidylcholine or phosphatidylcholine in cardiac lymph from dogs after incubation at 4°C for 30 min and that there was very little hydrolysis after incubation at 37°C for 90 min. In this table, the independent variable is described in the three columns on the left and the dependent variable in the three columns on the right. The units of measurement (°C, min, and %) are placed below the column headings and thus are easy to see. Trends in this table read across the rows. Abbreviations are used to keep the title, column headings, and columns compact. The abbreviations are defined in footnotes. "ND" is used to indicate missing data and is defined in a footnote.

both because asterisks (or other symbols) distinguish differences more clearly than a column of *P* values does and because a column of *P* values adds unnecessary bulk to the body of the table.

It is unnecessary to identify differences that are not statistically significant. Keep in mind that tables are a visual medium. A * protruding from a column of aligned numbers is a clear visual sign of a statistically significant difference (Table 2). The absence of a * is a clear visual sign of no significant difference. Adding in other symbols, or NS (for "not significant"), just creates clutter (Table 6A). In addition, NS is uninformative: was the *P* value small (0.07, for example) or large (0.7)?

Indicating Missing Data. To indicate data that are missing, two systems are used. One system is to put a dash and a footnote symbol (for example, "—ᵃ") in place of the missing data and, in a footnote, to state "ᵃNot determined" or "ᵃNot detectable" or whatever (Table 5). The other system is to write "ND" in place of the missing data and to define ND in a footnote (Table 4). The dash plus footnote symbol is preferable because it is visually distinct and makes the data that are present easier to see (compare Tables 4 and 5). Do not leave

Table 5
Recovery of Apolipoprotein A-I and Cholesterol in Ultracentrifugal Fractions
Obtained from Media of Different Ionic Strengths

| | Recovery (%) | | | | | | | | |
| | Apolipoprotein A-I* | | | | | Cholesterol† | | | |
Medium	1.063-T	1.21-1-B	1.21-2-B	1.21-T	Total	1.063-T	1.21-1-B	1.21-2-B	1.21-T
H_2O-KBr	0.4	8.1	6.9	83.7	99.1	—‡	2.0	0.2	17.0
D_2O-KBr	0.4	16.1	7.2	71.6	95.3	—	2.0	0.5	16.0
D_2O-CsCl	0.4	17.1	13.2	58.9	89.6	—	2.0	0.5	19.0

Data are from one preparation but are typical of recoveries from 20 other preparations.
*Percent of total serum apolipoprotein A-I.
†Percent of total serum cholesterol.
‡Not determined.

Table 5 presents data that make three points: that recovery of apolipoprotein A-I from the 1.21-T fraction decreased as the ionic strength of the medium decreased, thus indicating increasing losses of apolipoprotein A-I; that these losses occurred concurrently with increasing recovery of apolipoprotein A-I in the 1.21-1-B and 1.21-2-B fractions; and that the cholesterol content was constant. In this table, the independent variable (medium) is listed in order of decreasing ionic strength. Dashes and a footnote symbol after the first dash are used to indicate missing data. The reason the data are missing is given in a footnote. Footnote symbols in the body of the table are placed from left to right and then down.

a blank space where there are no data because a blank space is ambiguous. It could mean "not determined" or "not detectable," or it could be an error.

Footnotes

Footnotes are phrases or sentences placed below the body of the table that explain items in the column headings, body, or title of the table. Footnotes for column headings can explain details such as experimental methods (see Table 2), the way a variable was calculated (see Table 4), or the meaning of an abbreviation (see Table 4).

In the body of the table, in addition to being used to explain details or to define abbreviations (see Table 1), footnotes can be used to substitute for a column of values that are all the same. For example, if all data are for 11 dialysis procedures, a column labeled n is not necessary. Instead, the value can be mentioned in a footnote, preferably in the same footnote that defines the data as means ± SD: "Data are means ± SD for 11 dialysis procedures." Not only is a footnote more efficient than a column labeled n followed by a string of 11s; it is also clearer because it tells what n is: 11 dialysis procedures. Generally, "n" is not a clear abbreviation in a column heading or in a footnote. It is always clearer to write "Number of Samples," "Number of Rabbits," or whatever for a column heading (see Table 2), or "in 25 samples," "for 16 rabbits," or whatever in a footnote (see Table 3).

Another use of footnotes in the body of the table is to explain statistically significant differences between data. The usual practice is to put a footnote symbol, such as *, after each value that is different and then in the footnote to state what values you are comparing and what the P value is. Two phrases

TABLE 6. *Cardiac variables before and after pulmonary microvasacular injury in seven dogs*

Variable	Before	After
End-diastolic dimensions		
LV SF (mm)	50.7 ± 7.1	49.4 ± 7.5*
LV AP (mm)	56.7 ± 5.2	56.0 ± 5.5
LV area (mm²)	2730 ± 630	2640 ± 670†
RV SF (mm)	36.5 ± 5.2	36.7 ± 4.9
RV chord (mm)	64.2 ± 10.8	64.2 ± 11.2
RV area (mm²)	2330 ± 430	2320 ± 440
End-systolic dimensions		
LV SF (mm)	43.0 ± 5.2	42.0 ± 6.0
LV AP (mm)	53.5 ± 4.4	53.3 ± 5.3
LV area (mm²)	2320 ± 460	2260 ± 560
RV SF (mm)	36.3 ± 3.3	37.6 ± 2.8
RV chord (mm)	60.3 ± 10.5	41.2 ± 10.6
RV area (mm²)	2190 ± 380	2300 ± 440†
End-diastolic pressures (mmHg)		
LV	13 ± 8	8 ± 6†
RV	13 ± 5	10 ± 7
PA	14 ± 4	24 ± 9*
Maximum pressure (mmHg)		
LV	113 ± 23	105 ± 28
RV	31 ± 9	38 ± 15‡
PA	29 ± 7	38 ± 13§

Values are means ± SD. LV, left ventricle; RV, right ventricle; PA, pulmonary artery; SF, septal-free wall; AP, antero-posterior. *$P < 0.01$, †$P < 0.05$, ‡ $P < 0.06$, § $P < 0.02$ vs. the "before" value.

Table 6 presents data that make the point that pulmonary microvascular injury caused significant decreases in the left ventricular septal-free wall dimension, left ventricular area, and left ventricular end-diastolic pressure. In this table, the dependent variables are listed down the first column on the left rather than across the top to save space. Because data are not aligned on the decimal point but only on the ±, the different magnitudes are not easy to see at first glance.

commonly used for explaining significant differences are "*significantly different from the control value, $P < 0.01$" and "*$P < 0.01$ vs. control" (or 0.02, or whatever; or vs. another treatment group, etc.). The important thing is *not* to write simply "*$P < 0.05$," because then the reader has to guess which values you are comparing. Although comparisons are often with control data, they can also be with values obtained after other treatments, so it is clearest always to state which values are being compared (see Tables 2, 3, 6).

The order of information in footnotes is the same as the order of information in a figure legend: first experimental details (in sentences), then definitions of abbreviations and symbols not defined earlier in the footnotes, and finally statistical details (see Table 2). One exception is that the statement of how data are summarized (for example, "Values are mean ± SD") frequently appears before definitions of abbreviations (see Tables 4 and 6).

Footnotes should be brief and few. They should not overbalance the body of the table.

TABLE 6A. *Cardiac variables before and after pulmonary microvasacular injury in seven dogs*

Variable	Before	After	P
End-diastolic dimensions			
LV SF (mm)	50.7 ± 7.1	49.4 ± 7.5	0.01
LV AP (mm)	56.7 ± 5.2	56.0 ± 5.5	NS
LV area (mm^2)	2730 ± 630	2640 ± 670	0.05
RV SF (mm)	36.5 ± 5.2	36.7 ± 4.9	NS
RV chord (mm)	64.2 ± 10.8	64.2 ± 11.2	NS
RV area (mm^2)	2330 ± 430	2320 ± 440	NS
End-systolic dimensions			
LV SF (mm)	43.0 ± 5.2	42.0 ± 6.0	NS
LV AP (mm)	53.5 ± 4.4	53.3 ± 5.3	NS
LV area (mm^2)	2320 ± 460	2260 ± 560	NS
RV SF (mm)	36.3 ± 3.3	37.6 ± 2.8	NS
RV chord (mm)	60.3 ± 10.5	41.2 ± 10.6	NS
RV area (mm^2)	2190 ± 380	2300 ± 440	0.05
End-diastolic pressures (mmHg)			
LV	13 ± 8	8 ± 6	0.05
RV	13 ± 5	10 ± 7	NS
PA	14 ± 4	24 ± 9	0.01
Maximum pressure (mmHg)			
LV	113 ± 23	105 ± 28	NS
RV	31 ± 9	38 ± 15	0.06
PA	29 ± 7	38 ± 13	0.02

Values are means ± SD. LV, left ventricle; RV, right ventricle; PA, pulmonary artery; SF, septal-free wall; AP, antero-posterior. NS, not significant.

> Table 6A illustrates how using a column of *P* values to show statistically significant differences, rather than using symbols as in Table 6, has less visual impact than symbols do and adds unnecessary bulk to the table.

Footnotes are usually identified by superscript symbols or superscript letters. One standard series of footnote symbols is *, †, ‡, §, ‖, ¶, #, **, ††, etc. (Table 5). Letters used to identify footnotes are in lower case: a, b, c, etc. (Table 1). When footnotes are used only to show statistically significant differences, sometimes the following series of symbols is used: $*P < 0.05$, $**P < 0.01$, $***P < 0.001$. Some journals do not use footnote symbols or letters for footnotes that apply to the entire table but only for footnotes that apply to a single item in the table.

Footnote symbols or letters are placed in sequence from left to right and then down, the same as the direction in which we read (Table 5).

The Size of Tables

Tables should contain neither so many data as to be overwhelming nor so few data as to be unnecessary. The goal is to make tables a size in between these extremes.

Sometimes an excessively large or excessively small table is necessary or desirable. For example, a large table may be needed to give background data for a large number of subjects or to give individual experimental data for all subjects, animals, or specimens. A small table may be desirable to present data for the most important point in the paper, even if the values would take up less space in the text, because a table has more visual impact.

Nevertheless, in general, a table should have enough data to be more efficient than presenting the data in the text, should be small enough to be readable, and should be as compact as possible without sacrificing clarity. The solution to a table that has very few data is usually to omit the table and to write the values in the text. Some solutions to a table that is too large are to omit unnecessary columns or rows of information, to keep the title, column headings, and footnotes brief, and, if necessary, to break the table into two smaller tables. (For an excellent example of one clear table created from two excessively large tables by omitting unnecessary rows of data and redesigning the remaining information, see "Tables with Several Simultaneous Faults" in Woodford, Chap. 10, Design of Tables and Figures.) In particular, if the purpose of the table is to make a point, do everything in your power to make the table as small as possible so that the point is apparent, not buried in all the numbers.

To omit unnecessary columns of information,

Omit a column of less important data (for example, confirmatory data).

Omit a column of easily calculated data that are not central to the point of the story. For example, if you report stroke volume, heart rate, and minute volume (which equals stroke volume times heart rate), one of those variables could probably be omitted.

Omit a column that contains only one value; report that value in the text.

Omit a column in which all or most values are the same; put the information in a short footnote or in the text. For example, if $n = 10$ for all data, state that in a footnote: "Data are for 10 lambs." If all values in a column are essentially the same as baseline, report the baseline value in the text and say that the experimental values were not different from baseline: "Heart rates did not differ significantly from the baseline value of 84 beats/min."

Omit a column of P values; put symbols after the values that are different.

To keep column headings brief and thus save space in the table, use short terms or abbreviations in the column headings and subheadings, and explain the abbreviations in footnotes if necessary. Because of the need to save space, more abbreviations are used in tables than in the text. For example, in the column heading "Cyclic GMP Concn," "concn" is used instead of "concentration" and GMP is used instead of "guanidine monophosphate." Another possibility is "[Cyclic GMP]." In the column heading "Recovery (% of total)," "%" is used instead of "percent." "Concn" and "%" do not need to be defined. But if an abbreviation, even a standard abbreviation, such as "FRC," is used as a column heading, define it in a footnote ("FRC, functional residual capacity"). If the abbreviation is not defined in a footnote, readers who do not know the meaning (and there are always some readers in this category) have to search through the text to find the definition, which is inconvenient. [*Exception*: Abbreviations that are more familiar than the words they stand for do not need to be defined; for example, DNA (deoxyribonucleic acid). GMP may be another example.] Definitions are needed only in the first table in which the abbreviations appear. In later tables, use a footnote to refer readers to the table where the abbreviations are defined, for example, "Abbreviations as in Table II."

Although column headings should be brief, they do not necessarily have to be written as abbreviations. If space permits writing out the name of a variable in a column heading, do so. For example, "heart rate" never needs to be abbreviated.

Also, try to use the shortest and the fewest footnotes possible. An excess of footnotes is not an improvement over long headings. Thus, in Table 3, the column headings are long and the footnotes are brief and few.

In addition to omitting unnecessary data and keeping column headings and footnotes brief, avoid repetition of information within a table. For example, if the title says "in 10 Lambs," you do not need a column labeled "Number of Lambs" or a footnote saying "Data are for 10 lambs."

If after trying all these ways of shortening a table you still have an excessively large table, consider dividing the large table into two smaller tables. Be careful to keep data that are to be compared in one table.

Format of Tables

A variety of formats is used for tables, depending on the journal. One detail that is standard is that three horizontal lines are used to separate the parts of a table: one above the column headings, one below the column headings, and one below the data (Tables 1, 3, 6). If there are any subheadings, short horizontal lines are used to group the subheadings under the appropriate headings (Tables 2, 4, 5).

In addition, some journals use horizontal lines between rows of data; other journals use vertical lines between columns of data; still other journals use both horizontal and vertical lines between rows and columns. These extra lines give the table a cluttered look; usually rows and columns can be clearly separated by adequate spacing. Nevertheless, follow the practice of the journal to which you are submitting your paper.

Most other details of format for tables vary from journal to journal. Some of these details are the use of a roman or an arabic table number; centering or flush left placement of the table number, title, column headings, and data; the use of capital letters and italics; the placement of footnotes; and the type of footnote symbols used. The variety of format details is illustrated in part in the tables in this chapter. For your papers, follow the practice of the journal you are submitting your paper to.

TELLING A STORY

Creating a Sequence of Figures and Tables

In addition to each figure and table being clearly designed and the legends for figures and the titles and footnotes for tables being clearly written, the figures and tables taken together should form a clear sequence that tells the story of the paper. To create a clear sequence, design the figures to be as parallel as possible, design the tables to be as parallel as possible, write figure legends of parallel figures in parallel form, and write titles and footnotes of parallel tables in parallel form. Thus, each figure and table will prepare the reader for the next figure or table.

For example, in a paper showing that pulmonary venous blood flow (but not mitral inflow) as assessed by transesophageal pulsed Doppler echocardiography accurately estimates mean left atrial pressure as an indicator of left ventricular performance, three tables and five figures were used. One table and one figure were used for methods. The table listed the characteristics of the patients in the study. The figure, the velocity-time profiles of pulmonary venous flow and mitral inflow, showed how the velocity-time integrals were measured.

The remaining tables and figures presented data for three lines of evidence. For the first line of evidence, Table 2 listed the data showing the correlations between mean left atrial pressure and all the Doppler variables for both pulmonary venous flow and mitral inflow. In addition, Figure 2, a scattergram, showed the correlation between mean left atrial pressure and the most strongly correlated pulmonary venous flow variable. For the second line of evidence, Figure 3, two scattergrams, showed the correlations between *changes* in mean left atrial pressure and *changes* in the most strongly correlated pulmonary flow variable and in the most strongly correlated mitral inflow variable. For the third line of evidence, Table 3 listed values for all the variables measured at both normal and elevated mean left atrial pressures, showing that values were different at elevated mean left atrial pressures. In addition, Figures 4 and 5, velocity-time profiles, showed primary evidence of changes in pulmonary venous flow patterns (Figure 4) and mitral inflow patterns (Figure 5) at elevated mean left atrial pressures, again indicating the relation between mean left atrial pressure and pulmonary venous flow.

In these three tables and five figures, parallel design and parallel titles were used whenever possible. For example, in the two results tables, the variables are listed in the first column on the left and the appropriate data are in the columns on the right. In addition to this parallel design, the titles of the two tables are as parallel as possible: Table 2. Correlation of Doppler Variables with Mean Left Atrial Pressure; Table 3. Hemodynamic, Doppler, and Two-Dimensional Echocardiographic Variables in Patients with Normal and Elevated Mean Left Atrial Pressure. For the two correlation figures and for the two velocity-time profiles showing the effect of increasing mean left atrial pressure, the legends are parallel:

Fig. 2. Correlation of the systolic fraction of pulmonary venous flow with mean left atrial pressure. *r*, correlation coefficient; SEE, standard error of the estimate; *n*, number of study periods. The curved lines are 95% confidence intervals for the mean value of systolic fraction.

Fig. 3. Correlation of changes in the systolic fraction of pulmonary venous flow (top) and changes in the ratio of peak early to peak late diastolic mitral inflow (Δ peak early/late) (bottom) with changes in mean left atrial pressure (Δ mean LAP). Abbreviations as in Fig. 2.

Fig. 4. Effect of increased mean left atrial pressure on pulmonary venous flow patterns. (etc.)

Fig. 5. Effect of increased mean left atrial pressure, estimated by pulmonary capillary wedge pressure (PCWP), on mitral inflow patterns. (etc.)

Because of the parallel designs of the figures and of the tables and the parallel form of the table titles and of the figure legends, the story of the paper is clear from looking at the figures and tables. For another example of figures and tables that tell the story of the paper, see Chapter 12, The Big Picture, Exercise 12.1.

Relating the Figures and Tables to the Text

In addition to the figures and tables forming a clear sequence, they must clearly and accurately show what the text states. That is, the point illustrated in a figure or a table must be the point stated in the text. For example, if the text describes an apparatus, the important features of the apparatus must be immediately visible in the figure. Similarly, if the text says that when X was done, Y increased, then in the figure Y should look as if it increased. If the increase is not obvious, the figure is unconvincing. Also, if some values from graphs or tables are restated in the text, the name of the variable (and all other key terms), the unit of measurement, and the values should be the same in the text and in the graph or table.

Number of Figures and Tables

Finally, use the fewest figures and tables needed to tell the story. The reader can pull the story together more easily from 5 or 6 figures and tables than from 15 or 16.

Do not present the same data in both a figure and a table. However, it is OK, for example, to have a table or a figure summarizing data for all the experiments in a series and a figure showing primary evidence, such as a polygraph recording, for a single experiment.

**SUMMARY OF
GUIDELINES
FOR FIGURES
AND TABLES**

FIGURES

Figures are usually used to clarify methods or to present evidence that supports
the results.
Design figures to have strong visual impact.

Design

Draw drawings and diagrams in black on white and keep them simple.
Make primary evidence of high quality.

> For halftone figures (for example, micrographs), make the photograph
> sharp and clear.
>
> For photographs of patients, cover facial features to prevent identification
> when possible, and use A, B, etc., to refer to patients, not the patients'
> initials.
>
> For micrographs:
>
>> Ensure that contrast is sufficient to make the features of interest
>> clear.
>>
>> Make the photograph just enough larger than the features of interest
>> to give a sense of where they are in their context.
>>
>> Make labels brief, few, and just big enough to be readily visible.
>>
>> To show magnification, use either a scale bar on the figure (for a
>> general journal) or a number in the legend (for a specialty journal).
>>
>> Use thin white lines to separate micrographs grouped into plates.
>>
>> Number each micrograph in the lower left corner. Use a black num-
>> ber inside a white circle outlined by a black line.
>
> For gel electrophoretograms, label the gels and the important fractions.
> Labels should not overwhelm the data.
>
> For polygraph recordings:
>
>> If you remove grid lines, add vertical scales and horizontal scales
>> or scale markers. Be sure the scales and scale markers are ac-
>> curate.
>>
>> Label each axis with the name of the variable followed by the unit
>> of measurement in parentheses. Use uppercase and lowercase let-
>> ters for the name of the variable; use International System (SI)
>> abbreviations for the units of measurement.
>>
>> Label each scale marker with the unit it represents.
>>
>> Align horizontal axis labels on the left. Do not let axis labels pro-
>> trude into the column of scale numbers.

Use the appropriate type of graph to display the type of data you have.

> A line graph is a two-axis graph on which curves, data points, or both
> show the relation between two variables. Scale each axis accurately.
>
> A scattergram is a two-axis graph that plots individual data points and
> fits a mathematical function to the points to show how strongly two
> variables are correlated.
>
> A bar graph is a one-axis graph for comparing amounts or frequencies
> for classes of a discontinuous or a "relative-scale" variable. In bar graphs,
> the axis must include zero.
>
> An individual-value bar graph is a variation on vertical bar graphs in
> which individual data points are shown either in addition to or instead
> of the mean. For paired data, lines can be drawn to show the direction
> of change.
>
> A histogram is a two-axis graph that shows a single frequency distribution
> by means of a series of contiguous rectangles. The rectangles in a
> histogram should be of equal widths.

A frequency polygon is a two-axis graph that uses data points joined by lines to show two or more overlapping frequency distributions or a single distribution. Data points are plotted at the midpoint of each class and the lines joining the data points are extended to the baseline to complete the distribution.

Ensure that each figure is easy to read.

After the graph is reduced to fit the journal's column, letters should be large enough (at least 1.5 mm high) to be legible.

Symbols should be large enough to be seen and easy to distinguish. The easiest data point symbols to distinguish are ● and ○.

Draw figures to emphasize the data. In line graphs:

Make curves the darkest lines;

Make axis labels less dark;

Make axes, tick marks, error bars, keys, and curve labels the least dark.

Ensure that each figure makes a clear point.

Figure Legends

A figure legend has four parts:

Title

The title is the first item in the figure legend; it does not appear in the figure.

The title should be a brief phrase that identifies the specific topic of the figure. The title should contain no excess details and no abbreviations.

For drawings, diagrams, and primary evidence, the title should identify the type of figure if necessary and the apparatus, concept, or biological specimen shown. For example, "Fig. 1. Bright-field light micrograph of a segment of a bacterial filament."

For a graph, the standard title is "Effect of X on Y in Z" or "Y in response to X in Z," where X is the independent variable, Y is the dependent variable, and Z is the species, the material, or both. For experiments that have no independent variable, the standard title is "Y in Z." The title may also include the point of the graph. For example, "Inhibition of Y by X in Z."

For composites, provide a title for the entire figure and identify the parts of the composite either within the title or in separate subtitles.

Experimental Details

Give just enough experimental details to permit the reader to understand the figure. In legends for graphs, do not simply repeat the information in the axis labels.

Write experimental details in sentences.

It is unnecessary to say "For details, see Methods."

Definitions

Symbols, line or bar patterns, and abbreviations that are not defined in the figure or earlier in the legend should be defined after experimental details are given. Definitions can be written as phrases or as sentences.

If the same symbols, line or bar patterns, or abbreviations are used in more than one figure, define them in the legend for the first relevant figure only. In succeeding legends, refer the reader to that legend. For example, "Abbreviations as in Fig. 1."

Statistical Information

State whether data points or bars represent individual or mean values and whether error bars represent standard deviations, standard errors of the mean, confidence intervals, or ranges.

State the sample size (n).

Avoid writing "$n = 12$." Write "12 samples," "12 dogs," or whatever.

For data in bar graphs that have been analyzed by a statistical test, state which values were compared by statistical analysis and the significance value. For example, "* significantly different from the control value, $P < 0.01$."

Other information may be included in a figure legend.

A figure legend may include statements pointing out an unusual or an interesting feature.

A figure legend should not include results as such. However, for graphs, results can be indicated by stating the point in the title. For figures that show primary evidence, results can be indicated by pointing out a feature on the figure ("Note . . .").

If you republish figures that have already been published, you must first obtain permission from the copyright holder (usually the publisher) and from the author. Give credit to the source by citing the reference at the end of the figure legend. For example, "From Fraser (1975), with permission." Give the complete reference in the reference list. You must obtain permission whether you use all of the original figure, part of the figure, or a modified version of the figure.

TABLES

Tables are usually used to present background information related to methods or to present data.

Tables of data either present individual data for all subjects, animals, or specimens studied or make a point.

Tables should be arranged to have clear visual impact.

The Title

Make the title a short phrase that states the topic or the point of the table.

For titles of tables that give background information or that present data for experiments that have only dependent variables, use the form "Y in Z."

For titles of tables that present data for experiments that have both independent and dependent variables, use the form "Effect of X on Y in Z" or "Y during X in Z."

Keep titles brief by using a category term in place of the names of two or more variables.

Use the same terms in the title and in the column headings.

Column Headings

Give each type of information its own column and its own column heading.

To subdivide a column heading into two or more categories, use subheadings.

Put the unit of measurement (usually in parentheses) after or below the name of the variable in the column heading.

Use International System (SI) abbreviations.

Choose units that eliminate unnecessary zeros.

Avoid using multipliers as a way of eliminating unnecessary zeros.

The Body of the Table

In the columns on the left, list the items for which data are given; list these
items in a logical order according to the experimental design (for example,
in increasing or decreasing order). In the columns on the right, present the
data. For experiments that have both independent and dependent variables,
the column(s) on the left are the independent variable(s) and the column(s)
on the right are the dependent variable(s).

Present control data first (that is, in the top row).

If sample sizes (n) are different, list them in a column between the independent
and the dependent variables.

Arrange data to reveal trends down a column or across a row or to permit easy
comparison between adjacent columns or rows. Put standard deviations (SD),
standard errors of the mean (SEM), confidence intervals (CI), or ranges either
to the right of the means or below the means, depending on whether readers
need to read down the columns or across the rows, respectively.

Present data to the fewest possible decimal places; have the same number of
decimal places in all values for one variable; have the same number of
decimal places in the SD as in the mean.

Align all values in each column on the decimal point, and if you give SDs or
SEMs after a ± to the right of the means, also align all values on the ± so
that the data will be easy to compare.

For excessively wide tables, either place SDs below means, switch the independent and dependent variables (run the dependent variables down the
first column on the left), see if the journal will run the table across two
pages, or run the table the length of the page rather than the width of the
page. The disadvantage of switching the independent and dependent variables is that the values will not align neatly on the decimal point, so the
magnitude of individual numbers will not be immediately obvious.

To indicate statistically significant differences between data, use a symbol
(such as *) after the value that is different and define the symbol in a footnote.

To indicate missing data, use a dash followed by a footnote symbol (for example,
"—ᵃ"), and in a footnote write "ᵃNot determined," "ᵃNot detectable," or whatever, or write "ND" in place of the missing data and define ND in a footnote.
A dash is visually more effective than ND is. Do not leave a blank space
when data are missing because a blank space is ambiguous.

Footnotes

Use footnotes to explain items in the column headings, body, or title of a table,
such as experimental details or abbreviations, and to substitute for a column
of values that are all the same, such as n. For example, "Data are mean ±
SD *for 11 dialysis procedures.*"

Use footnotes to explain statistically significant differences. Two common forms
are "*significantly different from the control value, $P < 0.01$" and "*$P <
0.01$ vs. control." Do not write only "$P < 0.01$" because that does not indicate
which values are being compared.

Put information in footnotes in the same order as information in a figure
legend: first experimental details (in sentences), then definitions of abbreviations and symbols, and finally statistical details (except put "Values are
mean ± SD" before definitions of abbreviations).

Keep footnotes brief and few.

Use superscript symbols or superscript lowercase letters to identify footnotes.
One standard series of footnote symbols is *, †, ‡, §, ‖, ¶, #, **, ††, etc. A

series of symbols sometimes used to show statistically significant differences is $*P < 0.05$, $**P < 0.01$, $***P < 0.001$.

Place footnote symbols or letters in sequence from left to right and then down.

The Size of Tables

Avoid making tables so large as to be overwhelming or so small as to be unnecessary. However, a large table may be needed to present background data or individual experimental data.

If the purpose of the table is to make a point, keep the table as condensed as possible. To condense a large table, omit unnecessary columns or rows of information and keep the title, column headings, and footnotes brief. If necessary, break a large table into two smaller tables, keeping data that are to be compared in the same table.

Avoid repetition of information within a table.

Format of Tables

Use three horizontal lines: one above the column headings, one below the column headings, and one below the data.

Use a short horizontal line to group subheadings under a heading.

If the journal also uses other horizontal or vertical lines, add them.

Follow journal style for details such as roman or arabic table number; centered or flush left table number, title, column headings, and data; capital letters and italics; the placement of footnotes; the type of footnote symbols.

Telling a Story

To create a clear sequence of figures and tables that tells the story of the paper, make the figures and their legends as parallel as possible, and make the tables and their titles and footnotes as parallel as possible.

Check that each figure and each table clearly and accurately shows what the text states.

Check that values repeated in the text are accurate.

Use the fewest figures and tables needed to tell the story.

Do not present the same data in both a figure and a table. However, primary evidence (for example, a polygraph recording) may be shown in addition to a figure or a table of summarized data.

■ *Exercise 8.1:* *DESIGN OF FIGURES AND TABLES AND THEIR RELATION TO THE TEXT*

1. *Assess the design of the figure and table below and also how well they relate to the text.*
2. *Assess the figure legend and the table title.*
3. *Redesign the figure and the table, and revise the legend, table title, and text as necessary.*

The <u>questions</u> this paper asks are, "How severe is cigarette smoke-induced bronchoconstriction, and what mechanisms are involved?"

Results

Inhalation of cigarette smoke into the lungs of anesthetized dogs caused 2- to 8-fold increases in airflow resistance of the total respiratory system depending on the dose of smoke inhaled (Fig. 2). Airflow resistance increased rapidly after the start of smoke inhalation; the maximum was reached within 1 min. Airflow resistance remained increased transiently, decreased to one-half the maximal value within 4 min (Table I), and returned to baseline before the next dose 20 min later (Fig. 2).

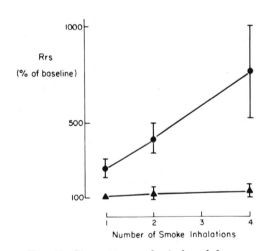

Fig. 2. Cigarette smoke-induced bronchoconstriction in 5 anesthetized dogs. Data are means ± SE before (▲) and after (●) 1, 2, or 4 tidal-volume inhalations of cigarette smoke. Inhalations were separated by 20 min.

Table I

Time course of bronchoconstriction after inhalation of two tidal volumes of cigarette smoke in 5 dogs

Dog No.	Airflow Resistance (% of baseline)			
	½ min	1 min	2 min	4 min
1	482	582	109	264
2	347	276	175	166
3	323	195	141	151
4	610	333	305	314
5	133	107	210	57
mean ± SD	379 ± 179	299 ± 180	188 ± 75	190 ± 101

■ *Exercise 8.2: TABLE DESIGN AND RELATION TO THE TEXT*

1. Assess the title and the arrangement of the table below.
2. Also compare the table with the relevant results (paras. 2 and 3 of Results).
3. Then <u>revise</u> the table to make the point clearer.

The <u>question</u> this paper asks is, "Do peritoneal dialysis and hemodialysis have similar effects on plasma cholesterol metabolism in patients with end-stage renal disease?"

Results

1 The concentrations of plasma total and free cholesterol and the phospholipid content were significantly lower in the hemodialysis patients than in the peritoneal dialysis patients or the control group (Table I). These lower values were partly reflected by the lower concentrations of high-density lipoprotein (HDL) and the lower HDL cholesterol in the hemodialysis patients.

2 Consistent with the lower HDL concentrations, apo A-I was much lower in the hemodialysis patients than in the control group, whereas the value for the peritoneal dialysis patients was intermediate (Table II). Apo A-II concentrations were very similar in all three groups. Apo B and apo E were in the normal range in both groups of patients. Apo D was slightly higher in the two groups of patients than in the controls.

3 The ratio of high-density lipoprotein and low-density lipoprotein (expressed here as the ratio between their major apolipoproteins, apo A-I and apo B, respectively) was significantly lower in the hemodialysis patients than in the controls (Table II). Values were intermediate in the peritoneal dialysis patients.

Table II. Plasma Apoprotein Levels
in Renal Disease and Control Subjects

	Hemodialysis	Controls	CAPD
Apo A-I *(mg/dl)*	102 ± 17	163 ± 23	123 ± 20
		(P < 0.0005)	
Apo A-II *(mg/dl)*	34.8 ± 6.5	36.4 ± 2.0	36 ± 4
Apo B *(mg/dl)*	89 ± 14	98 ± 32	94 ± 8
Apo D *(mg/dl)*	6.7 ± 1.3	5.6 ± 1.2	9.5 ± 1.0
		(P < 0.0005)	
Apo E *(mg/dl)*	6.8 ± 0.8	7.3 ± 1.6	7.5 ± 0.9
Apo A-I/Apo B	1.15 ± 0.18	1.7 ± 0.6	1.3 ± 0.2
	(0.005 < P < 0.010)		

Values represent means ± standard deviation from 15 hemodialysis, 6 peritoneal dialysis, and 10 control subjects.

CHAPTER 9

REFERENCES

PURPOSES

The purposes of including references in scientific research papers are to give credit to the ideas and findings of others and to direct readers to sources of further information.

SELECTING REFERENCES

Whereas review articles, which pull together and interpret a large body of information, cite a large number of references, a research report cites only immediately relevant references. When deciding which references to include in a research paper, select the most valid, the most available, and the fewest references.

Valid

The references generally considered most valid are journal articles, because journal articles undergo a review process before being accepted for publication, although the validity of the review process has yet to be established (Lock, *A Difficult Balance*). Other valid references include books, Ph.D. theses, and some conferences proceedings (those for which papers are reviewed). References considered less valid include abstracts for meetings, because abstracts do not contain enough information to permit assessment of the work, and some conference proceedings (those for which papers are not reviewed). These less valid references should be used primarily to credit the source of an idea, not to support a conclusion or an argument. Similarly, personal communications and unpublished data or unpublished observations should be used only for such purposes as supporting the results of preliminary studies or citing parallel results in another species. Because these "references" cannot be obtained and assessed, they do not constitute strong evidence and therefore should not be used to support conclusions or arguments.

Available

The most available references for most readers are journal articles. Books are also generally available. Ph.D. theses and proceedings of meetings take more trouble to find. When Ph.D. work is published in journals, cite the journal article rather than the thesis.

Journal articles that have not yet been published but that have been accepted for publication are referred to as being "in press" (American) or "in the press" (British). These articles can be located fairly easily by searching the appropriate journal beginning about the time the paper in which the "in press" reference is cited was accepted. When citing an "in press" paper, include the title of the journal followed by the words "in press."

Articles that have not yet been accepted are not available and therefore should not be included in the reference list. Even if the journal permits references such as "submitted" and "in preparation" in the reference list, work that has not yet been accepted should not be included in the reference list. Instead, it should be referred to in the text either as a personal communication (for work done by others) or as an unpublished observation (for work done by one or more of the authors). The year of the personal communication or observation should be included. Before citing a personal communication, check with the author. The information you thought you heard may not be what the author thought he or she said, or the results may not have been repeatable. Some journals require written confirmation of all personal communications.

Few

To keep your references to the fewest necessary, select, as appropriate, the first, the most important, the most elegant, and the most recent. Cite review articles where possible. Also, keep in mind that references cited in the papers in your reference list can lead readers to articles that you do not cite in your paper.

ACCURACY

Accuracy of the References

The references in the reference list must be accurate. A grossly inaccurate reference can be difficult or impossible to find. An inaccurate spelling of a name creates ambiguity in indexes (for example, is B. W. Goetzman the same person as B. W. Goetzmann?) (To do your part to keep indexes of the biomedical literature clear, use the same name and initials throughout your career. If you change you name in your private life, do not change it or hyphenate it in your professional life. Similarly, do not add or drop initials. For example, if your name is R. J. Gordon but your friends call you John, do not change your publishing name to J. Gordon part way through your career.)

The accuracy of every reference in the reference list is the author's responsibility. For every reference you cite, check the citation against the journal (first choice) or against a reprint or a photocopy (second choice). Build up a data base of verified references. Thus you will have to verify each reference only once.

To verify the citation of a journal article, check the following details:

Spelling of authors' names
Authors' initials
Title of the paper, including the subtitle if any
Journal
Year of publication
Volume

First page number
Last page number

One major source of inaccurate references is copying a reference from someone else's reference list (or even your own list). Since you should not cite a reference that you have not read, at least in part, you should not need to copy references from other people's lists. However, if you must cite an idea from an article you cannot find, make clear that you did not see the original article by using the following form of citation:

Example 9.1 Reference for an Article You Could Not Find

Powell JA. Title. Plugers Archiv 1972;XX:xx–xx (cited by Jones RE. Title. J Appl Physiol 1977;XX:xx–xx).

Accuracy of the Information

Not only must the references be accurate, but the information you cite must be accurate also. If you quote from a published paper, use quotation marks, and check that every word and punctuation mark is exactly as it was in the original. If you paraphrase the ideas, check that your statement is accurate and fair—one that the author would accept. After you finish writing the paper, read the articles you cited once again, to make sure that your statements do not misrepresent the authors' ideas.

Correlation of the Reference List and the Text

Finally, every reference in the text must be included in the reference list and every reference in the reference list must be cited in the text. Computer programs that do not permit discrepancies between references in the text and in the reference list are available. Otherwise, check this correlation yourself.

INCORPORATING REFERENCES INTO THE TEXT

Introducing Referenced Material in the Text

There are two ways to cite others' ideas in the text. One emphasizes the science:

Example 9.2 Citation Emphasizing Science

Glucagon may influence hepatic regeneration (23).

The other emphasizes the scientists:

Example 9.3 Citation Emphasizing Scientists

Bucher and Swaffield (23) reported that glucagon may influence hepatic regeneration.

Keep in mind that authors' names are not transition words. It is usually easier to keep the story going in a paragraph if you do not begin a sentence with authors' names. Also, avoid mixing the two types of citation in one paragraph unless you have a particular reason for doing so.

Referring to Authors of Other Papers

When referring to the authors of a paper, be careful to include all authors and then, in later sentences, to use the appropriate pronoun. For a paper by one author, use that author's name: "developed by Libanoff (4)." For a paper by two authors, use both authors' names every time: "Barrington and Finer (16) treated nine infants." For a paper by three or more authors, use the first author's name followed by the Latin term "et al.," which means "and others." Some journals prefer English terms such as "and others" or "and colleagues." "Et al." or a similar term must be used every time the authors of the paper are mentioned. It is never appropriate to refer to the paper only by the name of the first author: "Jackson et al. (12) reported. . . . Jackson (12) also found . . . ." Note that there is no comma between the first author's name and "et al." There is a period after "al.," which is an abbreviation for "alii."

The appropriate pronoun for Jackson et al. is "they," not "he." Thus, "Jackson et al. reported. . . . He also found. . ." is not possible. The appropriate wording is "Jackson et al. reported. . . . They also found. . . ."

Where to Place Reference Citations

Generally, place reference citations after the idea you are referring to (see Example 9.2 above) or after the names of the authors if the names are included in the text (see Example 9.3 above). Do not put reference citations in the middle of an idea (reference 29 in Example 9.4 below) or after general indications of a published work, such as "in a recent study" or "has been reported" (reference 16 in Example 9.4).

Example 9.4 Placement of Reference Citations

In the rat, the concentration of nuclear receptors in the brain decreases during the first 2 weeks after birth (30), whereas the receptor concentration in liver nuclei increases (**29**) during this period. In addition, a temporal correlation has been reported (**16**) between the T_3 binding capacity of nuclei and the activity of fatty acid synthetase in fetal rabbit lung.

Revision

In the rat, the concentration of nuclear receptors in the brain decreases during the first 2 weeks after birth (30), whereas the receptor concentration in liver nuclei increases during this period (**29**). In addition, a temporal correlation has been reported between the T_3 binding capacity of nuclei and the activity of fatty acid synthetase in fetal rabbit lung (**16**).

Placing reference citations after ideas does not necessarily mean that references will come at the end of the sentence. For example, it is important to distinguish between your ideas and the work of others. Thus, if you draw a conclusion based on another author's findings, put the citation after the author's finding, not after your conclusion (Example 9.5).

Example 9.5 Placement of Reference Citations

The potential for malignant transformation in lichen planus requires that caution be exercised in the long-term use of steroids (**12**).

Revision

The potential for malignant transformation in lichen planus (**12**) requires that caution be exercised in the long-term use of steroids.

Similarly, when you have several references for several points in one sentence, it is more useful to cite each reference after the appropriate point than to group all the references together at the end of the sentence, especially when the reference list does not include titles of articles.

Example 9.6   Placement of Reference Citations

Left atrial pressure dynamics have been shown to be inversely related to pulmonary venous blood flow in dogs and humans and also to influence mitral inflow (**8–12**).

Revision

Left atrial pressure dynamics have been shown to be inversely related to pulmonary venous blood flow in dogs (**8–10**) and humans (**8, 11**) and also to influence mitral inflow (**12**).

SYSTEMS FOR CITING REFERENCES

Citing References in the Text

Two main systems are used for citing references in the text: author and year (Example 9.7) and number (Example 9.8). The numbers used in the text are printed as superscripts or as numbers in parentheses or brackets.

Example 9.7   Author and Year Citation

The relationship is described by a power function ($y = ax^b$) with an exponent less than 1 (Jones et al. 1983, Brown 1984).

Example 9.8   Number Citation

The relationship is described by a power function ($y = ax^b$) with an exponent less than 1 (4, 5).

Order of References Cited for One Point

In the text, when more than one reference is cited for a point, the references are listed in chronological order when possible. For references cited by name and year, chronological order is always used. For references cited by number, numerical order is always used. Chronological order can be used simultaneously with numerical order on first citation of a group of references, as in Example 9.8 (4 = Jones et al. 1983, 5 = Brown 1984).

Arrangement of References in the Reference List

In the reference list, for the author and year system, references are listed in alphabetical order. The references are not numbered. For the number system, references are numbered in the order in which each reference is first cited in the text. If a reference appears only in a table or a figure legend, the reference is numbered according to where the table or figure is first cited in the paper. In some journals that use numbers in the text, the references in the list are alphabetized and then numbered.

Style of References in the Reference List

Most journals maintain individual styles for their references. Reference styles vary on such details as whether titles of articles are included, whether last page numbers are included, where authors' initials are placed (before or after the last name), where the year of publication is placed (after the authors' names, after the journal title, at the end of the reference), and how items are punctuated. You should consult the journal's instructions to authors and reference lists in three or four papers of a recent issue of the journal to which you are submitting your paper to see what style the journal uses for references.

A single style for references has been adopted by a large number of journals. This style is sometimes referred to as the Vancouver style because the meeting at which the style was adopted was held in Vancouver, British Columbia. The style is described in a document called "Uniform Requirements for Manuscripts Submitted to Biomedical Journals" and is published in *Annals of Internal Medicine*, February 1988, volume 108, pp. 258–265 and in *The British Medical Journal*, 6 February 1988, volume 296, pp. 401–405. The document is updated periodically. Computer programs that put references in the Vancouver style are available.

The Vancouver style of references for journal articles is as follows:

Example 9.9   Vancouver-Style Reference

You CH, Lee KY, Chey RY, Menguy R. Electrogastrographic study of patients with unexplained nausea, bloating and vomiting. Gastroenterology 1980; 79:311–4.

The purpose of having a single style is for the convenience of authors. The journals that have adopted the Uniform Requirements will all accept papers in which the references are typed in the style prescribed. However, some journals change the references to a different style for publication.

SUMMARY OF GUIDELINES FOR REFERENCES

References give credit to the ideas and findings of others and direct readers to sources of further information.

Select the most valid, the most available, and the fewest references.

> Valid: journal articles, books, Ph.D. theses, reviewed conference proceedings.
>
> Less valid: abstracts for meetings, unreviewed conference proceedings.
>
> Available: journal articles either published or in press, books.
>
> Less available: Ph.D. theses, conference proceedings.
>
> Not available: journal articles submitted or in preparation; do not include these in the reference list; cite them in the text as personal communications or unpublished observations.
>
> For the fewest references, select the first, most important, most elegant, and most recent papers. Use review articles when possible.

References must be accurate in every detail: authors' names, authors' initials, title of the paper, title of the journal, year of publication, volume number, first and last page numbers.

Quotations must be exact.

Paraphrases must be accurate and fair.

Every reference in the text must be in the reference list, and vice versa.

When naming the authors of a paper in the text, include all authors. For papers by three or more authors, use the form "Jackson et al." and the pronoun "they" (not "he").

Put reference citations after the idea you are citing or after the authors' names if names are included.

If you draw a conclusion based on another author's findings, put the citation after the author's finding, not after your conclusion.

For several references in one sentence, cite each reference after the appropriate point rather than grouping all references at the end of the sentence.

Use either authors and years or numbers to identify references in the text, whichever the journal requests.

For more than one reference for one point, cite references in chronological order.

In the reference list, use alphabetical order when authors and years are cited in the text. Use numerical order according to first citation in the text when numbers are used for citations, unless the journal prefers alphabetical order.

Follow the journal's style for details in the reference list. If the journal has adopted the Vancouver style, use it.

■ *EXERCISE 9.1: ACCURACY OF REFERENCES*

In a list of references from a paper you are working on, a paper you have published, or a paper published by another author, verify the accuracy of each reference by checking the reference against the original journal article or a photocopy of the journal article.

Check the following information:

1. *Authors*
   a. *Are all authors included?*
   b. *Are they listed in the right order?*
   c. *Are all names spelled correctly?*
   d. *Are all the initials correct?*

2. *Title*
   a. *Is the title complete, including the subtitle if any?*
   b. *Is every word and every punctuation mark exactly the same as in the original?*

3. *Journal*
   a. *Is the journal correct?*
   b. *Is it abbreviated correctly?*

4. *Volume: Correct?*

5. *Pages: Are both the first and the last page numbers correct?*

6. *Year: Correct?*

SECTION IV

THE OVERVIEW

In Sections I–III, we saw how to choose words and arrange them in clear sentences and paragraphs (Section I), how to write each section of a biomedical research paper to tell a clear story (Section II), and how to design figures and tables and present references clearly (Section III). In Section IV, we turn our attention to providing a clear overview of the story. In Chapter 10 (The Abstract) and Chapter 11 (The Title), our central concern will be to provide the overview alone, with a bare minimum of details. In Chapter 12 (The Big Picture), we will consider how to provide the overview together with all the necessary details.

The abstract and the title provide an overview to two groups of readers. One group reads only the title or the title and the abstract. This group includes readers who have access only to sources such as *Index Medicus, Current Contents*, abstract journals, or abstracting services. The other group of readers reads not only the title and the abstract but also the paper. Therefore, just as figures and tables need to tell the story of the paper both for readers who do not read the text and for readers who do, so the abstract and the title need to tell the story both for readers who do not read either the text or the figures and tables and for readers who read the whole paper. The next two chapters explain how to write abstracts and titles that will be clear to both groups of readers. Abstracts for both results papers and methods papers are included.

In the paper as a whole, both the overview and the details need to be clear. Chapter 12 illustrates how to provide a clear overview in addition to presenting all the necessary details.

CHAPTER 10

THE ABSTRACT

FUNCTION

The function of the abstract of a scientific research paper is to provide an overview of the paper. The overview should present the main story and a few essential details of the paper for readers who read only the abstract and should serve as both a clear preview and a clear, accurate recapitulation of the main story for readers who read the paper. Thus, the abstract should make sense both when read alone and when read with the paper.

The abstract should be neither vague and general on the one hand nor fussily detailed on the other. Rather, it should be specific and selective. As its name suggests, an abstract (*ab*, out + *trahere*, to pull) should select (pull out) the highlights from each section of the paper.

Sometimes the overview in the abstract is clearer than the overview in the text. The reason is usually either that part of the overview is omitted in the text or that the details in the text obscure the overview. Although the author should make every effort to weave a clear overview into the text so that the text does not become all trees and no forest, an advantage of having a clear, concise overview in the abstract is that it can compensate for some lapses in the overview in the text.

ABSTRACTS OF RESULTS PAPERS

Content

The abstract of a results paper should state concisely the question that was asked, what was done to answer the question, what was found that answers the question, and the answer to the question. In addition, the abstract may begin with a sentence or two of background information to help the reader understand the question and may end with a sentence stating an implication of the answer or a speculation based on the answer. Because the abstract must make sense when read alone, as well as when read in conjunction with the paper, the abstract should not include citations of the scientific literature or citations of figures or tables.

Question

State the question you asked. If you asked more than one question, you may not be able to include in the abstract all the questions you asked. In this case, state only the most important question(s) in the abstract.

What Was Done

Name the species or population and the material you studied. If necessary, include the condition of the animals or subjects, such as anesthetized.

State the experimental approach or the protocol. Include both the independent and the dependent variables. Mention only important details of materials and methods.

What Was Found

Include only results that answer the question. Give data, if at all, only for the most important results. Give percent change rather than exact data when possible. Do not include figures or tables.

Answer

State the answer to the question. Be sure that the answer answers the question you asked. Do not write vague statements such as "The causes of this response are discussed."

Background

If readers would wonder why you are asking your question, begin the abstract with a sentence or two of background information. The background information should be the same as that given at the beginning of the Introduction, only briefer.

Implication or Speculation

If part or all of the importance of your paper is the implication of the answer or a speculation based on the answer, include a sentence stating the implication or speculation at the end of the abstract, as in Example 10.1.

Example 10.1

^{A}Background

^{B_1}Question

^{B_2,} ^{C}What was done

^{D,} ^{E}What was found

^{F}Answer

^{G}Implication

^{A}In patients with heart disease, left ventricular diastolic performance is evaluated clinically by inserting a Swan-Ganz catheter to measure pulmonary capillary wedge pressure as an estimate of left atrial pressure. ^{B_1}To determine whether pulmonary venous flow and mitral inflow assessed less invasively, by transesophageal pulsed Doppler echocardiography, accurately estimate mean left atrial pressure, ^{B_2}we prospectively studied 27 consecutive patients undergoing cardiovascular surgery. ^{C}We correlated Doppler variables of pulmonary venous flow and mitral inflow with simultaneously measured mean left atrial pressure and changes in pressure assessed by left atrial or pulmonary artery catheters. ^{D}We found that the most strongly correlated pulmonary venous flow variable, the systolic fraction of pulmonary venous flow, correlated more strongly with mean left atrial pressure ($r = -0.86$) than did the most strongly correlated mitral inflow variable, the ratio of peak early diastolic to peak late diastolic mitral flow velocity ($r = 0.75$). ^{E}Similarly, changes in the systolic fraction of pulmonary venous flow correlated more strongly with changes in mean left atrial pressures ($r = -0.79$) than did changes in the ratio of peak early diastolic to peak late diastolic mitral inflow velocity ($r = 0.65$). ^{F}We conclude that pulmonary venous flow assessed by transesophageal pulsed Doppler echocardiography accurately estimates mean left atrial pressure. ^{G}We suggest that this technique may offer a relatively noninvasive means of estimating mean left atrial pressure in patients with heart disease.

In this abstract, sentence A gives background information, B_1 states the question, and B_2 and C state what was done to answer the question [the prospective design and the population (B_2) and the experimental approach (C)]. Sentences D and E state what was found. Minimal data are given. The answer, stated in the second-to-last sentence (F), answers the question asked in B_1. A clinical implication that relates to the patients described at the beginning of the abstract is stated at the end of the abstract (G).

Organization

Overall Organization

The overall organization of the abstract is the same as the organization of the text: background (if any), question, what was done, what was found, answer, implication or speculation (if any). However, the abstract is often streamlined in one way: often only the species or the population, their condition, the material, and maybe a brief overview of the experimental approach are given in the statement of what was done. The details of what was done—specific independent and dependent variables, doses, methods—are given in the sentences that tell what was found. This organizational strategy avoids repetition (see Example 10.2 below).

Although the overall organization of the abstract follows the organization of the paper, the abstract does not give equal weight to all sections of the paper. The abstract includes much of the Introduction (background, the question, experimental approach, species or population, their condition, material) but only a few details from methods (specific independent and dependent variables, doses, methods), only key results and key data from Results, figures, and tables, and only the answer and maybe an implication or a speculation from the Discussion.

Organization of Results

If you include two or more results in your abstract, arrange them in a logical order, such as most to least important or least to most important. When organizing from most to least important, describe control results last, if you include them at all.

Example 10.2

A_1 *Question*

A_2 *What was done*

B–E What was found

F Answer

A_1To determine whether lesions of the nucleus tractus solitarium alter pulmonary artery pressures and pulmonary lymph flow without altering the systemic circulation, A_2we measured pressures and lymph flow in 6 halothane-anesthetized sheep in which we created lesions of the nucleus by bilateral thermocoagulation. BWe found that pulmonary artery pressure rose to 150% of baseline and remained elevated for the 3-h duration of the experiment. CPulmonary lymph flow doubled within 2 h. DSystemic and left atrial pressures did not change. ESham nucleus tractus solitarium lesions and lesions lateral to the nucleus produced no changes. FThese experiments demonstrate that lesions of the nucleus tractus solitarium alter pulmonary artery pressures and pulmonary lymph flow independently of the effects on the systemic circulation.

In this abstract, the question is stated at the beginning of the first sentence (A_1) and is followed by a statement of what was done (dependent variables measured, sample size, species, their condition, and how the independent variable was created) at the end of the sentence (A_2). To streamline the abstract, other details of what was done are included in the statements of what was found. Thus, the duration of the experiment (3 h) and the specific dependent variables of the systemic circulation (systemic and left atrial pressures) are mentioned only when the results are given (sentences B and D). Similarly, the control maneuvers are mentioned only at the beginning of the sentence stating control results (E). Results are reported in a logical order (most to least important): experimental results first (B–D) and control results last (E). In addition, variables that changed (B, C) are reported before variables that did not change (D)—also a logical order. Note also that the details of what was found are in the same order as the details in the question: first pulmonary artery pressures, next pulmonary lymph flow, and last systemic circulatory variables. Data are given as a percentage ["150% of baseline" (B)] and as a proportion ["doubled" (C)] rather than as exact values. The answer is stated in the last sentence (F) and answers the question as it was asked (using the same key terms, the same verb, and the same point of view).

Writing

Continuity

To provide clear continuity throughout the abstract, repeat key terms, use the same order for details, keep the same point of view in the question and the answer, and use either parallel form or consistent point of view for comparisons and other parallel ideas (see Example 10.3 below).

Signaling Topics

Abstracts are conventionally written as one paragraph. Therefore, it helps the reader if you signal the parts of an abstract for a results paper both visually, by starting a new sentence, and verbally, by stating the topic at the beginning of the sentence. Thus, begin a new sentence for the question, for what was found, and also for the answer. Signal what was found by "We found that" or something similar. Signal the answer by "We conclude that" or "Thus" or something similar. The question and what was done can usually be in one sentence, for example, "To determine X, we. . . ." However, if the sentence gets too long, you can state the question and what was done in separate sentences. Possible signals of the question and of what was done are "We asked whether. . ." (question) and "To answer this question, we. . ." (what was done) (as in Revision B of Example 10.7 below).

If your abstract includes an implication, be careful to distinguish between the answer and the implication by using clear signals and appropriate verbs. For answers, in addition to the signals "We conclude that" and "Thus," you can use "These findings show that," "These results indicate that," or "Therefore." Use a definite verb in the answer. For example, "We conclude that X causes Y" ("we conclude that" is the signal of the answer and "causes" is a definite verb). For implications, use signals such as "These results suggest that" or "We suggest that" followed by a hedged verb. For example, "These results suggest that X may play a role in Y" ("these results suggest that" is the signal of the implication and "may play" is a hedged verb). For the clearest

THE ABSTRACT **261**

distinction between answers and implications, also put them in separate sentences (as in Example 10.1 above).

Some journals do not permit "we" in the abstract. In these journals, signals for the question, what was done, and what was found are problematic. Possible signals are as follows. Question and what was done: "To determine Q, X was injected into Z and Y was assessed" (that is, use passive voice to describe what you did). Question alone: "This study asks whether. . . ." What was done alone: "To answer this question, X was injected into Z and Y was assessed" or "For this study, X was injected into Z and Y was assessed" (passive). What was found: "The findings were that. . ." (but not "The findings show that. . .," which is a signal of the answer). Answer: "Thus," "Therefore," or "This study shows that. . . ." Implication: "These results suggest that. . . ." Some of these signals are long and cumbersome, but they are the best you can do when you cannot use "we."

Verb Tense

Verb tenses in the abstract should be the same as those in the paper: present tense for the question and the answer; past tense for what was done and what was found.

Sentence Structure

Write short sentences. Avoid noun clusters. If your technical terms are composed of several words, as in Example 10.1 above, writing short sentences may be difficult.

Word Choice

Use simple words. For the sake of foreign readers and readers who work in other fields, avoid jargon.

Abbreviations

Avoid abbreviations wherever possible. You should use standard abbreviations for units of measurement (International System abbreviations), and you can use standard, widely accepted abbreviations such as DNA. But semistandard and nonstandard abbreviations make reading a chore and should therefore be avoided. If you must use a nonstandard abbreviation that is not widely accepted, define it the first time you use it in the abstract, for example, "glutamate pyruvate transferase (GPT)." Some specialty journals permit abbreviations that are standard in their specialty to be used without definition in the abstract and in the paper. This practice makes reading difficult for newcomers to the specialty.

For those who like numerical guidelines, one abbreviation (other than a unit of measurement) is no problem, two abbreviations are OK, three are borderline. Reading becomes geometrically more difficult after that. If you cannot avoid abbreviations altogether, try to have only one abbreviation in an abstract and certainly no more than three.

Length

Most journals limit the length of the abstract (usually to 250 words or less). "Uniform Requirements for Manuscripts Submitted to Biomedical Journals" (see Literature Cited) specifies 150 words or less. If no limit is stated, make your abstract no longer than the abstracts in recent issues of the journal.

Do not include unimportant details or unnecessary words just to fill up space. If you can summarize your paper in fewer words than the maximum allowed, do so.

If you are tempted to add more and more detail, keep in mind that the abstract will become more and more unreadable; the trees will overshadow the forest. That is the exact opposite of what you want. The overview is easiest to see in a short abstract, so keep your abstract short. In no case should your abstract be more than 250 words, even if the journal publishes longer abstracts.

In your effort to keep the abstract short, do not write in the style of a telegram; that is, do not omit necessary "a's," "an's," and "the's."

Example 10.3

A₁ Question

A₂, B What was done (details)

C–E What was found

F Answer

A₁ To determine whether 4 drugs used in the treatment of asthma inhibit the toluene diisocyanate-induced late asthmatic reaction and the associated increase in airway responsiveness to methacholine, *A₂* we assessed these variables in 24 sensitized subjects divided into 4 groups of 6 subjects each. *B* Either slow-release verapamil (120 mg twice a day), cromolyn (20 mg 4 times a day via spinhaler), slow-release theophylline (6.5 mg/kg twice a day), or beclomethasone aerosol (1 mg twice a day) was administered for 7 days, each to one of the 4 groups, according to a double-blind, crossover, placebo-controlled study design. *C* We found that neither placebo, verapamil, nor cromolyn inhibited the large increase in forced expiratory volume in the first second (FEV_1) or the increase in airway responsiveness to methacholine after exposure to toluene. *D* Slow-release theophylline partially inhibited the increase in FEV_1 but had no effect on airway responsiveness to methacholine. *E* Beclomethasone inhibited both variables. *F* Thus, only the high-dose inhaled steroid beclomethasone effectively inhibits toluene diisocyanate-induced late asthmatic reactions and the associated increases in airway responsiveness to methacholine.

This abstract follows the guidelines for content and organization of abstracts. Note that results (C–E) are presented in the order of least to most effective (least to most important). Thus, either the order of most to least important, as in Example 10.2, or the order of least to most important, as in Example 10.3, can be used for results.

This abstract also follows most of the guidelines for writing. Continuity is strong because of repetition of key terms (inhibit, verapamil, cromolyn, theophylline, beclomethasone, toluene, late asthmatic reaction, increase in airway responsiveness to methacholine, FEV_1), consistent order of the drugs in what was done (B) and what was found (C–E), and consistent point of view for what was found (C–E).

What was found is signaled by "We found that" at the beginning of a new sentence. The answer is signaled by "Thus" at the beginning of a new sentence.

Verb tenses are appropriate: present tense for the question ("inhibit") and the answer ("inhibits"); past tense for what was done ("assessed," "was administered") and what was found ("inhibited," "inhibited," "had," "inhibited").

Word choice is as simple as possible. Only one abbreviation is used (FEV_1). Although it is a standard abbreviation in respiratory physiology, it is defined.

The abstract is reasonably short (181 words) and the overview is clear.

However, the sentences, especially sentences A and B, are rather long (A, 44 words; B, 57 words; mean, 30.2 words per sentence). One way to shorten the sentences (and the abstract) slightly without omitting any information is to condense the sentence that states what was done (B) and name the drugs and the doses only in the sentences that state results, as in the revision.

Revision

A_1 *Question*

A_2, B *What was done (overview)*

C–E *What was found*

F *Answer*

A_1To determine whether 4 drugs used in the treatment of asthma inhibit the toluene diisocyanate-induced late asthmatic reaction and the associated increase in airway responsiveness to methacholine, A_2we assessed these variables in 24 sensitized subjects divided into 4 groups of 6 subjects each. BSubjects in each group received one drug for 7 days according to a double-blind, crossover, placebo-controlled study design. CWe found that neither placebo, slow-release verapamil (120 mg twice a day), nor cromolyn (20 mg 4 times a day via spinhaler) inhibited the large increase in forced expiratory volume in the first second (FEV_1) or the increase in airway responsiveness to methacholine after exposure to toluene. DSlow-release theophylline (6.5 mg/kg twice a day) partially inhibited the increase in FEV_1 but had no effect on airway responsiveness to methacholine. EBeclomethasone aerosol (1 mg twice a day) inhibited both variables. FThus, only the high-dose inhaled steroid beclomethasone effectively inhibits toluene diisocyanate-induced late asthmatic reactions and the associated increases in airway responsiveness to methacholine.

Putting the details of what was done in what was found shortens the abstract by 10 words (171 vs. 181). It also shortens sentence B considerably (20 vs. 57 words) and thus makes the overview of what was done clearer. Although sentence C is now longer (48 vs. 33 words), mean sentence length is shorter (28.5 vs. 30.2 words per sentence).

Common Problems in Abstracts of Results Papers

Deviations From the Standard Form

Deviations from the standard form of the abstract for results papers obscure the overview we expect to get when we read an abstract. Typical deviations include omitting the question, stating the question only vaguely, and stating an implication instead of an answer.

Question Omitted. If the question is omitted, we read the abstract blindly, with little or no understanding of the purpose of the maneuvers and the measurements or of the possible meaning of the results. We understand the abstract only at the end and then have to reread it to fit the details into the picture.

Example 10.4

A–E *What was done*

F, G *What was found*

ASeventy-two rabbits were separated into groups to receive either verapamil in 1 of 3 doses, subcutaneous verapamil, other drugs (metoprolol, hydralazine, or both), or no drug daily for 10 weeks. BThe rabbits also received a high-cholesterol diet. CSerum concentrations of verapamil, cholesterol, and triglycerides were measured twice during the the study. DBlood pressure, heart rate, and weight were measured every 2 weeks. EThe percent of the aorta covered by atheromatous plaque was assessed at the end of the study. FWe found that in the 60% of the rabbits given oral verapamil that had detectable serum concentrations of this drug, the percent of the aorta covered by atheromatous plaque was much less than in any other group (27% vs. 50–77%) even though cholesterol concentrations were higher. GHowever, blood

H Answer

pressure in rabbits given oral verapamil was no different from that of other groups. *H*Thus, protection from atherosclerosis by verapamil in the cholesterol-fed rabbit is not the result of lowering of blood pressure.

In this abstract, we get a clear idea of "what was done, what was found, what was concluded," which is one idea of what the standard form of an abstract is. But we do not have a sense from the beginning of what the question was, and therefore we do not know why verapamil and the other drugs were given, why the rabbits received a high-cholesterol diet, or why cholesterol, triglycerides, blood pressure, heart rate, weight, and atheromatous plaque were measured. Not until sentence E does the word "atheromatous" appear, and not until the last sentence of the abstract do we see the point of what was done and what was found. Reading this abstract is like being led through a maze without having any idea of where we are going. This is not a comfortable feeling. To enlighten the reader from the beginning, state the question at the beginning of the abstract, and think of the structure of the abstract not as "what was done, what was found, what was concluded," but as "question, what was done, what was found, answer."

Revision

A₁ Question

A₂-E What was done

F, G What was found

H Answer

*A₁*To determine whether lowering blood pressure is the mechanism by which verapamil provides protection from atherosclerosis in rabbits fed cholesterol, *A₂*we separated 72 rabbits into groups to receive either verapamil in 1 of 3 doses, subcutaneous verapamil, other drugs (metoprolol, hydralazine, or both), or no drug daily for 10 weeks. *B*The rabbits also received a high cholesterol diet. *C*Serum concentrations of verapamil, cholesterol, and triglycerides were measured twice during the study. *D*Blood pressure, heart rate, and weight were measured every 2 weeks. *E*The percent of the aorta covered by atheromatous plaque was assessed at the end of the study. *F*We found that in the 60% of the rabbits given oral verapamil that had detectable serum concentrations of this drug, the percent of the aorta covered by atheromatous plaque was much less than in any other group (27% vs. 50–77%) even though cholesterol concentrations were higher. *G*However, blood pressure in rabbits given oral verapamil was no different from that of other groups. *H*Thus, lowering blood pressure is not the mechanism by which verapamil protects cholesterol-fed rabbits from atherosclerosis.

In this revision, adding the question clarifies from the beginning why verapamil was given, why the rabbits were fed a high-cholesterol diet, and why cholesterol, blood pressure, and atheromatous plaque were measured. The other details included are not explained. They are indirectly related to the question: the other drugs are used for comparison, triglycerides are the other serum lipid besides cholesterol, large changes in heart rate could have secondary effects on atherosclerosis, and weight indicates whether the rabbits were eating and thus getting cholesterol. For greatest clarity, these secondary details should either be explained or omitted from the abstract. Note that the answer has been rewritten to make the point of view the same in the question and the answer.

Stating the Question Vaguely.   A second deviation from the standard form of the abstract is stating the question vaguely. In a question stated vaguely, only the dependent variable is named, for example "Y was studied." But for questions that have both an independent and a dependent variable, the independent variable must also be included in the question. For questions that have only a dependent variable, the specific aspect of the dependent variable studied must be named. To ensure that the question is specific, check it against the answer: use the same key terms for the independent variable (if any) and the dependent variable. Also, keep the same point of view. It is not absolutely necessary to use a verb to state the question. For example, the question can be in the form "to determine the effects of X on Y in Z." But for a more specific question that anticipates the answer, use a verb in the question—the same verb as in the answer. For example, if the answer is "X impairs Y in Z," the specific question is "to determine whether X impairs Y in Z," not "to determine the effects of X on Y in Z."

Example 10.5

A_1 *Vague question*
  (What was done)

A_2 *Study subjects*
B, C *What was found*

D *Comparison*

E_1 *Answer*

E_2 *Implication*

A_1 Plasma cholesterol metabolism was studied A_2 in young, nonobese, normolipidemic men who smoked moderately (24 ± 5 (SD) cigarettes/day) and in a matched nonsmoking normal control group. B In the smokers, both net transport of cholesterol from cell membranes into plasma ($P < 0.001$) and the ratio of the rate of cholesteryl ester transfer to the amount of low- and very-low-density lipoprotein ($P < 0.05$) were decreased. C In addition, apoprotein E was increased in smokers' plasma ($P < 0.05$) whereas apoprotein A-I, the major apoprotein of high-density lipoprotein, was decreased ($P < 0.05$). D This pattern of abnormalities has previously been observed in several other groups of subjects at increased risk for atherosclerotic vascular disease (diabetics, dysbetalipoproteinemics, and hyperbetalipoproteinemics). E_1 These data indicate that cigarette smoking causes abnormal metabolism of plasma cholesterol in young men, E_2 which could partly explain the high incidence of atherosclerotic vascular disease in older male smokers.

Like Example 10.4, this abstract is easy to read, and we have a clear idea of what was done, what was found, and what was concluded. But even though a question appears to be stated, we do not have a clear overview from the beginning. The reason is that the question (A_1) is stated vaguely. Only the dependent variable (plasma cholesterol metabolism) is named. The independent variable (cigarette smoking) is hidden in the description of the study subjects (A_2). Furthermore, the specific topic—abnormal metabolism—is missing. To have a specific question that anticipates the answer ("cigarette smoking causes abnormal metabolism of plasma cholesterol in young men"), the question would have to be "to determine whether cigarette smoking by young men causes abnormal metabolism of plasma cholesterol," not "plasma cholesterol metabolism was studied." Stating the question specifically, as in the revision below, prepares for the answer more clearly. Similarly, the first sentence should prepare the reader to hear the implication about atherosclerotic vascular disease in the last sentence.

Two other common flaws also appear in this abstract. One is that P values are included but no data are given. P values alone are not useful. If you want to give a quantitative idea of the data without presenting actual values such as mean and standard deviation, give percent change. If you do give a P value, also give the mean, standard deviation, and sample size (n) (see Example 10.7 below).

In addition, in the last sentence, the term "data" is used, but, as we have just seen, no data are given. "Data" in sentence E should be changed to "results" or "findings," which are generalizations based on data. (See Chap. 6: "Results and Data" under "Content.")

Revision

A_1 *Specific question*
A_2 *Implied ultimate question*
A_3 *What was done*
B, C *What was found*

^{A_1}To determine whether cigarette smoking by young men causes abnormal metabolism of plasma cholesterol ^{A_2}indicative of atherosclerotic vascular disease, ^{A_3}we compared plasma cholesterol metabolism in young, nonobese, normolipidemic men who smoked moderately (24 ± 5 (SD) cigarettes/day) with cholesterol metabolism in a matched nonsmoking normal control group. ^{B}We found that in the smokers, both net transport of cholesterol from cell membranes into plasma and the ratio of the rate of cholesteryl ester transfer to the amount of low- and very-low-density lipoprotein were decreased. ^{C}In addition, apoprotein E was increased in smokers' plasma whereas apoprotein A-I, the major apoprotein of high-density lipoprotein, was decreased. ^{D}This pattern of abnormalities has previously been observed in several other groups of subjects at increased risk for atherosclerotic vascular disease (diabetics, dysbetalipoproteinemics, and hyperbetalipoproteinemics). ^{E_1}These results indicate that cigarette smoking causes abnormal metabolism of plasma cholesterol in young men, ^{E_2}which could partly explain the high incidence of atherosclerotic vascular disease in older male smokers.

D *Comparison*

E_1 *Answer*

E_2 *Implication*

In this revision, the question is made specific by adding the independent variable ("cigarette smoking"), the specific topic ("abnormal metabolism of plasma cholesterol"), and the verb "causes." In addition to these specific details, the first sentence includes "indicative of atherosclerotic vascular disease," which implies the ultimate question behind the question asked in this paper and thus prepares for the implication stated after the answer (sentence E_2). Finally, *P* values are omitted and "data" is changed to "results" (E_1).

Some people may prefer to state the question more generally ("To determine the effect of cigarette smoking by young men on the metabolism of plasma cholesterol") because it is more objective sounding. But if you really suspected that cigarette smoking might cause abnormal metabolism of cholesterol, you should state the question specifically. Although a general question is better than a vague question, a specific question is best, because a specific question prepares the reader for the specific answer.

Answer Not Stated.   A third deviation from the standard form of the abstract is that even though the question is stated, the answer is not. Instead an implication is stated. Considering that the function of the abstract is to provide an overview of the story and that the answer is the culmination of the story, not stating the answer undermines the abstract. Furthermore, most readers do not realize that the answer is missing, so they could be confused without knowing it. For a clear abstract that has an unmistakable message, the answer must be stated (and clearly signaled).

Example 10.6

A *Background*
B_1 *Question*

B_2 *What was done*

C *What was found*

D *Implication*

^{A}Digestion of low-density lipoprotein in vitro by the specific endoprotease kallikrein produces two fragments from B-100: K_1 and K_2. ^{B_1}To determine whether these fragments arise from the same point of cleavage as the naturally occurring fragments of B-100, B-74 and B-26, ^{B_2}we used kallikrein to digest low-density lipoprotein from human plasma and compared the resulting fragments, K_1 and K_2, with B-74 and B-26. ^{C}We found that not only the molecular weight and the stoichiometry but also the amino terminal amino acid sequence in K_1 and K_2 precisely matched those in B-74 and B-26. ^{D}These findings strongly suggest that kallikrein is the agent responsible for the formation of B-74 and B-26 in human low-density lipoprotein.

In this abstract, we see the overview from the beginning and can easily follow the story until the last sentence. Although the abstract ends by stating a closely related implication of the findings, that is not what we were expecting. We were expecting the answer to the question. The implication can be added after the answer, but it should not be stated instead of the answer.

Revision

A Background
B₁ Question

B₂ What was done

C What was found

D Answer

E Implication

A Digestion of low-density lipoprotein in vitro by the specific endoprotease kallikrein produces two fragments from B-100: K_1 and K_2. *B₁* To determine whether these fragments arise from the same point of cleavage as the naturally occurring fragments of B-100, B-74 and B-26, *B₂* we used kallikrein to digest low-density lipoprotein from human plasma and compared the resulting fragments, K_1 and K_2, with B-74 and B-26. *C* We found that not only the molecular weight and the stoichiometry but also the amino terminal amino acid sequence in K_1 and K_2 precisely matched those in B-74 and B-26. *D* We conclude that fragments K_1 and K_2 arise from the same point of cleavage as the naturally occurring fragments B-74 and B-26. *E* These findings strongly suggest that kallikrein is the agent responsible for the formation of B-74 and B-26 in human low-density lipoprotein.

In the revision, the answer has been added (D), thus making the story complete and clear. In addition, because the answer uses the same key terms, the same point of view, and the same verb as in the question, it is easy to see that the answer answers the question asked. Furthermore, the answer is a missing step in the logic. Once the answer is stated, it is easier to understand the implication.

In summary, to ensure that your abstract provides a clear overview (1) state the question you asked, (2) make the statement of the question specific rather than vague or general (name both the independent and the dependent variables, using the same key terms and the same point of view as in the answer, and, to anticipate the answer, use a verb in the question—the same verb as in the answer), and (3) state the answer to the question, making sure that the answer answers the question asked.

Excessive Length

Another common problem in abstracts for results papers is excessive length. Although many journals request abstracts no longer than 250 words, and other journals have shorter limits, many published abstracts are well over 250 words. Even those that are less than 250 words may be longer than necessary. Example 10.7 is a clearly written abstract, but at 271 words it is 121 words longer than what the journal requested.

Example 10.7   *(271 words)*

A, B Background

C₁ Question

C₂–E What was done

A Delayed closure of the ductus arteriosus after birth has been observed in newborn infants who have critical pulmonic stenosis and in newborn lambs that have experimental pulmonic stenosis. *B* This delayed ductal closure may be caused by decreased ability of the muscle to contract when exposed to oxygen or by increased production of or sensitivity to prostaglandin E_2 (PGE_2), the endogenous ductus arteriosus vasodilator. *C₁* To determine the cause of the delayed ductal closure in fetal lambs that have experimental pulmonic stenosis, *C₂* we operated on 10 fetal lambs of gestational ages 70 to 77 days (term is 148 days) and placed a band around the pulmonary artery. *D* Catheterization at

*F–H*What was found

137 to 142 days showed severe pulmonic stenosis. *E*We then studied isolated rings of ductus arteriosus from these lambs. *F*We found that the oxygen-induced increase in muscle tension was significantly less in rings of ductus arteriosus from 10 lambs with pulmonic stenosis than in rings from 6 control lambs (2.55 ± 0.38 vs. 4.03 ± 0.51 g/mm^2, $P < 0.03$). *G*There was no difference between the two groups either in the amount of PGE$_2$ released by the rings or in the sensitivity (expressed as median effective dose) of the rings to PGE$_2$.

*I*Answer

*H*There was also no difference in the increase in tension when endogenous PGE$_2$ was inhibited by indomethacin. *I*We conclude that delayed closure of the ductus arteriosus in fetal lambs that have experimental pulmonic stenosis is not caused by increased production of or sensitivity to PGE$_2$ in the ductus arteriosus (as it is in premature lambs) but rather is the result of decreased ability of the ductus arteriosus to contract when exposed to oxygen.

The revision below cuts 92 words from the original version, thus more nearly approaching the requested length of 150 words. The revision retains the essential information and omits less important details. Specifically,

> The two sentences of background (A and B of the original version) are condensed into a single sentence (A of the revision).
> The definition of prostaglandin E$_2$ as a vasodilator (end of B) is omitted (A).
> Experimental preparation for the independent variable (C$_2$, D) is omitted and sentences C–E are combined into a single sentence that states the question and the experimental approach for the independent and dependent variables (B).
> Data (F) are omitted; instead percent change is given (C).
> The statement of how sensitivity to PGE$_2$ is expressed (G) is omitted (D).
> Confirmatory results (H) are omitted.
> The negative conclusion and the comparison with premature lambs (I) are omitted.

Revision A   (179 words)

*A*Background

*B₁*Question
*B₂*What was done

*C, D*What was found

*E*Answer

*A*Delayed closure of the ductus arteriosus in newborn infants who have critical pulmonic stenosis may be caused by decreased ability of the muscle to contract when exposed to oxygen or by increased production of or sensitivity to prostaglandin E$_2$ (PGE$_2$). *B₁*To determine the cause of delayed ductal closure in fetal lambs that have experimental pulmonic stenosis, *B₂*we induced pulmonic stenosis in 10 fetal lambs at ages 70–77 days (term is 148 days) and then, at 137–142 days, studied isolated rings of ductus arteriosus from these lambs. *C*We found that the oxygen-induced increase in muscle tension in rings of ductus arteriosus from 10 lambs with pulmonic stenosis was only 65% of that in rings from 6 control lambs. *D*There was no difference between the two groups either in the amount of PGE$_2$ released by the rings or in the sensitivity of the rings to PGE$_2$. *E*We conclude that delayed closure of the ductus arteriosus in fetal lambs that have experimental pulmonic stenosis is caused by decreased ability of the ductus arteriosus to contract when exposed to oxygen.

Even though the original, longer abstract is quite readable, the shorter revision gets the overview across more clearly. Thus, for the clearest overview, condense long abstracts. To condense a long abstract, in addition to omitting unnecessary words, condense background and omit less important information, such as definitions, experimental preparation, details of methods, exact data, confirmatory results, and comparisons with previous results.

To condense this abstract further, to the requested length of 150 words, you have to omit some important information. Revision B omits the background statement (A) entirely, thus losing the relation of the study to human illness, and also omits the length of term (B_2). In addition, Revision B changes "rings of ductus arteriosus" to "ductal rings" in the statements of what was done and what was found, makes sentence D active, changes "sensitivity of the rings" to "rings' sensitivity," changes "we conclude that" to "thus," and uses "results from" instead of "is caused by" in the question and answer.

Revision B   (151 words)

A Question

B What was done

C, D What was found

E Answer

^{A}We asked whether delayed closure of the ductus arteriosus in fetal lambs that have experimental pulmonic stenosis results from decreased ability of the muscle to contract when exposed to oxygen or from increased production of or sensitivity to prostaglandin E_2 (PGE_2). ^{B}To answer this question, we induced pulmonic stenosis in 10 fetal lambs at ages 70–77 days and then, at 137–142 days, studied isolated ductal rings from these lambs. ^{C}We found that the oxygen-induced increase in muscle tension in ductal rings from 10 lambs with pulmonic stenosis was only 65% of that in rings from 6 control lambs. ^{D}Neither the amount of PGE_2 released by the rings nor the rings' sensitivity to PGE_2 differed between the two groups. ^{E}Thus, delayed closure of the ductus arteriosus in fetal lambs that have experimental pulmonic stenosis results from decreased ability of the ductus arteriosus to contract when exposed to oxygen.

Note on Using Abbreviations.   The solution to condensing this abstract was not to use abbreviations instead of words. Using abbreviations makes reading more difficult for most readers, the difficulty increasing geometrically for each new abbreviation used. For an example, see the last example in Exercise 1.1 in Chapter 1.

Note on Counting Words.   Count every word. For example, in sentence D of Example 10.7, "catheterization" counts as one word and "at" counts as one word. Count abbreviations as one word. Thus, "PGE_2" is one word and "vs." is one word. For numbers and units of measurement, count each number as one word and each abbreviation as one word: "255" is one word, "0.38" is one word, "g" is one word, and "mm^2" is one word. For P values, count P as one word and the number (here 0.03) as one word. Do not count $\pm$, $<$, /, or similar symbols.

Excessive Detail

A similar but more serious problem than excessive length in an abstract is excessive detail. The difference between an excessively long abstract and an excessively detailed abstract is that an excessively long abstract is readable but an excessively detailed abstract is not. The details ("trees"), such as long lists of variables, numerous data, several P values, and repetition of statistical terms, such as "significantly" and "mean $\pm$ SD," obscure the overview (forest). The solution is to omit almost all the detail. Use category terms instead of listing all the variables; report data only for the most important results, or give percent change instead of exact data; omit P values; omit "significantly"; use "(mean $\pm$ SD)" only once. Include only enough detail to show that your study was well designed and that your evidence is strong. Omit other details so that the trees do not overshadow the forest.

Exceptions

Some journals request a form different from the one described above for abstracts of results papers. Follow the form requested by the journal. For example, *Science* requests abstracts that "include a sentence or two explaining to the general reader why the research was undertaken and why the results should be viewed as important. The abstract should convey the main point of the paper and outline the results or conclusions." Thus, the question, results or conclusions, and their importance are emphasized, methods are minimized, and data are omitted. The abstracts are often quite short and easy to read. Example 10.8 below from *Science* follows this form.

Example 10.8

A Implied question
B Importance

C_1 What was done
C_2 What was found

A The existence of spontaneous neural activity in mammalian retinal ganglion cells during prenatal life has long been suspected. B This activity could play a key role in the refinement of retinal projections during development. C_1 Recordings in vivo from the retinas of rat fetuses between embryonic days 17 and 21 C_2 found action potentials in spontaneously active ganglion cells at all the ages studied.

Annals of Internal Medicine requests a specific structured form for abstracts of structured studies. Rather than having a single paragraph, these abstracts contain a sequence of short paragraphs, each preceded by a subheading. Some paragraphs contain phrases rather than sentences (see "Study Objective," "Design," and "Setting" in Example 10.9 below). Although these abstracts tend to be longer than single-paragraph abstracts, they are clear, and each type of information is easy to find.

Example 10.9

Study Objective: To determine the association between current use of non-aspirin nonsteroidal anti-inflammatory drugs and fatal peptic ulcers or upper gastrointestinal hemorrhage in the elderly.

Design: Nested case control study using a linked Medicaid-death certificate database.

Setting: Tennessee Medicaid enrollees aged 60 and greater from 1976 to 1984.

Patients: One hundred twenty-two patients ("the cases") had a terminal hospitalization and a peptic ulcer or upper gastrointestinal hemorrhage confirmed by hospital chart review. Population controls ($n = 3897$) were matched to potential cases by age, sex, race, calendar year, and nursing home status.

Measurements and Main Results: The 122 patients ("cases") more frequently filled a prescription for a non-aspirin nonsteroidal anti-inflammatory drug within 30 days before onset of illness than did controls (34% vs. 11%; adjusted odds ratio, 4.7; 95% CI, 3.1 to 7.2). This association between current use of nonaspirin nonsteroidal anti-inflammatory drugs and fatal peptic ulcer disease was consistent in three age groups, women and men, whites and non-whites, and community and nursing home dwellers. There was no significant association between case status and previous use of nonaspirin nonsteroidal anti-inflammatory drugs (adjusted odds ratio, 1.9; 95% CI, 0.7 to 4.7).

Conclusions: The findings of this study add to the growing evidence that nonaspirin nonsteroidal anti-inflammatory drugs can increase the risk for clinically serious peptic ulcer disease in the elderly.

ABSTRACTS OF METHODS PAPERS

Content

Methods papers are papers that describe new or improved methods, apparatus, or materials.

The abstract of a methods paper should include the following information: the name or the category term of the method, apparatus, or material; the purpose; the species or population; the key features of the apparatus or material or how the method or apparatus works, or both; the advantages; how the method, apparatus, or material was tested; and how well it works.

Name

If the method, apparatus, or material has a name, use the name in the abstract. Otherwise, use a category term such as "method" or "apparatus," or, if possible, add an adjective that states a key feature of the method before the category term. For example, instead of "a system for measuring oxygen consumption continuously in fetal sheep has been developed" ("system" is a category term), the authors wrote "a *microcomputer-based* system for measuring oxygen consumption continuously in fetal sheep has been developed." The adjective "microcomputer-based" indicates a key feature of the system, thus giving a clearer idea of what the system is than would the category term "system" alone.

In addition to naming the method or stating its category, you can indicate that a method is an improved version of an existing method by adding "improved" before the name or the category term. It is not usually necessary to indicate that a method is new, but it is OK to do so.

Purpose

The purpose is usually stated in the verb form "for doing X," though "to do X" may also be used. In the example above, the purpose is stated in the form "for doing X": "a microcomputer-based system *for measuring* oxygen consumption continuously in fetal sheep."

Species

The species or population that the method, apparatus, or material applies to should be included unless the species is either all humans or humans and other species. In the example above, the species is stated—fetal sheep.

Key Features and How the Method Works

Key features of the apparatus or the material, how the method or apparatus works, or both are included to give the reader an idea of what the method, apparatus, or material is.

Advantages

Advantages are included to convince the reader that a new method is a good one or that an improved method is better than existing methods. The advantages of an improved method should solve the problems of the existing methods. Stating the advantages is important so that the reader knows why the method is needed.

How It Was Tested and How Well It Works

How the method was tested and how well it works are included to convince the reader that the method is reliable, accurate, or whatever.

Organization

The information in an abstract for a methods paper should be organized essentially in the order just stated (see Example 10.11 below). Specifically, the abstract should always begin with the name of the method followed by its purpose and the species and then by its key features or how it works. However, the order of the final three items (advantages, how the method was tested, how well it works) may be changed if necessary (see Example 10.10).

More than one kind of information can be included in one sentence. Specifically, the name of the method, its purpose, and the species are virtually always in one sentence, and how the method was tested and how well it works are often in one sentence (see Examples 10.10 and 10.11).

Verb Tense

In the sentence that names the method, the verb is in past tense (actually, present perfect tense) or present tense, depending on the verb used. For example, "An improved method *has been developed*" (done in the past, so past tense) or "An improved method *is described*" (still true, so present tense). Verbs in sentences that describe the method and its advantages are in present tense. For example, "The system *includes* . . ."; "The method *cuts* short and *simplifies* the conventional procedure . . ."; "Additional advantages of the method *are*. . . ." Verbs in sentences telling how the method was tested and how well it works are in past tense. For example, "the flowmeter accurately *measured* a wide range of tidal volumes."

Writing

Principles for continuity, sentence structure, word choice, abbreviations, and length in abstracts for methods papers are the same as those for results papers.

Example 10.10

A_1 *Name*
A_2 *Purpose*
A_3 *How it works*
B *Advantages*
C_1 *How it was tested*
C_2 *How well it works*
D, E *Advantages*

A_1 An improved method has been developed A_2 for isolating alveolar type II cells A_3 by digesting lung tissue with elastase and "panning" the resultant cell suspension on plates coated with IgG. B This method provides both high yield and high purity of type II cells. C_1 In 50 experiments in rats, C_2 we obtained 35 ± 11 (SD) $\times 10^6$ cells/rat, $89 \pm 4\%$ of which were type II cells. D In addition, type II cells isolated by "panning" adhere more rapidly and completely in tissue culture than do cells isolated by centrifugation over discontinuous density gradients of metrizamide. E Finally, the method is reproducible and easily adapted to isolating type II cells for species other than rats.

This abstract begins by using a category term ("method") to identify the method and describes it as improved (A_1). Next the purpose is stated (A_2) followed by a concise description of how the method works (A_3). All of this information is in one sentence. The species is not stated because although the study was done in rats (see sentence C), the method also applies to humans and other species (see sentence E). Sentence B states two advantages of this method (high yield and high purity). Sentence C tells how the method was tested (C_1) and then gives data that support the high yield and the high purity, thus indicating how well the method works (C_2). Sentence D states two advantages over another method, thus supporting the claim that the method is an improvement (A_1). Sentence E states two final advantages.

Continuity is clear because key terms are repeated ("method" in A, B, and E; "panning" in A and D; "type II cells" in A, B, C, D, and E) and because transition words are used ("in addition," "finally"). The sentences are short (mean, 22 words per sentence). Words are as simple as possible, and only one abbreviation is used—IgG (immunoglobulin G). It is not defined because it is considered a standard abbreviation. The abstract is short (110 words) and the overview is clear.

Example 10.11

A_1 *Name*
A_2 *Purpose*
A_3 *Population*
B, C *Key features*

D *Advantage*

E_1 *How it was tested*
E_2 *How well it works*

A_1 We have designed a new endotracheal flowmeter A_2 to measure tidal volume, phasic and mean airway pressure, inspiratory time, and end-tidal PCO_2 and PO_2 A_3 in intubated infants. B The flowmeter is light (11 g) and adds minimal dead space (1.0 ml) and resistance (2 cm H_2O/110 ml per s) to the infant's airway. C The volume signal ($\leq$ 10 ml) is linear to 7 Hz, and end-tidal gases can be measured at respiratory rates of 90 breaths/min. D This flowmeter is particularly valuable for evaluating rapid mechanical ventilation of very-low-birth-weight infants. E_1 In 125 studies in 50 infants weighing 740–1500 g, E_2 the flowmeter accurately measured a wide range of tidal volumes.

This abstract describes a new apparatus. The first sentence states the name of the apparatus (endotracheal flowmeter) (A_1), identifies it as new (A_1), states its purpose (A_2), and names the population the apparatus applies to (A_3). The next two sentences (B, C) describe key features of the flowmeter and include a number of specific details. Sentence D states an advantage. The last sentence tells how the flowmeter was tested (E_1) and how well it works (E_2).

Continuity is clear from repetition of the key term "flowmeter" (in A, B, D, and E) and consistent point of view ("flowmeter," in B, D, and E). The sentences are short (mean, 22.6 words/sentence). Words are as simple as possible. Two standard abbreviations are used (PCO_2, partial pressure of carbon dioxide; PO_2, partial pressure of oxygen). The abstract is brief (113 words) and the overview is clear.

INDEXING TERMS

Use of Indexing Terms

Some journals ask authors to supply a list of indexing terms (also called key words) to guide indexers in selecting terms for the journal's index. Indexing terms are sometimes printed after the abstract or after the title in the journal's table of contents.

Principles for Selecting Indexing Terms

Indexing terms should name important topics in your paper. Select terms that you would look up if you were trying to find your own paper and that would attract the readers you hope to reach.

When selecting indexing terms, use current terms. Some journals request that authors select indexing terms from the medical subject headings (MeSH) listed in the January issue of *Index Medicus*. However, MeSH terms usually lag behind terms used in the most recent research, so you may need to use indexing terms that are not yet included in MeSH. For example, the term "acquired immunodeficiency syndrome" was needed for at least a year before it appeared in MeSH.

In addition, when selecting indexing terms, use the most specific terms possible. For example, in a paper about erythromycin, "erythromycin" should be given as an indexing term, not the more general term "antibiotics." Indexers can easily extrapolate from the specific ("erythromycin") to the general ("antibiotics") if necessary, but they cannot easily extrapolate from the general to the specific.

Note that indexing terms can be phrases as well as single words. Thus, a phrase such as "blood coagulation disorders" is a possible indexing term.

Note also that because indexers can easily pick indexing terms out of the title of the paper, some journals ask authors to supply only indexing terms that are not in the title.

Finally, words used as indexing terms do not have to be in the paper. For example, in the paper "Regional Differences in Pleural Lymphatic Albumin Concentration in Sheep," the indexing term "capillary exchange" does not appear in the paper.

ABSTRACTS FOR MEETINGS

Functions

The functions of abstracts for meetings are first to show that you have a valuable contribution and second to lure an audience to your talk.

Content

To fulfill these functions, abstracts for meetings should follow the same guidelines as abstracts of papers except that abstracts for meetings are likely to include more details of methods and to display data in a table or a graph. The reason for including more methods details and data is that this extra information helps the selection committee and the people attending the meeting evaluate the validity of the work. In addition, abstracts for meetings are more likely to include implications than are abstracts of papers, to indicate the importance of the work.

Amount of Detail and Use of Abbreviations

Resist the temptation to cram as many methods details, data, and statistical details as possible into an abstract for a meeting. Excess details make the abstract unreadable because the trees overshadow the forest. It is better to give one good result than to give a lot of data. If the result is good, the abstract will be accepted. If not, data will not help; data just show that you did a lot of work.

Also resist the temptation to use abbreviations so that you can add more details. Using a lot of abbreviations makes the abstract unreadable because the reader has to concentrate on breaking the code.

Finally, keep in mind that even a detailed abstract for a meeting cannot replace the paper. For all practical purposes, abstracts for meetings self-destruct after a year. If the paper is not published eventually, the details and data (as well as the conclusions) in the abstract cannot be used because there is no way of validating them.

Thus, the judicious use of details and abbreviations, not the maximal use, shows that your contribution is valuable and lures an audience to your talk.

Presentation of Data and Results

Data included in an abstract for a meeting, unlike data in an abstract of a journal article, are sometimes presented in a table or a graph. The table or graph should be designed clearly, the same as a table or graph for a paper. The only differences are that in abstracts no title is given for tables and no legends are included for graphs.

When you include a table or a graph in an abstract for a meeting, be careful not to omit the statement of the results that the data support. Omitting the results obscures the overview (see Example 10.12). For greatest clarity, the table or graph should be placed after the sentence that states the results that the data support, not instead of the results sentence.

Example 10.12

CROMOLYN SODIUM FAILS TO PREVENT HYPOXIA-INDUCED PULMONARY VASOCONSTRICTION IN NEWBORN AND YOUNG LAMBS. Author Number One, Author Number Two, Author Number Three, and Author Number Four. Department of Pediatrics, University of XXX, City, State

Leukotrienes, which are found in a variety of pulmonary cell types including mast cells, have been suggested to mediate hypoxia-induced pulmonary vasoconstriction. Cromolyn sodium, a stabilizer of mast cell membranes, has been reported to prevent hypoxia-induced pulmonary vasoconstriction in adult sheep and young lambs, presumably by preventing the release of leukotrienes. We were unable to reproduce these results not only in newborn lambs but also in young sheep. Six newborn lambs were instrumented to measure pulmonary (PAP) and systemic (SAP) arterial pressures and cardiac output (Q). After baseline measurements, vehicle was infused and responses to alveolar hypoxia were recorded. After return to baseline, cromolyn sodium (3 mg/kg/min) was infused for 10 min before and continued during alveolar hypoxia and responses were recorded. Studies were done at 4-7 d (newborn) and again at 15-18 d (young sheep).

Treatment	PAP (mmHg)		SAP (mmHg)		Q (L/min/kg)	
	Newborn	Young	Newborn	Young	Newborn	Young
Baseline	15±2	20±7	79± 6	90±10	0.24±0.07	0.31±0.09
Hypoxia	28±3*	31±9*	76± 4	88± 9	0.29±0.11	0.41±0.08
Cromolyn	19±4	25±6	79±10	83±11	0.22±0.06	0.25±0.07
Crom + Hypox	31±5†	35±6†	80± 6	92±13	0.25±0.08	0.39±0.13†

Mean ± SD; *$P < 0.05$ vs. baseline; $^\dagger P < 0.05$ vs. cromolyn (ANOVA). Cromolyn sodium at 5 mg/kg/min, in 2 lambs, produced similar results. The results of this study contradict previous reports that cromolyn sodium prevents hypoxia-induced pulmonary vasoconstriction and thus question the importance of mast cells in producing hypoxia-induced pulmonary vasoconstriction.

Two major problems in the way this abstract is written make the overview unclear:

1. The question is not stated at the beginning. Instead the answer is given (third sentence). Substituting the answer for the question is disorienting because the answer can be misread as background information.
2. The results are not stated. Only data are shown (in the table). Thus, when we read the sentence below the table ("Cromolyn sodium at 5 mg/kg/min, in 2 lambs, produced similar results"), we do not know what the results are, unless we have figured them out for ourselves. The reader should not have to figure out the results. The author should state them.

In addition, the omission of some important details further obscures the clarity of this abstract.

3. Only one of the two doses tested is mentioned in what was done, so we do not expect results for a second dose.
4. The sample size and the dose are missing from the footnote of the table.
5. The implication at the end of the last sentence says nothing about leukotrienes. Thus, the expectation raised by the first word of the abstract (a very powerful position) and emphasized by the last word of the second sentence is not fulfilled.

Finally, the inclusion of some secondary details partly obscures the point of the abstract by drawing attention away from the important details.

6. The statistical comparisons in the table are not directly relevant to the results that answer the question. These comparisons show that hypoxia indeed induced pulmonary vasoconstriction, as reflected by increases in pulmonary arterial pressure. However, the crucial comparison is between pulmonary arterial pressures for hypoxia alone and for cromolyn plus hypoxia. The point is that the values were not significantly different.
7. Systemic arterial pressure and cardiac output are not strictly necessary for answering the question, but they are included in the table to show that the changes in pulmonary arterial pressure did not result from changes in systemic arterial pressure or from changes in cardiac output.

In the revision, the question is stated and the results are stated. In addition, the second dose tested is mentioned in what was done, the sample size and the dose are added to the footnote of the table, and "leukotriene release" is added to the last sentence. These changes make the abstract clearer. The statistical comparisons and the data for systemic arterial pressure and cardiac output, though of secondary importance, are retained to show the validity of the results. Finally, to keep the abstract the same length as the original version, "which are found in," "a variety of," and "have been suggested to" in the first sentence have been shortened to "released by," "various," and "may." In the second sentence, "a stabilizer of mast cell membranes" has been changed to the noun cluster "a mast cell membrane stabilizer." In what was found, "we" is used instead of passive voice, and "six" at the beginning of the sentence becomes "6" within the sentence. In the sentence before the table, "the" has been omitted before "pulmonary arterial pressure responses." In the last sentence, "these" has been changed to "our" and "previous" before "reports" has been omitted.

Revision

CROMOLYN SODIUM FAILS TO PREVENT HYPOXIA-INDUCED PULMONARY VASOCONSTRICTION IN NEWBORN AND YOUNG LAMBS. Author Number One, Author Number Two, Author Number Three, and Author Number Four. Department of Pediatrics, University of XXX, City, State

Leukotrienes, released by various pulmonary cell types including mast cells, may mediate hypoxia-induced pulmonary vasoconstriction. Cromolyn sodium, a mast cell membrane stabilizer, has been reported to prevent hypoxia-induced pulmonary vasoconstriction in adult sheep and young lambs, presumably by preventing release of leukotrienes. We tried to reproduce these results in newborn (4-7 d) and young (15-18 d) lambs. We instrumented 6 newborn lambs to measure pulmonary (PAP) and systemic (SAP) arterial pressures and cardiac output (Q̇). After baseline measurements, we infused vehicle and recorded responses to alveolar hypoxia. After return to baseline, we infused cromolyn sodium at 2 doses (3 mg/kg/min (6 lambs) and 5 mg/kg/min (2 lambs)) for 10 min before and then during alveolar hypoxia and recorded responses. We found no differences between pulmonary arterial pressure responses to hypoxia with and without cromolyn sodium at either dose at either age.

Treatment	PAP (mmHg)		SAP (mmHg)		Q̇ (L/min/kg)	
	Newborn	Young	Newborn	Young	Newborn	Young
Baseline	15±2	20±7	79± 6	90±10	0.24±0.07	0.31±0.09
Hypoxia	28±3*	31±9*	76± 4	88± 9	0.29±0.11	0.41±0.08
Cromolyn	19±4	25±6	79±10	83±11	0.22±0.06	0.25±0.07
Crom + Hypox	31±5†	35±6†	80± 6	92±13	0.25±0.08	0.39±0.13†

Mean ± SD for 6 lambs given 3 mg/kg/min cromolyn.

*P < 0.05 vs. baseline; †P < 0.05 vs. cromolyn (ANOVA).

Our results contradict reports that cromolyn sodium prevents hypoxia-induced pulmonary vasoconstriction and thus question the importance of leukotriene release from mast cells in producing hypoxia-induced pulmonary vasoconstriction.

SUMMARY OF GUIDELINES FOR ABSTRACTS

FUNCTION

The abstract should provide an overview of the main story and a few essential details.

The abstract should be clear both to readers who read the paper and to readers who do not read the paper.

ABSTRACTS OF RESULTS PAPERS

Content and Organization

State
> the question you asked.
> what you did to answer the question:
>> the species or population and the material you studied, and their condition if necessary.
>> the experimental approach or the protocol, including both the independent and the dependent variables.
> what you found that answers the question, including
>> only the most important results, in a logical order.
>> a minimum of data.
>> percent change rather than exact data when possible.
>> critical details of methods not mentioned earlier.
> the answer to the question. Be sure the answer answers the question asked.

If useful, also include
> background, at the beginning of the abstract.
> an implication or a speculation, at the end of the abstract.

Writing

Write the abstract as one paragraph.

Use the techniques of continuity to make the paragraph flow.

Use signals to indicate the parts of the abstract:
> Signal what you found by "We found that" or something similar.
> Signal the answer by "We conclude that" or "Thus" or something similar.
> Signal implications by "We suggest that" or something similar.

The question and what was done can usually be written in one sentence in the form "To determine X, we. . . ." If the question and what was done are in separate sentences, use signals such as "We asked whether . . ." (question) and "To answer this question, we . . ." (what was done).

Use appropriate verb tenses:
> Use present tense verbs for the question and the answer.
> Use past tense verbs to state what was done and what was found.
> Use a cautious present tense verb for implications (for example, "may mediate").

Be careful not to omit the question, not to state the question vaguely, and not to state an implication instead of the answer.

To ensure that the question is specific rather than vague, check the question against the answer: use the same key terms for the independent and dependent variables; keep the same point of view; and, to anticipate the answer, use the same verb in the question as in the answer.

If you give a P value, also give data (for example, mean $\pm$ SD) and the sample size (n).

Write short sentences. Avoid noun clusters.

Use simple words. Avoid jargon. Avoid abbreviations.

Keep the abstract short.

> Omit less important information (experimental preparation, confirmatory results, comparisons with previous results, data for less important variables, definitions, background, implications).
>
> Omit details [unnecessary details of methods, exact data (give percent change), P values, "significantly"].
>
> Avoid repetition (use a category term in what was done and name the variables in what was found; state "mean $\pm$ SD" only once).
>
> Use active voice instead of passive voice.
>
> Omit unnecessary words (use "Thus" instead of "We conclude that"; use an adjective or an apostrophe instead of an "of" phrase: for example, "*ductal* rings" instead of "rings of ductus arteriosus," "*rings'* sensitivity" instead of "sensitivity of the rings"; but do not omit "a," "an," or "the" when they are necessary).

Exceptions

If the journal to which you are submitting a paper requests a different form for the abstract, follow the requested form.

ABSTRACTS OF METHODS PAPERS

State

> the name or the category of the method, apparatus, or material.
> the purpose.
> the species or population.
> the key features, how it works, or both.
> the advantages (to indicate why the method is needed).
> how it was tested.
> how well it works.

Always begin with the first four items. The order of the last three items may be changed if necessary.

To indicate that the method is an improved version of an existing method, add "improved" before the name of the method. It is not usually necessary to indicate that a method is new, but it is OK to do so.

State the purpose in the form "for doing X" or "to do X."

Include the name, purpose, and species in one sentence.

Usually include how the method was tested and how well it works in one sentence.

Use past tense (present perfect tense) or present tense to name the method, depending on the verb used (for example, "An improved method *has been developed*" or "An improved method *is described*"). Use present tense to describe the method and its advantages. Use past tense to state how the method was tested and how well it works.

INDEXING TERMS

Select terms that you would look up to find your own paper and that would attract the readers you hope to reach.

Select current, specific terms, preferably medical subject headings (MeSH), that name important topics in your paper.

Use phrases as well as single words.

If the journal asks you to supply only terms that are not in the title of the paper, do so.

If necessary, include a term as an indexing term even if the term does not appear in your paper.

ABSTRACTS FOR MEETINGS

The functions of abstracts for meetings are to show that you have a valuable contribution and to lure an audience to your talk.

To fulfill these functions, in general, abstracts for meetings should follow the same guidelines as abstracts of papers.

Exceptions:

It is OK to give more details of methods in an abstract for a meeting than in an abstract of a paper and to display data in a table or a graph so that the reader can evaluate the validity of the work.

Implications are included in abstracts for meetings more often than in abstracts of papers to indicate the importance of the work.

However,

Do not add excessive detail, or the trees will overshadow the forest.

Do not use a lot of abbreviations, or the abstract will be unreadable.

Design the table or graph carefully, but omit the title of the table and the legend for the graph.

Do not omit the statement of the results that the data in the table or the figure support; instead, place the table or figure after the statement of the results.

■ EXERCISE 10.1: THE CONTENT OF ABSTRACTS

1. Grade the following abstracts A (excellent), B (good), C (average), D (poor), or F (terrible). Support your grade with reasons. Note that abstract 1 is from a methods *paper and that abstracts 2 and 3 are from* results *papers. Use the appropriate criteria to evaluate each type of abstract.*

2. Rewrite one or more of these abstracts.

1   *Intravenous Injection of Rats by the Use of a Novel Device*

*A*A novel "straitjacket" to immobilize rats for intravenous injection is described. *B*Its advantages include the incorporation of an injection unit, nontraumatic immobilization of the conscious rat, lack of physiological disturbance, exactness of dosage quantitation, feasibility of repeated attempts at insertion with only one venipuncture, and requirement of only a single operator.

Grade: _____

Reasons:

2   *Effects of Exposure to Ozone on Defensive Mechanisms of the Lung*

*A*Various components of the endogenous defense mechanism of the lung were studied by means of a unilateral lung exposure technique. *B*Low levels of ozone were found to decrease cellular viability, depress various intracellular hydrolytic enzymes (lysozyme, beta-glucuronidase, and acid phosphatase), and increase the absolute number and percent of polymorphonuclear leukocytes within pulmonary lavage fluid. *C*All these effects were dose related and were found only in the single lung exposed to ozone and not in the contralateral lung simultaneously breathing ambient air. *D*The responses were found to be the result of a direct toxicity of this pollutant rather than a generalized systemic response. *E*It was concluded that the observed effects could be responsible for the increased mortality of animals given a bacterial challenge following ozone exposure.

Grade: _____

Reasons:

3 *Pulmonary Mechanics and Gas Exchange in Seated Normal Men with Chest Restriction*

A Lung volumes, static pressure-volume curves, maximal expiratory flow-volume curves, right-to-left intrapulmonary shunts ($\dot{Q}s/\dot{Q}t$), and perfusion relative to the alveolar ventilation and perfusion ratio ($\dot{V}A/\dot{Q}$) were determined in seated normal men before chest strapping while breathing air (C_{air}) and during chest strapping while breathing air (S_{air}) or 100% oxygen (SO_2). *B* With S_{air} and SO_2, mean vital capacity was reduced by 44% from control. *C* Elastic recoil pressure [Pst(L)] of the lung at 50% control total lung capacity (TLC) increased significantly ($P < 0.05$) from 4.64 ± 0.39 cm H_2O (mean $\pm$ SE) to 7.00 ± 0.47 cm H_2O with S_{air} and to 7.24 ± 0.70 cm H_2O with SO_2. *D* Maximal expiratory flow at 50% of control TLC increased significantly ($P < 0.05$) from 3.22 ± 0.25 L/s (mean $\pm$ SE) to 5.84 ± 0.69 L/s with S_{air} and to 5.50 ± 0.68 L/s with SO_2. *E* With S_{air}, no significant increase in $\dot{Q}s/\dot{Q}t$ from control was observed. *F* With SO_2, mean $\dot{Q}s/\dot{Q}t$ increased significantly ($P < 0.05$) from 0 to 2.2 ± 0.9% of the cardiac output. *G* It is therefore unlikely that the development of atelectasis, as indicated by an increase in $\dot{Q}s/\dot{Q}t$, accounts for the increase in Pst(L) with S_{air} and SO_2. *H* Current evidence suggests that either change in alveolar surface compliance or distortion of the lung or both are responsible for the increased recoil pressure but that neither mechanism alone appears to explain it totally.

Grade: _____

Reasons:

■ *EXERCISE 10.2: LENGTH OF ABSTRACTS*

The abstract below is from <u>Science</u>, which does not use the standard format for abstracts. However, it does limit the length of abstracts—to 45–55 words. The abstract below has 69 words. Shorten this abstract without omitting any of the ideas. Keep in mind the principles of word choice (Chap. 1) and sentence structure (Chap. 2).

Abstract

The disposition of morphine was investigated by means of radioimmunoassay after a single intravenous dose (10 mg/70 kg) was administered to 10 adult normal male subjects who had not received other drugs for 2 weeks preceding the study. A multiphasic decline in serum concentrations of morphine occurred. Detectable blood concentrations of morphine, or of a metabolite, or of both persisted for 48 hours after a single intravenous dose.

Number of Words in Revised Version: _____

Revised Version:

CHAPTER 11

THE TITLE

FUNCTIONS

Titles of biomedical journal articles have two functions: to identify the main topic or the main point of the paper and to attract readers.

CONTENT OF TITLES FOR RESULTS PAPERS

Stating the Topic in the Title

The standard title of a biomedical research paper is a phrase that identifies the topic of the article, which is the same as the topic of the question. For a results paper, the topic includes three pieces of information: the independent variable(s) that you manipulated, if any (X), the dependent variable(s) you observed or measured (Y), and the species or population and the material on which you did the work (Z). The species studied must always be included in the title, whether or not the species is included in the question and the answer. If necessary, two other pieces of information may also be included: the condition of the animals or subjects during the study and the experimental approach. No other information should be included.

Titles for Papers That Have Both Independent and Dependent Variables

For studies that have both independent and dependent variables, the standard form of the title of a biomedical research paper is

Effect of X on Y in Z.

Example 11.1

	X		Y		Z

Effect of β-Endorphin on Breathing Movements in Fetal Sheep

Note that in this standard form, the species, population, or material studied comes at the end of the title.

When the species studied is humans, the species is often omitted from the title, as in Example 11.2, although it is OK to include "humans" in the title, as in Example 11.19 below.

Example 11.2

Effect of Membrane Splitting on Transmembrane Polypeptides

However, when the species is a subpopulation of humans, the species is always included in the title.

Example 11.3

Effects of Esmolol on Airway Function <u>in Patients Who Have Asthma</u>

For the negative implication to work (no species in the title implies that the species is humans), the species must always be included in the title when the work was done on animals.

Titles for Papers That Have Only Dependent Variables

For studies that have only dependent variables, the standard form of the title is

$$Y \text{ in } Z,$$

where Y is the dependent variable(s)—that is, the variable(s) observed or measured—and Z is the species or population and the material on which the work was done.

Example 11.4

     Y   *Z*

<u>Blood Supply</u> of the <u>Caudal Mediastinal Lymph Node in Sheep</u>

Other Information in the Title

In addition to these essential pieces of information (X, Y, and Z), the title of a results paper may sometimes include the condition the subjects or the animals were in during the experiments (Example 11.5) or the experimental approach (Example 11.6), if these details are important.

Example 11.5

Effect of Hypoproteinemia on Fluid Balance in the Lungs of <u>Awake</u> Newborn Lambs

Example 11.6

Microvascular Pressures <u>Measured by Micropuncture</u> in Lungs of Newborn Rabbits

Stating the Point in the Title

Traditionally, the title of a biomedical research paper states the topic of the paper. But if the paper comes to a strong, unambiguous conclusion supported by strong, unequivocal evidence, the title of the paper can state the point, that is, the answer to the question. The point can be stated either in a phrase or in a sentence.

Stating the Point in a Phrase

In a phrase title, the point is expressed by either an adjective or a noun placed before the dependent variable at the beginning of the title. The adjective or noun is based on the verb used in the question and answer. For example, if the question of the paper is "to determine whether the metabolic rate in rats *is reduced* during radio-frequency irradiation" and the answer to the question is yes, then this point can be expressed by the adjective "reduced" in the title, as in Example 11.7.

Example 11.7

<u>Reduced</u> Metabolic Rate in Rats During Radio-Frequency Irradiation

In Example 11.8 below, the point is expressed by the noun "alteration" before the dependent variable. The question was to "determine whether protein-calorie malnutrition *alters* lung mechanics."

Example 11.8

<u>Alteration of</u> Lung Mechanics by Protein-Calorie Malnutrition in Weaned Rats

Sometimes both an adjective and a noun are used to state the point, as in Example 11.9.

Example 11.9

<u>Hypoxia-Induced Alterations of</u> Vascular Reactivity to Norepinephrine in Isolated Perfused Lung from Cats

Stating the Point in a Sentence

Another way to state a point in the title is to use a sentence. In a sentence, the point is expressed by a verb in present tense, as in Example 11.10.

Example 11.10

Verapamil and Diet <u>Halt</u> the Progression of Atherosclerosis in Cholesterol-Fed Rabbits

Using a sentence to state a point is stronger than using a phrase is, as you can see by reading the list of titles in a journal's table of contents. It is the sentence titles that will jump out at you. The reason a sentence title is stronger is that verbs convey action more powerfully than nouns (or adjectives) do. Thus, the same title stated as a phrase and as a sentence will sound stronger as a sentence. (Compare "Arrested Progression of Atherosclerosis by Verapamil and Diet in Cholesterol-Fed Rabbits" with Example 11.10.)

Perhaps because of the strength of sentence titles, whether to use a sentence as a title is still controversial. In fact, some journals do not permit sentences to be used as titles. So even though sentence titles are a strong, clear way to state the message of a paper, use sentence titles cautiously.

CONTENT OF TITLES FOR METHODS PAPERS

The title of a methods paper should indicate whether the paper describes a method, an apparatus, or a material, should state its purpose, and should name the species or population the method is used for. In addition, the title may indicate whether the method is new or improved.

Name

To indicate whether the paper describes a method, an apparatus, or a material, use the name in the title if the method, apparatus, or material has a name.

Example 11.11

<u>Endotracheal Flowmeter</u> for Measuring Tidal Volume, Airway Pressure, and End-Tidal Gas in Newborns

Example 11.12

<u>Monoclonal Antibodies</u> as Probes for Distinguishing Unique Antigens in Secretory Cells of Heterogeneous Exocrine Organs

If the method does not have a name, use a category term such as "method" or "apparatus" in the title.

Example 11.13

A <u>Method</u> for Purifying the Glycoprotein IIb-IIIa Complex in Platelet Membrane

Purpose

To state the purpose, the verb form "for doing X" is used. Thus, in Examples 11.11 and 11.13 above, "for measuring" and "for purifying" are the verb forms used to state the purpose. Example 11.12 above uses a slightly modified form— "as probes for distinguishing." Both forms are clear indicators of purpose.

However, using "for" without an "ing" verb after it makes the title unclear.

Example 11.14

A Double-Catheter Technique <u>for</u> Caudally Misdirected Catheters in the Umbilical Artery

In this title, it is not clear what the technique is for.

Revision

A Double-Catheter Technique <u>for Avoiding</u> Caudally Misdirected Catheters in the Umbilical Artery

Adding the "ing" verb makes the purpose clear: "for avoiding."

Species

As in titles of results papers, the species that the method is used for is often omitted when the species is humans (Examples 11.12–11.14) or humans and other species (Example 11.16 below). However, the species is always stated when the species is not humans or is a specific subpopulation of humans (Examples 11.11 above and 11.15 below).

New or Improved

If a paper describes a new method, the title usually does not need to include the word "new" (see examples above) or its fancy alternative "novel." However, the title may include the most important feature or the most important advantage of the method. In Example 11.14 above, "double-catheter" is the most important feature of the new method.

If a paper describes an improved method, the title should, if possible, state what the improvement is by naming either the most important feature or the most important advantage of the improved method. In Example 11.15 below, "noninvasive" is the most important advantage of the improved method.

Example 11.15

<u>Noninvasive</u> Method for Monitoring Blood Gases in the Newborn

If the most important feature or advantage cannot be named easily, the title should use the general term "improved."

Example 11.16

An <u>Improved</u> Method for Isolating Type II Cells in High Yield and Purity

HALLMARKS OF A GOOD TITLE

The hallmarks of a good title are that it accurately, completely, and specifically identifies the main topic or the main point of the paper, is unambiguous, is concise, and begins with an important term.

Accurate, Complete, Specific

To make a title accurate, use the same terms in the title as in the question and answer of a results paper or, for a methods paper, use the same name of the method, purpose, and species or population as stated in the paper. To make a title complete, include all the necessary information (see "Content of Titles for Results Papers" and "Content of Titles for Methods Papers" above). To make a title specific, use specific words. The terms in the title should be usable as indexing terms for indexes and searches.

Accurate

For a results paper, check that your title is accurate by comparing it with the question and answer. The independent variable, the dependent variable, the species or population, the material, the condition (if necessary), the experimental approach (if necessary), and the point (if stated) should be the same in the title as in the question and answer stated in the Introduction, Discussion, and abstract.

Example 11.17

Title: Neutrophil-Induced Injury of Epithelial Cells in the Pulmonary Alveoli of Rats

Question: To determine whether the injury of epithelial cells in the pulmonary alveoli that occurs in many inflammatory conditions is induced in part by stimulated neutrophils, we exposed monolayers of purified alveolar epithelial cells from rats to stimulated human neutrophils and measured cytotoxicity using a ^{51}Cr-release assay.

Answer: We conclude that stimulated neutrophils induce injury in epithelial cells in the pulmonary alveoli.

For a methods paper, the name of the method, its purpose, and the species or population (if included) should be the same in the title as in the Introduction, Discussion, and abstract.

Example 11.18

Title: A Method for Purifying the Glycoprotein IIb-IIIa Complex in Platelet Membrane

Abstract: We have developed a method for the rapid purification of the glycoprotein IIb-IIIa complex in platelet membrane.

Complete

In a paper that makes two or more points, it may be difficult to make the title complete. If you cannot create a title that reflects all the points, select the most important point for the title. Similarly, if a study manipulated several independent variables or assessed several dependent variables and no category terms are available that include them all, select the most important independent and dependent variable for the title. Keep in mind that, just as the abstract cannot replace the paper, so the title cannot replace the abstract. Announcing the main point of the paper is stronger than trying to fit all the details into the title.

Specific

Two words that often make a title unspecific are "and" and "with." "And" is not a problem when it is used to join parallel terms, such as *"Cardiovascular and Metabolic* Effects of Halothane in *Normoxic and Hypoxic* Newborn Lambs." But "and" is a problem when it is used to join the independent and the dependent variables in the form "X and Y in Z" instead of the standard form "Effect of X on Y in Z." The problem is that "and" does not indicate any relationship between X and Y.

Example 11.19

Airway Caliber <u>and</u> the Work of Breathing in Humans

This title is not specific. What is the relationship between airway caliber and the work of breathing in humans? The title becomes specific when rewritten in the standard form "Effect of X on Y in Z."

Revision

<u>Effect of</u> Airway Caliber <u>on</u> the Work of Breathing in Humans

"With," as we saw in Chapter 1: Word Choice, is nearly always unclear because it is not specific. Therefore, avoid "with" wherever possible, except in its standard uses after certain verbs, such as "compared with," "measured with," "treated with," etc.

Example 11.20

Bronchoconstriction, Gas Trapping, and Hypoxia <u>with</u> Methacholine in Dogs

In this example, the relationship of methacholine to bronchoconstriction, gas trapping, and hypoxia is not clear. The solution is to change "with" to a more specific word.

Revision

Bronchoconstriction, Gas Trapping, and Hypoxia <u>Induced by</u> Methacholine in Dogs

Although "with" should be avoided, one use of "with" that is permissible is to describe patients, as in "patients with amiodarone-induced pulmonary toxicity" (Example 11.28 below). Still, "patients who have amiodarone-induced pulmonary toxicity" is clearer and should be used when space permits.

Unambiguous

To make a title unambiguous, follow the principles of sentence structure and word choice. In particular, avoid noun clusters and misplaced adjectives, and do not use abbreviations.

Noun Clusters

A noun cluster can be ambiguous alone, as in Example 11.21, or when preceded by an adjective, as in Example 11.22.

Example 11.21

Effects of Alveolar Pressure on <u>Lung Angiotensin-Converting Enzyme Function</u> in Rabbit Lungs in Vivo

In this title, it is not immediately clear that the effects are on function because the word "function" comes at the end of a long cluster. To make clear that the effects are on function, "function" should come immediately after "on." "Lung" can be omitted because it is stated again later in the title.

Revision

Effects of Alveolar Pressure on <u>the Function of Angiotensin-Converting Enzyme</u> in Rabbit Lungs in Vivo

Example 11.22

A <u>Delivery-Independent Blood Flow Effect</u> on Fatigue of the Skeletal Muscles

This title is ambiguous because it contains a cluster ("blood flow effect") preceded by an adjective ("delivery-independent"). Because two nouns come after the adjective, either one ("blood flow" or "effect") could be delivery independent.

Revision

A Delivery-Independent <u>Effect of Blood Flow</u> on Fatigue of the Skeletal Muscles

By untangling the noun cluster, this revision makes clear that it is the effect that is delivery independent and also that the effect described is the effect of blood flow. This clarity is achieved by having only one noun ("effect") after the adjective.

Misplaced Adjectives

For greatest clarity, an adjective should come immediately before or immediately after the word it modifies. For example, "*altered* permeability"; "rats *ventilated with ozone*." An adjective is misplaced when other words come between the adjective and the word it modifies. Thus, in Example 11.22 above, we could say that "delivery-independent" is misplaced. It should come immediately before "effect," as in the revision. In Example 11.23, "induced by" is misplaced.

Example 11.23

Alterations in Pulmonary Fluid Balance <u>Induced by</u> Positive End-Expiratory Pressure

In this title, it sounds as if *pulmonary fluid balance* is induced by positive end-expiratory pressure, but the intended meaning is that the *alterations* are induced by positive end-expiratory pressure. One way to make the meaning clear is to change "alterations in" to "altered."

Revision A

<u>Altered</u> Pulmonary Fluid Balance Induced by Positive End-Expiratory Pressure

Another solution is to use a time word such as "during" or "after" instead of the causal term "induced by."

Revision B

Alterations in Pulmonary Fluid Balance <u>During</u> Positive End-Expiratory Pressure

Abbreviations

Do not use abbreviations in titles. Titles are often read out of context, for example, in *Index Medicus* or *Current Contents*, so even if an abbreviation is well known in a particular specialty, it could be confusing to readers from other specialties.

Example 11.24

Quantification of the Effect of the Pericardium on the LV Diastolic PV Relation in Dogs

Revision

Quantification of the Pericardium's Effect on the Left Ventricular Diastolic Pressure-Volume Relation in Dogs

In the revision, to accommodate the words that LV and PV abbreviate, "effect of the pericardium" is condensed to "pericardium's effect." The revised title, containing no abbreviations, is clear to all readers. The original title is clear only to those who work in this field.

Two categories of abbreviation are acceptable in titles. One is abbreviations that are better known than the words they stand for, such as DNA (deoxyribonucleic acid). The other category is abbreviations for chemicals, such as N_2O_5 (dinitrogen pentoxide). Nevertheless, if you have space, write the words, especially short, familiar words such as "oxygen."

If you are unsure of whether an abbreviation will be clear, write the words.

Concise

Short titles have more impact than long titles do, so make your title as short as possible without sacrificing accuracy, completeness, specificity, or clarity. That is, make the title concise. Sometimes, just to include all the necessary details a title will need to be rather long. Nevertheless, try to keep your title shorter than 100 characters and spaces. Longer titles begin to fall apart under their own weight. Some journals have even shorter limits. Whatever the journal's limit, keep in mind that the aim is not to fill the space allowed. The aim is to convey the topic or the point of your paper accurately, completely, specifically, and unambiguously. If you can devise a short title that fulfills these criteria, do so.

Two ways to make titles concise are by omitting unnecessary words and by compacting the necessary words as tightly as possible.

Omitting Unnecessary Words

Omit nonspecific openings such as "Nature of" and "Studies of."

Example 11.25

Pharmacokinetic Studies of the Disposition of Acetaminophen in the Sheep Maternal-Placental-Fetal Unit

In this example, "pharmacokinetic studies of" is unnecessary. If "disposition" does not get the idea across, a more precise term, such as "pharmacokinetics," could be used.

Revision

Disposition of Acetaminophen in the Sheep Maternal-Placental-Fetal Unit

Omit nonspecific words elsewhere in the title.

Example 11.26

Alterations Induced by <u>Administration of</u> Chlorphentermine in Phospholipids and Proteins in Alveolar Surfactant

Revision A

Alterations Induced by Chlorphentermine in Phospholipids and Proteins in Alveolar Surfactant

Revision B

Chlorphentermine-Induced Alterations in Phospholipids and Proteins in Alveolar Surfactant

Usually omit "the" at the beginning of the title. Normally, "the" would appear at the beginning of a title in phrases such as "the effect of" or "the distribution of," but "the" is usually omitted from these phrases when they are at the beginning of a title, as in the revision of Example 11.25 above ("Disposition of").

However, do not omit "the" before singular nouns later in the title.

Example 11.27

Dynamics of Chest Wall in Preterm Infants

Revision

Dynamics of <u>the</u> Chest Wall in Preterm Infants

Compacting Necessary Words

In addition to omitting unnecessary words, at least three compacting techniques can be used to shorten titles.

Category Terms. One important compacting technique is to use a category term instead of details. Using a category term may seem to conflict with the recommendation to use specific words. But as Example 11.28 shows, it is possible to be too specific.

Example 11.28

Electron Microscopic Demonstration of Lysosomal Inclusion Bodies in <u>Lung, Liver, Lymph Nodes, and Blood Leukocytes</u> of Patients with Amiodarone-Induced Pulmonary Toxicity

By naming four specific tissues, this title gives trees but not the forest. The text of the paper makes clear that lysosomal inclusion bodies have already been reported in the lungs and that the news in this study is that lysosomal inclusion bodies also appear in extrapulmonary tissues. By substituting the category term "extrapulmonary tissues" for liver, lymph nodes, and blood leukocytes and omitting "lung" we get the forest.

Revision

Electron Microscopic Demonstration of Lysosomal Inclusion Bodies in <u>Extrapulmonary Tissues</u> of Patients with Amiodarone-Induced Pulmonary Toxicity

If no category term exists, select the most important variable for the title (see "Complete" above).

Adjectives to Express a Point.   Another compacting technique is to use an adjective instead of a noun followed by a preposition to express a point, as in Revision A of Example 11.23 above ("altered" instead of "alterations in").

Noun Clusters.   A third compacting technique is to use noun clusters instead of prepositional phrases. This technique must be used carefully to avoid creating an ambiguous title (see "Unambiguous" above).

One way to create noun clusters that do not cause serious reading problems is to use the name of the species as an adjective, rather than at the end of the title.

Example 11.29

Renal Mechanism of Action of <u>Rat</u> Atrial Natriuretic Factor

The longer way of writing this title would be "Renal Mechanism of Action of Atrial Natriuretic Factor in Rats." The longer version is a bit clearer and also gives more emphasis to the species, so if you have the room to write "in rats," do so.

Important Word First

To attract readers, put an important word first in your title. For titles of studies that have both independent and dependent variables, either the independent or the dependent variable can be the most important word, depending on what will interest the intended audience the most. For example, in Examples 11.30 and 11.31 below, putting halothane anesthesia (the independent variable) first would be appropriate for anesthesiologists, and putting impaired pulmonary function (the dependent variable) first would be appropriate for neonatologists.

Example 11.30

Halothane Anesthesia Impairs Pulmonary Function in Newborn Lambs

Example 11.31

Impaired Pulmonary Function in Newborn Lambs Anesthetized with Halothane

Subtitles

A technique for putting an important word first is to use a main title followed by a subtitle. The main title states the general topic and the subtitle states the specific topic. Note that a subtitle is separated from the main title by a colon (:).

Example 11.32

Human Apolipoprotein B: Structure of the Carboxyl-Terminal Domains and Sites of Gene Expression

Relation of the Subtitle to the Main Title.   Various relations of the specific topic in the subtitle to the general topic in the main title are possible. One relation is to have the main title state the material studied and the subtitle state the dependent variables, as in Example 11.32 above. This relation is often used in titles that have only dependent variables (Y in Z). Another relation is to have the main title state the dependent variable and the subtitle state the experimental approach, as in Example 11.33.

Example 11.33

Pulmonic Valve Endocarditis: A Serial Two-Dimensional Doppler Echocardiographic Study

In these types of subtitle, the colon replaces a preposition that would appear in the standard form of the title. To reconstruct the standard title, begin with the subtitle, add the appropriate preposition, and end with the main title. In the reconstruction of Example 11.33, the preposition joining the two parts of the title is "of": "A Serial Two-Dimensional Doppler Echocardiographic Study *of* Pulmonic Valve Endocarditis."

Another relation of the subtitle to the main title is to have the main title state an independent variable and the subtitle state its function (Example 11.34).

Example 11.34

Angiotensin II: A Potent Regulator of Acidification in the Early Proximal Convoluted Tubule of the Rat

In this example, the colon replaces the verb "is." Thus, if Example 11.34 did not use a subtitle, it would read "Angiotensin II *Is* a Potent Regulator of Acidification in the Early Proximal Convoluted Tubule of the Rat."

Whatever the relation between the main title and the subtitle, a crucial element in the use of subtitles is that the relation between the subtitle and the main title must be obvious. That is, the preposition or the verb that the colon replaces must be easy for the reader to supply.

Subtitles for a Series of Papers.   Some authors use subtitles to present a numbered series of papers.

Example 11.35

Morphology of the Rat Carotid Sinus Nerve: I. Course, Connections, Ultrastructure

Morphology of the Rat Carotid Sinus Nerve: II. Number and Size of Axons

If the papers are published in the same journal (preferably in the same issue of the journal) and truly could not be combined into a single paper, numbered subtitles, as in Example 11.35 above, are OK. But if part I is published alone, there is always the possibility that part II will never be published.

If it is published, it should be in the same journal as part I. The safest policy is not to start a numbered series of papers.

The Use of Subtitles.   In general, titles in a standard form, either a phrase or a sentence, are clearer than titles that have subtitles, because the crucial link relating the subtitle to the main title is missing in titles that have subtitles. Therefore, avoid using subtitles. Use a subtitle only if it is the best way to put an important word first.

DETAILS

Word Choice

When stating the point in a title, distinguish between adjectives that modify quantitative words and adjectives that modify qualitative words. The adjectives "increased" and "decreased" or "reduced" should be used to modify quantitative words such as "metabolic rate" (that is, metabolic rate is measurable), as in Example 11.7 above. The adjectives "improved" and "impaired" should be used for qualitative words, that is, for words signifying concepts that can get better or worse, such as function or performance. For example, "*Improved* Regional Ventricular *Function* after Successful Surgical Revascularization." See also Example 11.31 above.

Determining the Length of a Title

To determine the length of a title, count both the characters and the spaces between words. "Characters" is a category term for letters and punctuation marks. Count each letter as 1, each punctuation mark as 1, and each space as 1—except count the space after a colon as 2. For example, the title "Human Apolipoprotein B: Structure of the Carboxyl-Terminal Domains and Sites of Gene Expression" has a total of 96 characters and spaces.

RUNNING TITLES

Running titles (or running heads) are short phrases that appear at the top or bottom of every page, or every other page, in a journal article. The purpose of a running title is to identify the article. Some journals use the authors' names instead, or on alternate pages.

Because space along the top or bottom of the journal page is limited, the running title is shorter than the title.

A running title should be recognizable as a short version of the title and should be short enough to fit in the space allowed.

For results papers, usually the running title names the independent and the dependent variables. For papers that have no independent variable, the running title names the dependent variable, as in Example 11.36. The species can usually be omitted.

Example 11.36

Title: Locus of Hypoxia-Induced Vasoconstriction in Isolated
                Ferret Lungs

Running Title: Locus of Hypoxia-Induced Vasoconstriction

It is not always possible to use the beginning of the title as the running title. Sometimes you can pick a phrase out of the middle (Example 11.37).

Example 11.37

Title: Three-Dimensional Reconstruction of Alveoli in the Rat
                Lung for Pressure-Volume Relationships

Running Title: Reconstruction of Alveoli in the Rat Lung

Another possibility is to pick words out of the title, keeping the same order, and create a new phrase (Example 11.38).

Example 11.38

Title: Cooling Different Body Surfaces During Upper and Lower
                Body Exercise

Running Title: Cooling during Exercise

Another way to create a running title is to pick out important key terms, usually the independent and dependent variables, and join them with "and." Although "and" should not be used this way in titles (see "Specific" above), it is OK in running titles, whose only use is to indicate that this is the same article as on the previous page.

Example 11.39

Title: Influence of the Pericardium on Right and Left Ventricular
                Filling in the Dog

Running Title: Pericardium and Ventricular Filling

For methods papers, the running title can name the method only or the method and the species or the population (as in Example 11.40) or can include both the category term or the name of the method and a shortened statement of its purpose (as in Example 11.41).

Example 11.40

Title: Endotracheal Flowmeter for Measuring Tidal Volume,
                Airway Pressure, and End-Tidal Gas in Newborns

Running Title: Endotracheal Flowmeter for Newborns

Example 11.41

Title: An Improved Method for Isolating Type II Cells in High
                Yield and Purity

Running Title: Improved Method for Isolating Type II Cells

<table>
<tr><td>

**SUMMARY OF
GUIDELINES
FOR TITLES**

</td></tr>
</table>

FUNCTIONS

To identify the main topic or the main point of the paper.
To attract readers.

CONTENT OF TITLES FOR RESULTS PAPERS

Include the following information:
- Independent variable(s) (X).
- Dependent variable(s) (Y).
- Species or population and material (Z). (The population can be omitted if the population is all humans.)

If necessary, also include the
- Condition of the animals or subjects during the study.
- Experimental approach.

State either the topic or the point.
- To state a topic, use the form "Effect of X on Y in Z" or, for papers that have no independent variable, "Y in Z."
- To state a point, use either
  - A phrase, expressing the point in an adjective or a noun (or an adjective and a noun) before the dependent variable, or
  - A sentence, expressing the point in a verb in present tense.

CONTENT OF TITLES FOR METHODS PAPERS

Include the following information:
- The name or the category of the method, apparatus, or material.
- Its purpose.
- The species or population the method is used for, unless the population is all humans or humans and other species.

If the method is new, the word "new" usually does not need to appear in the title.

If the method is an improvement, either the improvement or the word "improved" should be included in the title.

HALLMARKS OF A GOOD TITLE

A good title accurately, completely, and specifically identifies the main topic or the main point of the paper.
- For accuracy, use the same terms in the title as in the question and the answer (results paper) or the same name of the method, purpose, and species or population as stated in the paper (methods paper).
- For completeness, include all the necessary information (see "Content" above). If the title cannot reflect all the main topics or points in the paper, it should reflect only the most important ones.
- For specificity,
  - Use specific words that can also function as indexing terms.
  - Do not use the form "X and Y in Z."
  - Avoid "with."

A good title is unambiguous.
- Avoid noun clusters.
- Avoid misplaced adjectives.
- Do not use abbreviations. *Exceptions*: abbreviations that are more familiar than the words they stand for and chemical formulas.

A good title is concise.

> Keep titles as brief as possible, preferably less than 100 characters and spaces.
>
> Omit unnecessary words.
>
> > Omit nonspecific openings such as "Studies of."
> >
> > Omit other vague or uninformative words.
> >
> > Usually omit "the" at the beginning of the title.
>
> Compact the necessary words.
>
> > Use a category term instead of several details.
> >
> > Use an adjective instead of a noun followed by a preposition to express a point (for example, "altered" rather than "alteration in").
> >
> > Use a noun cluster if it is not ambiguous (for example, "rat lung").

A good title begins with an important word that will attract the intended readers.

> For results papers, usually either the independent or the dependent variable is the most important word.
>
> If necessary, use a main title (for the most important word) followed by a colon and a subtitle.
>
> > The main title states the general topic of the paper.
> >
> > The subtitle states the specific topic.
> >
> > Have a clear relation between the main title and the subtitle: the preposition or the verb that the colon replaces should be easy to supply.
> >
> > Avoid starting numbered series of papers.

DETAILS

Use "increased" and "decreased" to modify quantitative words such as "metabolic rate."

Use "improved" and "impaired" to modify qualitative words such as "function."

To determine the length of a title, count every letter as 1 character, every punctuation mark as 1 character, and every space between words as 1 character, except count the space after a colon as 2.

RUNNING TITLES

A running title is a short phrase that appears at the top or bottom of every page or every other page of a journal article.

A running title should be recognizable as a short version of the title.

For results papers,

> Pick key terms, usually the independent and dependent variables, out of the title to create a running title; the species can usually be omitted.
>
> Put words in the same order in the running title as in the title.
>
> If necessary, use the form "X and Y" for the running title.

For methods papers, the running title should state either the

> Name of the method.
>
> Name of the method and the species.
>
> Name of the method and the purpose.

■ *EXERCISE 11.1: TITLES*

1. Write a title for each of the three abstracts below.

2. Also write a running title for the second abstract.

3. Underline the question and the answer in each abstract.

Abstract 1

A Continuous positive airway pressure (CPAP) is used routinely to improve oxygenation in newborns who have intrapulmonary shunts, which result in hypoxemia that is refractory to usual oxygen therapy. **B** Although the cardiovascular and pulmonary effects of CPAP on newborns are well known, little information is available concerning the effect of CPAP on renal function in newborns. **C** Accordingly, we determined the effect of CPAP (7.5 cm H_2O) on urine flow, sodium excretion, and glomerular filtration rate in six newborn goats that were lightly anesthetized with methoxyflurane. **D** We found that CPAP decreased urine flow, sodium excretion, and glomerular filtration rate. **E** CPAP also decreased pulse pressure but did not change mean systemic arterial pressure or heart rate. **F** We conclude that CPAP can impair renal function in newborns without significantly altering renal perfusion pressure.

Journal of Pediatrics

Title: 100 characters and spaces or less

Abstract 2

A To determine whether sulfur dioxide and cold dry air interact in causing bronchoconstriction in people who have asthma, we measured specific airway resistance in seven asthmatic subjects before and after they performed voluntary eucapnic hyperpnea for 3 min while breathing each of four different gas mixtures. **B** The mixtures, which the subjects breathed through a mouthpiece in random order on four different days, were humidified room-temperature air, humidified room-temperature air containing 0.5 ppm SO_2, cold dry air, and cold dry air containing 0.5 ppm SO_2. **C** Each subject breathed at a rate and depth known from preliminary studies to cause little or no bronchoconstriction when the subject inhaled only 0.5 ppm SO_2 in humidified room-temperature air or only cold dry air. **D** We found that when given independently in the blinded study, 0.5 ppm SO_2 or cold dry air again caused insignificant bronchoconstriction. [E]However, when given together, the two stimuli caused significant bronchoconstriction, as indicated by an increase in specific airway resistance from 6.94 ± 2.85 to 22.35 ± 10.28 L · cm H_2O · L · s (mean $\pm$ SD) ($P < 0.001$). [F]Thus, cold dry air increases the bronchoconstriction induced by inhaled SO_2 in people who have asthma. [G]This increase suggests that people who have asthma may be more sensitive to the bronchoconstrictor effects of ambient SO_2 in cold dry environments than in warm moist environments.

Journal of Applied Physiology

<u>Title</u>: 85 characters and spaces or less

<u>Running Title</u>: 55 characters and spaces or less

Abstract 3

[A]In mice, the inhalation of airplane glue or toluene fumes slows the sino-atrial rate, prolongs the P-R interval, and sensitizes the heart to asphyxia-induced atrioventricular block. [B]In humans who sniff glue or solvents, similar mechanisms may be a cause of sudden death.

Science

<u>Title</u>: 100 characters and spaces or less

CHAPTER 12

THE BIG PICTURE

In Chapters 10 and 11 we saw that the abstract and the title of a biomedical research paper should provide a clear overview of the paper. The challenge in the paper (both in the text and in the figures and tables) is to make the overview clear while simultaneously presenting all the necessary details. The overview is important because it is the framework against which the details of the paper make sense and because, ultimately, it is what the reader wants to know.

To make the overview clear in the text, the message must be stated clearly and a story must run from the beginning to the end of the paper. To make the overview clear in the figures and tables, the figures and tables should be simple, clear, and parallel in design, and the number of figures and tables should be kept to a minimum. In addition, all parts of the paper and of the figures and tables must correlate, no important information should be omitted, and no unnecessary information or unnecessary repetition should be included.

The techniques for making the overview clear have all been presented in the previous chapters. Here they are gathered together in a single checklist.

CHECKLIST FOR THE BIG PICTURE

Goal

To provide a clear overview of the paper while simultaneously presenting all the necessary details; that is, to avoid losing the forest for the trees.

The Message

State the message of the paper (the answer to the question) in a single sentence.
Make all statements of the answer the same.
Make all statements of the question the same.
Make the answer answer the question asked: use the same key terms, the same verb, and the same point of view.

The Story

Incorporate the overview of the story into the paper. The overview =
   the question,
   what was done to answer the question,
   what was found that answers the question,
   the answer,
   how the question and answer fit in with previous work,
   why the question and answer are important.

In the **Introduction**, the story = the funnel to the question (known, unknown), the question, and the experimental approach. The "known" includes how the question relates to previous work and why the question is important.

In **Materials and Methods**, the story = what was done to answer the question.

   The protocol gives the overview; it includes
      the independent variable,
      the dependent variable,
      all controls.

   The purpose of each procedure indicates how that procedure helps answer the question.

   Subtitles signal topics of subsections visually. Topic sentences, transition phrases, and words at the beginning of subsections and paragraphs signal topics verbally.

In **Results**, the story = what was found that answers the question.

   Results stated prominently (at the beginning of the section and at the beginning of each paragraph) tell the story.

   Topic sentences, transition phrases, and words signal topics at the beginning of paragraphs in Results.

In the **Discussion**, the story has three parts:

   The beginning states the answer to the question and gives evidence that supports the answer.

   The middle explains and expands the answer, thus indicating how the answer fits in with previous work.

   The end restates the answer or states applications, implications, or speculations, thus indicating the importance of the answer, or does both.

   Topic sentences, especially transition topic sentences, at the beginning of every paragraph tell the story in the Discussion.

   Signals of the answer identify the answer at both the beginning and the end of the Discussion.

   For the individual stories in each paragraph, supporting sentences are organized to support the topic sentence, and the organization is indicated by the techniques of continuity.

In all sections of the paper,

   Organize from most to least important when useful (always in the Discussion; where appropriate in Methods and Results).

   Use **topic sentences** to state the overview whenever possible.

   Check that reading the first sentence or two of every paragraph reveals the story.

Ensure that the **figures and tables** together also tell the story of the paper.

   Design each figure and table to be simple and to make a clear point.

   Make all figures and all tables as parallel as possible in design.

When appropriate, show the main story of the paper in figures and background information in tables.

Keep the number of figures and tables to a minimum.

Correlation of Parts

Have no loose ends in the text.

There should be

no answer in the Discussion without a question in the Introduction,

no answer in the Discussion without a result in Results,

no result in Results without a method in Methods.

The independent and dependent variables in the question or experimental approach, or indicators of these variables, should be the ones we read about in the Methods, Results, and Discussion. If an indicator is used, the variable that it is an indicator of should be stated.

Series of variables in the question or the experimental approach should be in the same order in the Methods, Results, and Discussion.

If the Introduction begins with a general problem and the Discussion ends with an implication, the implication should relate to the problem.

Key terms should be the same throughout the paper.

Make the **figures and tables** and the text agree.

All variables in figures and tables should be in Methods and Results, and the key terms naming the variables should be the same.

Values restated in the text should be the same as those in figures and tables, and the units of measurement should be the same.

Each figure and table should show what the text says it shows.

For the **references**,

Every reference in the text must be in the reference list.

Every reference in the reference list must be in the text.

Every reference must say what you claim it says.

Make the **abstract** both reflect the paper accurately and be understandable by itself.

The question in the abstract should be the same as the question in the Introduction.

The answer in the abstract should be the same as the answer in the Discussion.

The experimental approach and experimental details in the abstract should be the same as those in the Introduction and Methods.

Results and data in the abstract should be the same as those in Results, figures, and tables.

Signals should be used for what was found, the answer, and any implications.

The overview in the abstract should be the same as the overview in the text.

Make the **title** reflect the paper accurately.

If the title indicates the topic of the paper, it should be the same topic as in the question.

If the title indicates the answer to the question, it should be the same answer as in the abstract and the Discussion.

The title should include

the independent variable,

the dependent variable,

the species,

the point, when possible.

Important Information to Include

Do not omit any important information. Include
    the question (in the abstract and in the Introduction).
    the answer (in the abstract and in the Discussion).
    the species
        in the title.
        in the abstract.
        in the question or the experimental approach (Introduction).
        in Methods.
        in Results.
        in the answer or the signal of the answer (Discussion).
        in at least the first figure legend.
        in at least the first table title.
    key aspects of the study design, methods, and data analysis (in
        Methods).
    all relevant results, whether or not they support your answer (in Re-
        sults), and supporting data (in figures, tables, or the text).
    alternative explanations of results (in the Discussion).
    discussion of any weaknesses in the study design, limitations of the
        methods, and the validity of assumptions (in Methods or the Dis-
        cussion).
    definitions of abbreviations.
    definitions of values after a "$\pm$" in tables and in the text.
    definitions of error bars in graphs.
    the sample size (n).
    sufficient information in figure legends and in footnotes of tables to
        make the figure or table understandable without reference to the
        text.
    important references.

The Trees Versus the Forest

Do not include any unnecessary information or unnecessary repetition.
"The more noise, the less message."
    Check that all information in the text and in the figures and tables
        relates closely to the question and answer.
    Make sentences, paragraphs, and each section of the paper concise.
    In the **Introduction,**
        Start close to the specific topic.
        Do not review the literature.
        Funnel as efficiently as possible to the question.
    In **Methods,**
        Omit details of well known methods that have already been reported;
            cite a reference.
        For methods that have been reported but are less well known, in-
            clude a brief description in addition to citing a reference.
    In **Results,**
        Give only the overview.
        Do not repeat data shown in figures and tables.
        Omit separate sentences describing methods or figures and tables.
    In **figures and tables,**
        Omit nonessential figures and tables and nonessential data.
        Do not present the same data in both a figure and a table.

In the **Discussion**,

> Do not begin by repeating the Introduction or writing a new Introduction.
>
> Do not begin with a summary of the results.
>
> Do not include tangential topics.

In the **reference list**,

> Have a sufficient number of references to give credit to others' work and to direct readers to sources of further information.
>
> Keep the number of references to a minimum.

In the **abstract**,

> Omit all noncrucial details and noncrucial data.
>
> Use percent change instead of exact values where possible.

In the **title**, omit every word and every detail that is not essential.

Avoid abbreviations.

Make your paper short, meaty, and clear.

■ *EXERCISE 12.1: SEEING THE BIG PICTURE*

1. *Using the "Checklist for The Big Picture" as a guide, <u>list the strengths and weaknesses</u> of the paper below. Be specific. You may find it helpful to outline the structure of the abstract, the Introduction, and the Discussion as done in previous exercises. You may also find it helpful to read this paper 2 or 3 times over 2 or 3 days.*

2. *<u>Rewrite</u>, <u>add overview</u>, <u>reorganize</u>, and <u>condense</u> where necessary to make the overview clearer. (If you have time, condense the description of the surgical preparation so that it really is brief—about one-third of its current length.)*

3. *Check that the <u>answer answers the question.</u>*

4. *<u>Redesign tables</u> and <u>redraw figures</u> to make them clearer.*

CHANGES IN THE PULMONARY CIRCULATION DURING BIRTH-RELATED EVENTS

Abstract

*A*At birth, there is a rapid and dramatic decrease in pulmonary vascular resistance, allowing pulmonary blood flow to increase and oxygen exchange to occur in the lungs. *B*Many events are occurring simultaneously, and those responsible for this decrease in resistance are uncertain. *C*To determine whether ventilation and oxygenation of the fetal lungs could cause this decrease in resistance, we studied chronically instrumented, near-term sheep fetuses *in utero*. *D*In 16 fetuses, we measured vascular pressures and injected radionuclide-labeled microspheres to determine pulmonary blood flow. *E*We found that ventilation of the fetal lungs with a gas mixture that produced no changes in arterial blood gases caused a large but variable increase in pulmonary blood flow, to 401% of control, no change in pulmonary arterial pressure, and a doubling of left atrial pressure. *F*Thus, pulmonary vascular resistance fell dramatically, to 34% of control. *G*Oxygenation caused a modest further increase in pulmonary blood flow and a decrease in mean pulmonary arterial pressure, so that resistance fell to 10% of control. *H*Cord occlusion caused no further changes in vascular pressures or blood flow, so resistance remained similar to oxygenation levels (11% of control). *I*The fetuses appeared to fall into 2 groups with respect to their response to ventilation: 8 of the 16 developed near maximal increases in pulmonary blood flow during ventilation *without* oxygenation, and the other 8 developed an average of only 20% of the maximal increase in blood flow during ventilation. *J*We could find no differences in the 2 groups of fetuses to explain their different responses. *K*We conclude that the changes in pulmonary vascular resistance and blood flow that occur at birth can be achieved by *in utero* ventilation and oxygenation. ^{L}Moreover, much of the vasodilatory response can be achieved without an increase in fetal pO_2. ^{M}Investigating the metabolic differences between fetuses that do and do not respond to ventilation alone may help to define the metabolic processes involved in pulmonary vasodilation at birth.

Introduction

^{A}In the circulation of both fetuses and newborns, the main role of the right ventricle is to deliver blood to the gas exchange circulation for uptake of oxygen and removal of carbon dioxide. ^{B}In the fetus, this delivery is achieved by virtue of the pulmonary vascular resistance being very high. ^{C}Right ventricular output is thus diverted away from the lungs and toward the placenta, through the ductus arteriosus (1–4). ^{D}Immediately at birth, as the lungs become the organ of gas exchange, pulmonary vascular resistance must fall dramatically, allowing pulmonary blood flow to increase and oxygen exchange to occur in the lungs. ^{E}If pulmonary vascular resistance does not fall, the syndrome of persistent pulmonary hypertension of the newborn occurs, often leading to death.

^{F}Which of the many events that occur at birth are responsible for the normal decrease in pulmonary vascular resistance is not fully understood. ^{G}Three major events of the birth process that could be responsible are ventilation, or rhythmic gaseous distension, of fetal lungs, oxygenation of the lungs, and occlusion of the umbilical cord. ^{H}Two of these events—ventilation and oxygenation—have been studied in acutely exteriorized fetal sheep. ^{I}Most of the studies suggested that oxygenation rather than ventilation of the fetal lungs is the major event responsible for the decrease in pulmonary vascular resistance (5–10). ^{J}However, the metabolic effects of acute anesthesia and surgery may have altered the pulmonary vascular response in these studies, because this response is considered to be at least partly mediated by vasoactive metabolites. ^{K}Although a change in oxygen or carbon dioxide concentration (11) or induction of a gas-liquid interface in the alveolus (12) each may directly affect pulmonary vascular resistance, production or inhibition of various metabolic agents probably plays a major role in the profound decrease in pulmonary vascular resistance at birth. ^{L}Alterations in concentration of bradykinins (10, 13), angiotensin (14, 15), acetylcholine (16), and histamine (17, 18) have all

been investigated, but metabolites of arachidonic acid have been most exten-
sively studied and are considered to be the principal agents involved. *M*Of
the prostanoids, PGI_2 is the most potent pulmonary vasodilator and is produced
in response to breathing (19) or mechanical ventilation (20, 21). *N*Conversely,
leukotrienes are potent pulmonary vasoconstrictors (22–24), and inhibition of
leukotriene synthesis dramatically augments pulmonary blood flow in fetal
sheep (25).

*O*The purpose of this study was to determine whether the sequential exposure of the fetus to gaseous ventilation, oxygenation, and umbilical cord
occlusion could decrease pulmonary vascular resistance to levels seen at birth.
*P*To remove the superimposed effects of acute anesthetic and surgical stresses
and of other components of the birth process, such as prenatal hormonal surges,
labor, delivery, and cold exposure, we studied near-term fetal sheep *in utero*
2–3 days after surgery.

Methods

Animals

1 Sixteen fetal sheep were studied at 134.9 $\pm$ 1.2 (SD) days of gestation
(term is about 145 days). The fetuses were of normal weight (3.6 $\pm$ 0.6 kg)
and had normal blood gases (see Results) and hemoglobin concentrations (10.9
$\pm$ 1.6 g/dl) at the onset of the study.

Surgical Preparation

2 The surgical protocol has been described previously (4, 26). Briefly, the
ewe underwent a midline laparotomy under spinal (1% tetracaine hydrochloride) and supplemental intravenous (ketamine hydrochloride) anesthesia. The
fetus also received local anesthesia (0.25% lidocaine hydrochloride) for each
skin incision. Through a small uterine incision, the fetal hind limbs were
exposed individually and polyvinyl catheters were advanced to the descending
aorta and inferior vena cava via each pedal artery and vein. Two catheters
were also advanced into the main umbilical vein via a peripheral tributary
localized from the same uterine incision. This incision was closed after placement of a large polyvinyl catheter in the amniotic cavity for zero pressure
reference. A second uterine incision was then made over the left chest. A left
lateral thoracotomy was performed and catheters were placed in the ascending
aorta via the internal thoracic artery and directly in the pulmonary artery

and left atrium using a needle-cannula assembly (27). An 8F multiple side-hole polyvinyl catheter was left in the pleural cavity for drainage. The thoracotomy was closed and a midline incision was made in the neck. The trachea was exposed and ligated proximally, and an endotracheal tube (4.5 mm ID) was inserted directly and advanced to the region of the carina. The tube was attached to two pieces of 12F polyvinyl tubing via a Y connector and filled with 0.9% NaCl solution. One piece of tubing was sealed and the other was connected to another 12F tubing that was placed in the amniotic cavity, to allow free drainage of tracheal fluid postoperatively. The neck incision was closed. The umbilical cord was then located and a silicone rubber balloon occluder was placed around it, just distal to the abdomen. Antibiotics (400 mg of kanamycin sulfate and 1 million units of penicillin G potassium) were instilled in the amniotic cavity and 0.9% warmed saline was added to replace loss of amniotic fluid. The uterine incision was closed. All vascular catheters were filled with heparin sodium (1000 units/ml), sealed, and exteriorized along with the other tubing to the left flank of the ewe. The abdominal incision was closed in layers and the ewe was returned to the cage for recovery. Antibiotics (400 mg of kanamycin sulfate and 1 million units of penicillin G potassium) were administered intravenously to the ewe and into the amniotic cavity daily.

Experimental Protocol

3 Four experiments were performed in the sequence presented below. Each experiment was performed at least 15 minutes after pressures and blood gases had stabilized.

Control

4 The ewe was placed in a study cage and allowed free access to alfalfa pellets and water. During all 4 experiments, after vascular catheters were connected to Statham P23Db strain-gauge transducers (Statham Instruments, Oxnard, CA), pressures were recorded continuously on a direct-writing polygraph (Beckman Instruments, San Jose, CA). For control experiments, fetal blood samples were obtained from the ascending aorta for determination of pH, pCO_2, and pO_2 (Corning 158 pH/blood gas analyzer, Medfield, MA), and of hemoglobin concentration and hemoglobin oxygen saturation (Radiometer OSM2 hemoximeter, Copenhagen, Denmark). Radionuclide-labeled microspheres (selected from [57]Co, ^{51}Cr, [153]Gd, [114]In, [54]Mn, [95]Nb, [113]Sn, [85]Sr, and [65]Zn), 15 μm in diameter, were then injected into the inferior vena cava while reference blood samples were withdrawn from the ascending aorta, descending aorta, and pulmonary artery at a rate of 4 ml/min. Fetal or maternal blood was then given to replace the blood loss.

Ventilation

5 The 2 polyvinyl tubes connected to the tracheal tube were opened and the tracheal fluid was allowed to drain by gravity. A mixture of nitrogen, oxygen, and carbon dioxide was balanced to match the fetal blood gases obtained during the control experiment. The gas mixture was approximately 92% nitrogen, 3% oxygen, and 5% carbon dioxide. Before ventilation was begun, this gas mixture was briefly allowed to flow through the polyvinyl tubing at a rate of about 10 L/min so that the fetus would not be exposed to high concentrations of oxygen at the onset of ventilation. The tubing was then connected to a specially designed respirator, and ventilation was adjusted as described previously (26). Ventilatory settings are presented in Table 1. After variables stabilized, blood samples were obtained as for the control and two sets of radionuclide-labeled microspheres were injected, one into the inferior vena cava and the other into the left atrium, during withdrawal of reference blood samples as described for the control. Replacement blood was then infused into the fetus.

TABLE 1. *Ventilatory settings for variables in the fetal sheep during ventilation, oxygenation, and umbilical cord occlusion*

Variable	Ventilation[a]	Oxygenation	Cord Occlusion
Respiratory rate (breaths/min)	50 ± 8 (15)[b]	57 ± 12 (13)	57 ± 13 (11)
Peak inspiratory pressure[c] (mmHg)	27 ± 10 (15)	26 ± 9 (14)	25 ± 9 (12)
End expiratory pressure[c] (mmHg)	3 ± 6 (15)	4 ± 6 (14)	4 ± 6 (12)

[a]During ventilation, fetuses received a mixture of nitrogen, oxygen, and carbon dioxide balanced to match their blood gases during the control experiment.
[b]Data are mean ± 1 SD for the number of fetuses given in parentheses. There were no statistically significant differences between experiments for any of the variables.
[c]Pressures are referenced to amniotic cavity pressure.

Oxygenation

6 The gas mixture was then changed to 100% oxygen and ventilation was continued. Carbon dioxide was not added to the oxygen because its addition in the first few studies increased fetal pCO_2. This increase probably occurred because placental blood flow fell during oxygenation (4), impairing carbon dioxide removal. After variables stabilized, microspheres were injected into the inferior vena cava and the left atrium, blood samples were obtained, and replacement blood was infused.

Umbilical Cord Occlusion

7   The balloon around the umbilical cord was fully inflated to occlude the umbilical blood vessels and thus abolish placental blood flow (4). After variables stabilized, the experimental protocol was repeated. In 4 of the 16 fetuses, cord occlusion could not be studied, because of a faulty balloon in 2 and the development of pneumothoraces, which led to cardiovascular decompensation, in 2.

8   Upon completion of the last experiment, the ewe was killed by injection of large doses of sodium pentobarbital and the fetus was removed from the uterus and weighed. The lungs were removed from the carcass, and the lungs and carcass were separately weighed and placed in formalin. They were then separately carbonized in an oven, ground into a coarse powder, and placed in plastic vials to a uniform height of 3 cm. Radioactivity of the lungs and reference blood samples was counted in a 1000-channel multichannel pulse-height analyzer (Norland, Fort Atkinson, WI). Specific activity of each isotope within a sample was calculated by the least-squares method (28).

Calculations

9   During the control experiment, because there is no left-to-right shunt through the ductus arteriosus (29), pulmonary blood flow was measured by injecting microspheres into the inferior vena cava and withdrawing blood samples from the pulmonary artery. This injection and withdrawal technique excludes bronchial flow. In 6 fetuses we also injected microspheres into the left atrium during the control experiment. We found that bronchial flow was relatively constant and quite small, always less than 3% of combined ventricular output. We then subtracted this value from the pulmonary blood flow measurements in the remaining experiments.

10   Upon ventilation, pulmonary vascular resistance falls and blood flow increases dramatically. Thus, a left-to-right shunt through the ductus arteriosus cannot be excluded. To measure pulmonary blood flow in the presence of a left-to-right shunt requires a technique that determines the contribution of left ventricular output to pulmonary blood flow. Therefore, during ventilation, oxygenation, and umbilical cord occlusion, we injected microspheres labeled with different radionuclides simultaneously into both the inferior vena cava and the left atrium and calculated pulmonary blood flow as the difference between combined ventricular output and the sum of blood flows to the fetal body and placenta (4). Combined ventricular output was calculated as the sum of left and right ventricular outputs. Blood flows to fetal body and placenta were calculated from the left atrial injections and reference blood withdrawals from the ascending and descending aorta (4).

11　Pulmonary vascular resistance was calculated as the difference between mean pulmonary arterial pressure and mean left atrial pressure divided by pulmonary blood flow. For the 6 fetuses in which we were unable to measure left atrial pressure for technical reasons, we used the mean values obtained from the other fetuses during the same experiment.

Analysis of Data

12　In this study, we assessed the sequential effects of ventilation, oxygenation, and umbilical cord occlusion. Determination of their independent effects was not possible because the order of the experiments could not be randomized. One reason is that we were concerned that oxygenation of the fetal lungs might induce multiple and perhaps irreversible metabolic and hemodynamic consequences, so that subsequent ventilation without oxygenation could not be studied. Another reason is that the umbilical cord cannot be occluded before oxygenation. Thus, the protocol is composed of 4 sequential experiments, each serving as the control for the next. Data from each of these experiments were analyzed by the Mann-Whitney U test, comparing only the data obtained during one experiment with data obtained during the experiment immediately preceding it. Statistical significance was considered present when the P value was ≤ 0.01. All data are presented as mean $\pm$ 1 SD.

Results

1　Systemic arterial blood gases and hemoglobin oxygen saturation were normal in the control experiment, and did not change during ventilation alone (Table 2). Oxygenation caused a large increase in pO_2 and hemoglobin oxygen saturation, but did not change pH or pCO_2. Cord occlusion did not change these

TABLE 2. *Ascending aortic pH, blood gases, and hemoglobin oxygen saturations during the experiments*

Variable	Control	Ventilation	Oxygenation	Cord Occlusion
pH	7.37 ± 0.06 (15)[a]	7.35 ± 0.07 (16)	7.34 ± 0.09 (16)	7.29 ± 0.15 (13)
pO_2 (mmHg)	18 ± 3 (15)	19 ± 4 (16)	215 ± 154* (16)	263 ± 168 (13)
pCO_2 (mmHg)	55 ± 6 (15)	54 ± 6 (16)	51 ± 10 (16)	58 ± 21 (12)
Hgb O_2 sat.[b] (%)	47 ± 13 (16)	46 ± 12 (16)	97 ± 6* (16)	95 ± 10 (16)

[a]Data are mean ± 1 SD for four sequential experiments on the number of fetal sheep given in parentheses.
[b]Hgb O_2 sat., hemoglobin oxygen saturation.
*Significantly different from the value during the immediately preceding experiment, $P \leq 0.01$.

variables significantly, but there was much greater variability in pCO_2 and pH, probably because of the inability of some fetuses to maintain adequate CO_2 exchange in the lungs, because of pulmonary immaturity.

2 Pulmonary blood flow in the control experiment (33 ± 17 ml/min/kg fetal body weight) was similar to that previously measured in chronically instrumented fetuses of similar gestational ages (2, 3), constituting 9% of combined ventricular output (Figure 1). It increased dramatically during ventilation alone, to 401% of control values (133 ± 94 ml/min/kg fetal body weight). The variability of this increase in pulmonary blood flow was marked, however, which led us to separate the fetuses into 2 groups, as described below. Oxygenation increased pulmonary blood flow further, to a mean of 623% of control (206 ± 64 ml/min/kg fetal body weight). Umbilical cord occlusion did not cause any further change in pulmonary blood flow (190 ± 69 ml/min/kg fetal body weight).

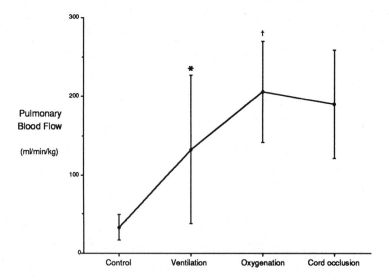

Figure 1. Pulmonary blood flow during sequential ventilation, oxygenation, and umbilical cord occlusion in the 16 fetal sheep. Data are mean ± 1 SD. * $P \leq 0.001$, † $P \leq 0.005$ vs. the experiment immediately preceding it.

3 Mean pulmonary arterial pressure was normal in the control experiment and did not change during ventilation (Table 3). There was a small but significant decrease in pressure during oxygenation. Because this decrease was similar to that seen in mean systemic arterial pressure, it can not be explained by partial closure of the ductus arteriosus. There was no further change in mean pulmonary or mean systemic arterial pressure after umbilical cord oc-

TABLE 3. *Mean vascular pressures during the experiments*

Pressure[a]	Control	Ventilation	Oxygenation	Cord Occlusion
Pulmonary arterial pressure (mmHg)	53 ± 8 (15)[b]	55 ± 9 (15)	$47 \pm 6^*$ (15)	48 ± 16 (12)
Systemic arterial pressure (mmHg)	52 ± 6 (15)	53 ± 6 (15)	$48 \pm 6^*$ (15)	58 ± 16 (12)
Left atrial pressure (mmHg)	4 ± 5 (12)	$9 \pm 4^*$ (10)	10 ± 5 (10)	9 ± 5 (7)

[a]Pressures are referenced to amniotic cavity pressure.
[b]Data are mean $\pm$ 1 SD for the number of fetal sheep given in parentheses.
*Significantly different from the value during the immediately preceding experiment, $P \leq 0.01$.

clusion. Left atrial pressure could be measured in only 10 fetuses for technical reasons. In association with the large increase in pulmonary blood flow during ventilation alone, mean left atrial pressure doubled (Table 3). It did not change further during oxygenation or cord occlusion. Pulmonary vascular resistance decreased dramatically (to 34% of control values) during ventilation alone (from 1.93 ± 1.31 to 0.66 ± 0.90 mmHg $\cdot$ min $\cdot$ kg/ml), decreased further during oxygenation (to 10% of control; 0.20 ± 0.77 mmHg $\cdot$ min $\cdot$ kg/ml), and did not change further after cord occlusion (11%; 0.22 ± 0.11 mmHg $\cdot$ min $\cdot$ kg/ml) (Figure 2).

Major vs. Minor Responders During Ventilation Alone

4 The individual changes in pulmonary blood flow were extremely variable (Figure 3). In some fetuses the majority of the increase occurred during ventilation alone, whereas in others there was almost no increase until oxygenation. This finding led us to separate the fetuses according to their response to ventilation and examine the reasons for this variability. We arbitrarily divided the fetuses into 2 groups: major responders, which showed an increase in pulmonary blood flow during ventilation alone that was at least 50% of the cumulative increase (the difference between pulmonary blood flow during control measurements and after cord occlusion), and minor responders, which

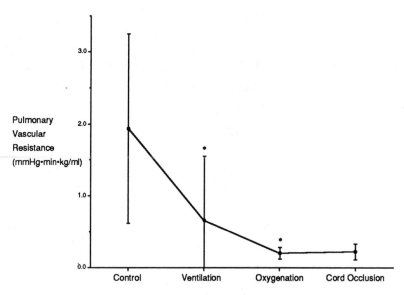

Figure 2. Pulmonary vascular resistance during sequential ventilation, oxygenation, and umbilical cord occlusion in the 16 fetal sheep. Data are mean ± 1 SD. * $P \le 0.001$ vs. the experiment immediately preceding it.

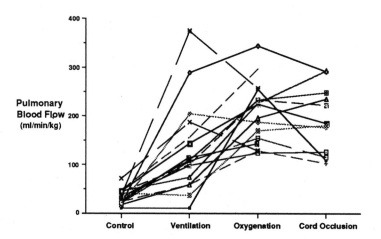

Figure 3. Individual changes in pulmonary blood flow in each of the 16 fetal sheep during sequential ventilation, oxygenation, and umbilical cord occlusion.

showed an increase of less than 50%. Interestingly, 8 fetuses were major responders and 8 were minor responders. The major responders had an increase in flow during ventilation that was equal to the cumulative increase (103 ± 52%), whereas the minor responders had a much smaller increase (20 ± 17%).

5 We examined the measured variables that could have caused this disparity between the major and minor responders (Table 4). None of those variables showed statistically significant differences between the 2 groups (Table 4). Indices of maturity and postoperative stability (gestational age, weight, and days after surgery), of initial pulmonary vascular tone (control pH and blood

TABLE 4. *Comparisons of variables in major and minor responders[a] during the control experiment and oxygenation*

Variable	Major responders		Minor responders	
Gestational age at study (days)	135 ± 1	(7)[b]	135 ± 1	(8)
Weight (kg)	3.5 ± 0.6	(8)	3.8 ± 0.6	(8)
Days after surgery	2.3 ± 0.7	(8)	2.0 ± 0.0	(8)
CONTROL				
pH	7.37 ± 0.07	(8)	7.39 ± 0.03	(7)
pO_2 (mmHg)	18 ± 2	(8)	18 ± 3	(7)
pCO_2 (mmHg)	55 ± 6	(8)	54 ± 6	(7)
Pulmonary blood flow (ml/min/kg)	33 ± 19	(8)	33 ± 15	(7)
Mean pulmonary arterial pressure(mmHg)	53 ± 12	(7)	53 ± 4	(8)
Combined ventricular output (ml/min/kg)	401 ± 84	(8)	378 ± 69	(8)
OXYGENATION				
pO_2 (mmHg)	215 ± 150	(8)	215 ± 168	(8)
pCO_2 (mmHg)	52 ± 11	(8)	49 ± 10	(8)
Pulmonary blood flow (ml/min/kg)	195 ± 76	(8)	217 ± 52	(8)

[a]Major responders had increases in pulmonary blood flow ≥ 50% of the cumulative increase during the study. Minor responders had increases < 50%.

[b]Data are mean ± 1 SD for the number of fetal sheep given in parentheses. No difference between groups was statistically significant.

gases and pulmonary blood flow and pressure), of ventricular function (combined ventricular output), and of adequacy of alveolar ventilation during oxygenation (blood gases and pulmonary blood flow during oxygenation) were remarkably similar. Adequacy of alveolar ventilation during ventilation alone (*without* oxygenation) could not be assessed, although there was no change in the method of ventilation in either group when oxygenation was established. Of those fetuses in which sex was recorded, the majority in both groups were female (6 of 7 of the major responders, 4 of 6 of the minor responders).

Discussion

1 *A*Three major events of the birth process are ventilation, or rhythmic gaseous distension of the lungs, oxygenation, and loss of the umbilical-placental circulation. *B*We found that ventilation and oxygenation together can account for the decrease in pulmonary vascular resistance, and thus for the large increase in pulmonary blood flow, that normally occur at birth. *C*Moreover, on average, nearly two-thirds of the increase in pulmonary blood flow occurred during ventilation alone.

2 ^{D}Our finding that about two-thirds of the decrease in pulmonary vascular resistance occurs during ventilation alone is much larger than the previously accepted value of about one-third (6). ^{E}The reason we found a larger decrease than previously accepted may be that previous studies were performed on acutely exteriorized fetuses (5, 6, 8–10). ^{F}An acute stress such as that caused by the anesthesia and surgery used to exteriorize a fetus can greatly alter production and inhibition of various metabolic agents. ^{G}Altered metabolite production and inhibition could have slowed the rate of decrease in pulmonary vascular resistance during the second phase of the decrease (30) in those studies. ^{H}Evidence for this possibility is that the prostaglandin synthesis inhibitor indomethacin has been shown to attenuate this slow second phase of the decrease, which lasts for 10–20 minutes after the rapid first phase (30). ^{I}(In contrast, the first phase, a rapid decrease that lasts for only 30 seconds, is not altered by indomethacin but may be altered by direct mechanical effects of ventilation: the establishment of a gas-liquid interface in the alveoli may decrease perivascular pressures and thus distend the small arterioles and decrease resistance (30).) ^{J}Further evidence that prostaglandin metabolites are important in the decrease of pulmonary vascular resistance is that prostaglandin I_2, a potent pulmonary vasodilator, is produced in response to either mechanical ventilation (20, 21) or breathing (19) in recently delivered fetal lambs. ^{K}In addition, the production of prostaglandin E_1, prostaglandin D_2, and bradykinin and the inhibition of leukotrienes C_4 and D_4 may affect pulmonary vascular resistance (31). ^{L}Thus, the variable but generally lesser effects of ventilation alone in the previous studies may be ascribed to the variable effects of the study protocols on the metabolic milieu of the pulmonary vascular bed.

3 ^{M}We also found great variability in the response of fetal pulmonary blood flow to the effects of ventilation alone. ^{N}In one-half of the fetuses, the mean increase in pulmonary blood flow during ventilation alone was maximal, whereas in the other half it was only about 20% of the cumulative response. ^{O}Interestingly, Cook et al. (11) found similar variability in their study of nitrogen and air ventilation: of the 6 fetuses studied, 2 showed no effect of nitrogen ventilation but a large effect upon changing to air, 2 showed a small effect of nitrogen and a larger response to air, and 2 showed a large increase in pulmonary blood flow during nitrogen ventilation with no further change upon exposure to air. ^{P}To explain these findings, Cook et al. noted that nitrogen had the greatest effect on the smallest fetuses. ^QHowever, we were unable to identify the reasons for the variability we found. ^RIt was not on a purely arithmetic basis. ^SThat is, the major responders did not begin with lower control flows or have lower maximal flows. ^TIn fact, the 2 groups had remarkably similar pulmonary blood flows both during control measurements and during ventilation with 100% oxygen. ^UThe groups were also not different in their overall maturity, with respect to either gestational age or weight. ^VIn addition, differences in pO_2 were not responsible for the differences between major and minor responders, since both during control measurements and during ventilation alone, the minor responders were neither more hypoxic nor more hypercapnic than the major responders. ^WLastly, adequacy of alveolar ventilation was probably not responsible for the difference between the groups. ^XAlthough we were not able to determine the adequacy of alveolar ventilation during ventilation alone, during oxygenation, pO_2 and pCO_2 values were similar in the 2 groups, without the method of ventilation having been changed in either group.

4 ^YThe marked difference between the pulmonary vasodilatory responses of the 2 groups of fetuses is thus unexplained, but this difference may have important implications for future studies. ^ZFirst, it may be important in uncovering the metabolic processes responsible for an incomplete decrease in pulmonary vascular resistance at birth. ^AASecond, evaluation of the concentrations and fluxes of the putative metabolic agents involved may demonstrate different fates of these agents in major and minor responders. ^BBHowever, careful evaluation of lung mechanics is critical in future studies to ensure that the differences between the responses of the pulmonary vascular bed are not caused solely by differences in pulmonary function. ^CCIn this regard, it would be of interest to determine whether static gaseous distension of the lungs (that is, distension without ventilation) can induce a similar decrease in pulmonary vascular resistance. ^DDStatic distension does increase lung compliance in fetal sheep (32) and has been shown to decrease pulmonary vascular resistance to some degree in acutely exteriorized fetal sheep (12).

5 ^EEIn summary, the changes in pulmonary vascular resistance and blood flow that are critical to the adaptation of the fetus to the postnatal environment can be achieved by *in utero* ventilation and oxygenation. ^FFMoreover, much of the vasodilatory response can be achieved without an increase in fetal pO_2.

*GG*This effect is variable. *HH*The variability is probably mediated in part by alterations in a variety of vasoactive metabolites. *II*By using an *in utero* preparation to investigate the metabolic differences between fetuses that do and do not respond to ventilation alone, the processes responsible for the syndrome of persistent pulmonary hypertension of the newborn may be better elucidated.

References

1. Reuss ML, Rudolph AM. Distribution and recirculation of umbilical and systemic venous blood flow in fetal lambs during hypoxia. J Dev Physiol 1980;2:71–84.
2. Anderson DF, Bissonnette JM, Faber JJ, Thornburg KL. Central shunt flows and pressures in the mature fetal lamb. Am J Physiol 1981;241:H60–6.
3. Heymann MA, Creasy RK, Rudolph AM. Quantitation of blood flow patterns in the foetal lamb *in utero*. In: Foetal and neonatal physiology: proceedings of the Sir Joseph Barcroft centenary symposium. Cambridge: Cambridge University Press, 1973:129–35.
4. Teitel DF, Iwamoto HS, Rudolph AM. Effects of birth-related events on central blood flow patterns. Pediatr Res 1987;22:557–66.
5. Lauer RM, Evans JA, Aoki H, Kittle CF. Factors controlling pulmonary vascular resistance in fetal lambs. J Pediatr 1965;67:568–77.
6. Dawes GS, Mott JC, Widdicombe JG, Wyatt DG. Changes in the lungs of the new-born lamb. J Physiol 1953;121:141–62.
7. Dawes GS. The pulmonary circulation in the foetus and newborn. In: Foetal and neonatal physiology: a comparative study of the changes at birth. Chicago: Yearbook Medical Publishers, 1968:79–90.
8. Cassin S, Dawes GS, Mott JC, Ross BB, Strang LB. The vascular resistance of the foetal and newly ventilated lung of the lamb. J Physiol 1964;171:61–79.
9. Assali NS, Kirschbaum TH, Dilts PV Jr. Effects of hyperbaric oxygen on uteroplacental and fetal circulation. Circ Res 1968;22:573–88.
10. Heymann MA, Rudolph AM, Nies AS, Melmon KL. Bradykinin production associated with oxygenation of the fetal lamb. Circ Res 1969;25:521–34.
11. Cook CD, Drinker PA, Jacobson HN, Levison H, Strang LB. Control of pulmonary blood flow in the foetal and newly born lamb. J Physiol 1963;169:10–29.
12. Colebatch HJH, Dawes GS, Goodwin JW, Nadeau RA. The nervous control of the circulation in the foetal and newly expanded lungs of the lamb. J Physiol 1965;178:544–62.
13. Campbell AGM, Cockburn F, Dawes GS, Milligan JE. Pulmonary vasoconstriction in asphyxia during cross-circulation between twin foetal lambs. J Physiol 1967;192:111–21.
14. Hyman A, Heymann M, Levin D, Rudolph A. Angiotensin is not the mediator of hypoxia-induced pulmonary vasoconstriction in fetal lambs [Abstract]. Circulation 1975;52 (Suppl II):132.
15. Davidson D, Stalcup SA, Mellins RB. Angiotensin-converting enzyme activity and its modulation by oxygen tension in the guinea pig fetal-placental unit. Circ Res 1981;48:286–91.
16. Lewis AB, Heymann MA, Rudolph AM. Gestational changes in pulmonary vascular responses in fetal lambs in utero. Circ Res 1976;39:536–41.

17. Cassin S, Dawes GS, Ross BB. Pulmonary blood flow and vascular resistance in immature foetal lambs. J Physiol 1964;171:80–9.
18. Goetzman BW, Milstein JM. Pulmonary vascular histamine receptors in newborn and young lambs. J Appl Physiol 1980;49:380–85.
19. Leffler CW, Hessler JR, Green RS. The onset of breathing at birth stimulates pulmonary vascular prostacyclin synthesis. Pediatr Res 1984;18:938–42.
20. Leffler CW, Hessler JR. Perinatal pulmonary prostaglandin production. Am J Physiol 1981;241:H756–9.
21. Leffler CW, Hessler JR, Terragno NA. Ventilation-induced release of prostaglandinlike material from fetal lungs. Am J Physiol 1980;238:H282–6.
22. Schreiber MD, Heymann MA, Soifer SJ. The differential effects of leukotriene C_4 and D_4 on the pulmonary and systemic circulations in newborn lambs. Pediatr Res 1987;21:176–82.
23. Hand JM, Will JA, Buckner CK. Effects of leukotrienes on isolated guinea-pig pulmonary arteries. Eur J Pharmacol 1981;76:439–42.
24. Morganroth ML, Stenmark KR, Zirrolli JA, et al. Leukotriene C_4 production during hypoxic pulmonary vasoconstriction in isolated rat lungs. Prostaglandins 1984;28:867–75.
25. Lebidois J, Soifer SJ, Clyman RI, Heymann MA. Piriprost: a putative leukotriene synthesis inhibitor increases pulmonary blood flow in fetal lambs. Pediatr Res 1987;22:350–4.
26. Iwamoto HS, Teitel DF, Rudolph AM. Effects of birth-related events on blood flow distribution. Pediatr Res 1987;22:634–40.
27. Iwamoto HS, Rudolph AM. Chronic renal venous catheterization in fetal sheep. Am J Physiol 1983;245:H524–7.
28. Baer RW, Payne BD, Verrier ED, et al. Increased number of myocardial blood flow measurements with radionuclide-labeled microspheres. Am J Physiol 1984;246:H418–34.
29. Assali NS, Sehgal N, Marable S. Pulmonary and ductus arteriosus circulation in the fetal lamb before and after birth. Am J Physiol 1962;202:536–40.
30. Leffler CW, Tyler TL, Cassin S. Effect of indomethacin on pulmonary vascular response to ventilation of fetal goats. Am J Physiol 1978;234:H346–51.
31. Heymann MA. Control of the pulmonary circulation in the perinatal period. J Dev Physiol 1984;6:281–90.
32. Ikegami M, Jobe A, Berry D, Elkady T, Pettenazzo A, Seidner S. Effects of distention of the preterm fetal lamb lung on lung function with ventilation. Am Rev Respir Dis 1987;135:600–6.

REACHING THE GOAL: SUGGESTIONS FOR WRITING

This book deals with what a clearly written biomedical research paper looks like when it is done. Getting a paper into clear final form is another matter. To help you move from a blank piece of paper to a finished manuscript based on the principles in this book, here are a few suggestions.

WRITING THE FIRST DRAFT

Writing the first draft is difficult. The reason is that you have only a rough idea of what you want to say. It is only as you are writing the first draft that you discover exactly what you want to say. So expect to spend a fair amount of time and energy writing your first draft.

To make writing the first draft as easy as possible,

- Reserve a block of time for writing (3–4 hours every day for 4 or 5 days).
- Write when your energy is high, not when you are tired.
- Surround yourself with everything you need to write efficiently (all the data, drafts of figures and tables, references, computer or paper, coffee . . .).
- Work in a quiet place where you will not be interrupted.
- Decide what journal you plan to submit your paper to and tailor the paper to that journal and its readers, at least approximately (for example, clinical journal, basic research journal, general journal) (see Huth, Chap. 1).

Starting is the hardest part. To get started, write the easiest section first. For many authors, the easiest section is Methods. For example, you may want to write Methods and Results first, then the Discussion, the Introduction, and the reference list, then figure legends and footnotes for tables, and finally the abstract and the title. However, it does not matter what order you write the paper in. All that matters is what the paper looks like when it is finished, so do what works for you.

You may not know exactly what to say as you begin. The exact words and even the exact sentences are not important at this stage. Say something and then keep moving. As you write, ideas will come to you. You can always cross out the first sentence or two or even the first paragraph or two.

Write as quickly as you can, with no thought of following any of the writing principles in this book or any other rules of writing. The goal of the first draft is to get something on paper or into the computer, to capture your ideas before they flee from your mind, so that you have something to work with. So once you have started, do not stop. To keep speed, use abbreviations, and if you cannot think of a word, leave a blank space; you can always fill it in later, if the sentence is still in the paper later. Do not worry about whether your subjects and verbs agree, whether you changed key terms, or whether your paragraphs have topic sentences. All of these things can be dealt with during the revisions.

It is a good idea to formulate your answer and your question before you start writing because the answer and question are the touchstones against which you decide what is in the paper and what is out, and also how to organize. However, keep in mind that your answer is likely to evolve as you write your Discussion. For example, you may find that you state the answer one way at the beginning of the Discussion and another way at the end. That is in fact a great benefit of writing a paper—discovering the precise way to formulate the answer. Once you have discovered your answer, reword the question to match it and then write an Introduction that leads to that question. If you cannot manage all this matching on the first draft, that is OK. You can work on it in the revisions.

When you write the abstract, look at the way you stated the question and answer in the Introduction and Discussion. The statements of the question and answer need to be the same throughout the paper, so take the easy path—do not write a new question and answer; just copy the ones you already wrote. Similarly, when you write the title, look at the question and answer. Use the same key terms. If you use a verb in the title, make it the same verb as in the answer. But again, if it is easier for you to write without looking at the rest of the paper, you can do this matching during the revisions.

If it helps you to work from an outline, whether it is short and simple or long and complex, do so. If you cannot work from an outline, do not. Do whatever works for you. But do have some idea, either mental or written, of what you are going to say first and what next before you start to write, particularly in the Discussion.

To make writing a paper less overwhelming, think of each section as a separate task. Once Methods is written, that is one task done, etc. Also, write less. For example, write a one-paragraph Introduction if possible, just 10 or 12 sentences. Twenty sentences take longer to write, and some of them (the ones that review the literature, for example) will need to be omitted, so try to save yourself the trouble of writing them in the first place. Similarly, in the Discussion, 6 or 7 paragraphs are often enough, so try not to write 10 or 15. One unnecessary paragraph is the paragraph of introduction at the beginning. Forget that. Start by answering the question. However, if it is easier for you to begin the Discussion by rewriting the introduction, or to begin the Results by writing "Figure 1 shows," do it. You can always cross them out later. The important thing on the first draft is to keep going.

Probably you will need 4 or 5 days to write the first draft, so do not be discouraged if you cannot finish in one day. When you find yourself spinning your wheels after 3 or 4 hours, stop, and start again the next day.

REVISING: USING THE CHECKLISTS

As soon as you finish the first draft, revise it. You will see a lot to change. As you revise, use the summaries provided earlier in this book for each section of the paper as checklists, or compose your own shorter checklists of details that you have particular trouble with. Once you are satisfied with the content and organization of each section, go back and check the summaries for the chapters on paragraph structure, sentence structure, and word choice. Pay particular attention to key terms and topic sentences. Finally, check the overall story in your paper, using the checklist for the big picture. It is usually at a fairly late stage that the topic sentences that create the overview of the story are added. In some paragraphs you may have written the supporting details first and the point last. This is the natural way to write, because you are discovering what you think. However, this organization makes reading difficult, so in the revision, move the point to the beginning of the paragraph (topic sentence) and put the supporting details after the topic sentence. At a late stage also look for all possible ways to condense your paper: omit unnecessary paragraphs, unnecessary details, and unnecessary words. To decide whether to include a paragraph, a sentence, or a word, think of yourself as the reader. "Would I want to read this paragraph?" "Would I *need* to read this paragraph?" Be honest. If the answer is no, omit the paragraph. Most readers prefer short, meaty, clear papers. Have the courage to make your paper short, meaty, and clear.

You will not be able to do all this revising on one draft, so revise in stages. Do as much as you can on the first revision. When you no longer see anything to change, put the paper in a drawer for a week or two—however long it takes for you to forget what you wrote. When you look at the paper again, you should see it with fresh, critical eyes: "Did I write that?" "What could that possibly mean?" Then you are ready to work on the second draft. Most authors need four or five drafts to get a paper ready to submit. However, do not spend forever writing one paper. Scientific research papers are working knowledge, not poems. The writing does not need to be perfect, just clear.

Before submitting a paper, make one last check of three details that are frequently overlooked:

- Does the answer answer the question, and do all statements of the answer and all statements of the question say the same thing?
- Is the species stated in the title, the abstract, the question or the experimental approach (Introduction), Methods, Results, the answer or the signal of the answer (Discussion), and at least the first figure legend and the first table title?
- Are summarized data presented with all three components: mean, SD, n?

For information on submitting a paper and seeing it through to publication, see Huth, Chapters 15–19.

THE REWARDS OF CLEAR WRITING

Over the years, as you continue writing papers, reviewing the checklists in this book, and getting critical comments from your colleagues, you should be able to write better and better first drafts and better and better final drafts, though the first draft of a paper in a new field of research will be difficult to write. In addition, as you gain experience in your field and confidence in your own expertise, you should be able to write papers that are not only clear but also lively. Both you and your readers will benefit as your command of writing increases. You will understand your science more deeply, will feel comfortable about your writing, and will have the satisfaction of getting your message across and telling a clear story. In addition, your readers will enjoy reading your papers because they will be able to see the forest and not just the trees. Finally, the scientific literature will benefit: it will be shorter, clearer, meatier, and livelier. All of these goals are worth reaching.

REVISIONS OF EXERCISES

CHAPTER 1

Summary of Guidelines for Word Choice

Words in scientific research papers should be

Precise.
Simple.
Necessary.
Familiar:
   No invented words.
   No jargon.
   Few if any abbreviations.

Exercise 1.1: Principles of Word Choice

  I. <u>Words in scientific research papers should be PRECISE.</u>
      (Strunk and White, II. 16, p. 21: Use definite, specific, concrete language.)

    1. greatly decreased; reduced by 80%.
       POINT: "Compromised" is imprecise: what happened to renal blood flow? "Drastically" is also imprecise. Science is quantitative; thus, a quantitative detail such as "by 80%" is clearer than a qualitative term such as "greatly."
    2. 5? 7? 9?
       POINT: "Several" is imprecise. How long is several hours? State the mean or a range.
    3. increase.
       POINT: A change could be either an increase or a decrease. From the first sentence we cannot tell whether the author meant increase or decrease. But from "further increase" in the next sentence we can see that the change in the first sentence must have been an increase. It is clearest to write "increase," not "change," in the first sentence.
    4. incubated in.
       POINT: "Exposed to" is imprecise. How were the cells exposed? Use a specific term.
    5. lambs.
       POINT: Keep the species in the reader's mind.
    6. <u>caused</u> OR <u>resulted in</u> OR <u>led to</u> an increase in microvascular pressure, OR <u>increased</u> microvascular pressure.
       POINT: "Was associated with" is imprecise. It indicates only that some connection exists. If you can specify what the connection is, you should do so.
    7. and, OR accompanied by.

8. during.

9. induced by.

10. , reaching.

11. plasma that contained heparin, OR heparinized plasma, OR heparin-containing plasma.

    POINT: "With" is the vaguest, most ambiguous word in English. Sentences 7–11 illustrate five different meanings of "with": addition, time, cause, supporting detail, and component, respectively. Because "with" can mean so many different things, it is clearest to use a precise term whenever possible. The reader should not have to guess what you mean. (Note: There are times when "with" is OK. For example, "compared with," "treated with.")

    In Example 11, "plasma that contained heparin" is the clearest wording. "Heparinized plasma" is also OK because "heparinized" is in the dictionary (Webster's Third). "Heparin-containing plasma" must have a hyphen; otherwise it means "heparin that contains plasma."

II. <u>Words in scientific research papers should be <u>SIMPLE</u></u>.
    (Strunk and White, V. 14, p. 76: Avoid fancy words.)

12. girls, boys, after, beginning.

    POINT: The only technical term in the sentence is "dialysis," which is a heavy word. To keep the sentence light and readable, make the other words as simple as possible. (Note that "female," "male," "following," and "initiation" are not "bad words"; they are just unnecessarily fancy in this sentence.)

13. used, before.

14. cell bodies.

15. toward the liver.

    POINT: Even though "perikarya" and "hepatopetally" are legitimate technical terms, the simpler terms "cell bodies" and "toward the liver" can be used here. Specialists will not be insulted by the use of the simpler terms, and people from other fields will understand the simpler terms more readily than they will the fancy ones.

III. <u>Words in scientific research papers should be <u>NECESSARY</u></u>.
     (Strunk and White, II. 17, p. 23: Omit needless words.)

16. After 4 h we abruptly ended the hemodialysis procedure.

    POINT: "Of hemodialysis" is unnecessary because it is implied by the rest of the sentence.

17. Oxygen uptake in response to drugs varied considerably.

    POINT: It is unnecessary to say that you examined a response. If you found a response, you must have examined it. Similarly, it is not necessary in this sentence to say that a response was found. If you say what the response was, this must be what you found.

18. Both <u>of these changes</u> were greater when the pericardium was closed.

    POINT: The repetition in this sentence is worse than unnecessary: it is confusing. We do not immediately recognize that the underlined words in the original second sentence refer to the effects described in the previous sentence. To indicate to the reader that these are the same effects, it is clearest to use a category term that encompasses both decreases and increases. The best category term here is "changes." In addition, add "these" to indicate that you mentioned the changes in the previous sentence.

IV. <u>Words in scientific research papers should be FAMILIAR.</u>

A. <u>Do not invent NEW VERBS (or other new words) if old ones will do the job.</u>
    (Strunk and White, IV. -ize, p. 50: Do not coin verbs. . . .)

    19. We <u>spun</u> OR <u>agitated</u> the tubes on a Vortex mixer.
    20. We <u>injected endorphins into</u> the dogs.
    21. We studied the effect of clonidine on the hindleg reflexes of rats whose spinal cords had been cut? destroyed? rats given a spinal injection? paralyzed? anesthetized?
    22. We <u>bled</u> the dogs.
    23. Sufficient dialyzed protein was added to 200 ml of gold <u>at the proper pH</u>.
        POINT: Although verbs are powerful words in English (see Chap. 2), coining new verbs can be dangerous. The new verbs may be either unclear or ungrammatical. To ensure that your writing is clear and grammatical, and thus incapable of being misunderstood, do not use made-up verbs.

        In the examples here, "vortex" is probably the most tempting coinage because it has a precise meaning as a noun (the rotation of fluid around an axis, such as water going down a drain). The meaning would be the same for the verb. However, not everyone is familiar with the noun, so they would not understand the verb either. "Endorphinized" is much less desirable because it gives no clue to its meaning. We can guess that endorphins are involved, but how are they involved? What does it mean to endorphinize a dog? Similarly, what does it mean for a rat to be spinalized? These two made-up verbs are extremely imprecise.

        Although "hemorrhaged" and "pH'd" are more understandable, they are ungrammatical. A dog can hemorrhage (that is, bleed excessively), but someone cannot hemorrhage a dog. ("Hemorrhage" is intransitive; that is, it does not take an object.) Similarly, gold cannot be "pH'd." Since pH is not a verb, it has no past participle to be used as an adjective.

B. <u>Do not use JARGON.</u>
    (Strunk and White, V. 21, p. 81: Prefer the standard to the offbeat.)

    24. After <u>inserting catheters into</u> a femoral artery and vein, OR
    After <u>inserting catheters into a surgically exposed</u> femoral artery and vein, OR
    After <u>surgical cannulation</u> of a femoral artery and vein,
    POINT: Although "cutdown" is in the dictionary (Webster's Third), as used here it is not what the word means or what the author intended. These facts bring up an important point: just because a word is in the dictionary does not mean that you have to use it.
    25. radioactive, radiolabeled.
    26. ventilated with, connected to.
    POINT: Jargon is imprecise and ambiguous and sometimes very far from the intended meaning.

C. <u>Do not use NONSTANDARD ABBREVIATIONS.</u>
    (Strunk and White, V. 19, p. 81: Do not take shortcuts at the cost of clarity.)

    27. Omit all the abbreviations. Omitting unnecessary variables in results will permit the names of the remaining variables to be written out in full. In addition, since there were no significant differences between

groups, sentences G–K can probably be condensed to "no significant differences were found between the means of any of these variables for the two groups." This revision shortens the abstract substantially and thus leaves plenty of room to write out all the words that are now abbreviated.

Comments on Guidelines for Word Choice

Precise

Your words should be as precise as your science.

Note that precise, definite, concrete, specific words evoke a mental image. For example, "dog" evokes much more of a mental image than "animal" does. Similarly, "pattern of discharge" evokes much more of a mental image than "response characteristics" does. Words that evoke mental images help make writing easy to read. Abstractions (such as "animal" and "characteristics") make reading difficult.

Simple

Use simple words.

The point is not that big, fancy words are bad and that little, simple words are good. The point is that you must use technical words, and these tend to be big, fancy, and heavy. Therefore, to keep your writing from being too heavy, choose simple words for the rest of the sentence. Simple words usually have few syllables. They are words you would say to a child. For example, most people would not say "utilize" to a child; they would say "use." Some fancy words and their simple equivalents are listed below.

Fancy, Heavy	Simple, Light
prior to	before
subsequent to	after
following	after
utilize	use
initiate	begin
initial	first

In general, if an idea is simple, do not make it complex. If an idea is complex, write it as simply as possible.

Necessary

Use the fewest words possible. The more noise, the less message. However, remember that brevity is not the first principle of word choice; it is the third principle. The point is to be as brief as possible consistent with clarity. If it takes more words to be clear, use more words. (For example, see Chap. 2, "Do Not Pile Nouns Into Noun Clusters.")

Familiar

Use familiar words. Do not use invented words, jargon, or abbreviations.

One argument against using invented words, jargon, and abbreviations is that they are unlikely to be familiar to many of your readers. In addition, invented words and jargon are often imprecise. For example, what does the invented word "endorphinized" mean, as in "we endorphinized the dogs"? For another example, some people always misread the jargon term "hot" in "scintillation fluid was added to the hot samples" as "heated" instead of "radioactive."

Abbreviations are deceptive. They make reading easier *if* you know them already. If the abbreviations are new to you, they make reading a chore. Since a sizable percentage of your readers may not recognize the abbreviations (for example, readers whose first language is not English, or graduate students and others new to the field), you should keep abbreviations to a minimum.

Guidelines for Using Abbreviations

Note: These guidelines are for abbreviations made of the first letter of each word or of each important syllable (for example, DNA, deoxyribonucleic acid). Standard abbreviations for units of measurement (Système International, or SI, units, for example, ml, kg, min) are internationally accepted and therefore can be used freely.

General

Avoid abbreviations, especially nonstandard and semistandard ones. Reading becomes geometrically more difficult as the number of abbreviations increases. As a rule, one abbreviation per paragraph is reasonable. Two are tolerable. Three start turning sense into alphabet soup. In any given paper, try to have no more than three abbreviations. Having no abbreviations is best.

Abbreviations make writing faster and give the writer a feeling of belonging to the club, but they make reading a chore, especially for people who do not work in the field and for people whose first language is not English. A special problem arises when a given combination of letters has one meaning in one field and another meaning in another field. For example, BPD means bronchopulmonary dysplasia in neonatology and biparietal diameter in obstetrics. When readers read in the other field, they automatically give the abbreviation their own meaning and have to make a conscious effort to assign the other meaning to the abbreviation. This extra effort slows down reading.

Remember, the goal is not to use abbreviations; the goal is clarity. Just because an abbreviation exists, that does not mean you have to use it.

Types of Abbreviations and Their Uses

Type	*Definition*	*Example*	*Use*
Standard	Recognized by scientists in all specialties	DNA (deoxyribonucleic acid) cAMP (cyclic adenosine monophosphate) EDTA (ethylenediaminetetraacetic acid)	Any journal
Semi-standard	Recognized by scientists in a given specialty	In respiratory physiology: TLC (total lung capacity) FRC (functional residual capacity) FEV_1 (forced expiratory volume in the first second)	Specialty journals (Treat semistandard abbreviations as nonstandard abbreviations in general journals)
Non-standard	Made up for a given paper	Group A, Group B IHE (isometric handgrip exercise)	Avoid

When to Use Abbreviations

Use abbreviations only when they are unavoidable. An abbreviation is unavoidable only when the term that the abbreviation stands for is *long or unwieldy and* the term appears a *great many* times in the paper. "Heart rate" is not long or unwieldy. "Norepinephrine" is not long or unwieldy. Five times is not many. Ten times is not many. If an abbreviation appears only 5 or 10 times in a paper, some readers have to keep looking up its meaning, which hinders reading. An abbreviation should be used often enough that the reader does not forget the meaning. One exception is that a very long term, such as tetradecanoylphorbal acetate (TPA), should be abbreviated even if it is used only once or twice more in the paper, preferably within one paragraph. Another exception is an abbreviation that is more familiar to the readers of the journal than is the term the abbreviation stands for, for example, DNA, HEPES buffer. Such abbreviations may be used freely.

Where to Use Abbreviations

in chemical formulas
in mathematical equations
in tables if space is limited
in the text only if they are unavoidable
not in titles of papers

How to Use Abbreviations

Define the abbreviation on first use by enclosing the abbreviation in parentheses after the term, for example, "deoxyribonucleic acid (DNA)."
    Use the abbreviation consistently thereafter, except:

Use the word in the first relevant table and the first relevant figure.
Use the word, not the abbreviation, in conclusions.

Use the abbreviation only in the defined meaning. For example, if "RV" means "right ventricle," it should not later be used to mean "right ventricular."
    Use the abbreviation only in the singular; add "s" or "'s" for the plural: "in six RVs."
    Do not use one abbreviation to modify another.

Example: Pre- and post-IHE FBF were similar in both groups.
Solution: Both before and after exercise, forearm blood flows were
                 similar in the two groups.

Avoid putting an abbreviation at the beginning of a sentence.

How to Avoid Abbreviations

Instead of an abbreviation, sometimes one word from a long term can be used. For example, "isometric handgrip exercise" can be called "exercise," instead of "IHE" (a nonstandard abbreviation), if only one type of exercise is mentioned in the paper.
    Similarly, to avoid repeating a long term that you have chosen not to abbreviate, use a pronoun and a category term when appropriate (for example, for "Basenji-Greyhound dogs," use "these dogs").
    To avoid "Group A," try to use a characteristic to name the group, for example "the hypotensive group."

In abstracts for meetings, use abbreviations only after you are sure you have condensed the information and the writing and have omitted unnecessary information and details as much as possible. More than three abbreviations in an abstract make reading a chore.

When inventing new words, try to invent short terms that do not need to be abbreviated. For example, "endorphins," was a good choice—far better than "opiate receptor blockers" would have been.

Creating Abbreviations

If you must create an abbreviation,

- Do not use a single letter as an abbreviation (for example, "E" for "epinephrine").
- Do not abbreviate single words (for example, "epinephrine").
- Avoid creating an abbreviation that spells a word (for example, "PEEP" for "positive end-expiratory pressure").
- Do not attach letters to an already existing standard abbreviation, because it is difficult to recognize the standard abbreviation within the new abbreviation.

> For example,
> Standard: REM sleep (rapid-eye-movement sleep)
> New: NREM sleep
> Better: non-REM sleep
>
> Standard: AV block (atrioventricular block)
> New: HGAVB
> Better: high-grade AV block

- Avoid using the same letter in two different abbreviations.

> Example: IH<u>E</u> (isometric handgrip <u>exercise</u>) and N<u>E</u> (norepi<u>nephrine</u>).
> Solution: Neither abbreviation is necessary. "Norepinephrine" is not a long, unwieldy word. "Isometric handgrip exercise" can be referred to as "exercise."

Suggestion

Try writing a paper or an abstract for a meeting without using any abbreviations. You may be pleasantly surprised.

Exercise 1.2: Words Carelessly Interchanged

1. affected.
2. concentration.
   COMMENT: "Level" is more general than "amount," "concentration," and "content." It is OK to use "level" instead of "amount," "concentration," or "content" if you have only one kind of level in your paper, but if you have, for example, both amounts and concentrations, or if you use "level" to mean "horizontal state or line," write the specific terms every time.
3. clogged.
4. consisted of. (Omit "no other drugs were used.")
5. increases.

6. improved.
7. speeds.
8. intervals, period.
9. variables.
10. regimens.
11. is.
12. various.

CHAPTER 2

Exercise 2.1: Express the Core of the Message in the Subject, Verb, and Completer

1. At the end of dialysis, the plasma acetate <u>concentration</u> *in* the adults **was** *almost double* that *in* the children.
   <u>COMMENT</u>: *Note that the subject, verb, and completer in the revised sentence give more of the message than do the subject, verb, and completer of the original sentence: "concentration was almost double" versus "adults ended dialysis." Also note that the same preposition ("in") is used before "adults" and "children"; "of" could be used instead of "in." Finally, if both the adults and the children underwent dialysis, that fact is clearest if "at the end of dialysis" comes at the beginning of the sentence, because a condition holds until you change it (see Chap. 3, "The Duration of a Signal" under "Signaling the Subtopics of a Paragraph").*
2. The patient's <u>symptoms</u> **did not change**.
   The patient's <u>symptoms</u> **were unchanged**.
3. After the <u>patient</u> **began** taking 6 g of aspirin daily, his/her <u>arthritis</u> **resolved**.
   <u>Aspirin</u> (6 g daily) **resolved** the patient's arthritis.
4. The <u>death rate</u> **decreased** progressively OR progressively **decreased**.
5. <u>Ethanol</u> **evaporates** from the mixture rapidly.
   Ethanol evaporates rapidly from the mixture.
6. <u>Potassium perchlorate</u> **was removed** by centrifugation of the supernatant liquid at $1400 \times g$ for 10 min. (*passive*)
   <u>Centrifugation</u> of the supernatant liquid at $1400 \times g$ for 10 min **removed** *potassium perchlorate*. (*active*)
   <u>We</u> **removed** *potassium perchlorate* by centrifuging the supernatant liquid at $1400 \times g$ for 10 min. (*one way to use "we"*)
   To remove potassium perchlorate, <u>we</u> **centrifuged** *the supernatant liquid* at $1400 \times g$ for 10 min. (*another way to use "we"*)
7. Blood <u>pH</u> **was measured** *by* OR *with* a Radiometer capillary electrode.
   <u>COMMENT</u>: *"By" implies that the machine made the measurement unassisted. "With" implies that the investigator manipulated the machine.*
8. The <u>lives</u> of uremic patients **have been prolonged** by improved conservative treatment and hemodialysis.
   <u>Uremic patients</u> **live longer** because of improved conservative treatment and hemodialysis.
   <u>Improved conservative treatment</u> and <u>hemodialysis</u> **have prolonged** the *lives* of uremic patients.

9. <u>Minute ventilation</u> and <u>respiratory frequency</u> **increased** abruptly in all dogs as exercise began.

   <u>Exercise</u> **increased** *minute ventilation* and *respiratory frequency* abruptly in all dogs.

   *COMMENT: Not "All <u>dogs</u> **increased** their minute ventilation and respiratory frequency abruptly as exercise began," because "dogs" is not the topic.*

10. We **analyzed** each <u>specimen</u> at least twice.

11. <u>Infusion of tyramine</u> **decreased** <u>cutaneous blood flow</u>.

12. These <u>agents</u> **act** by **inhibiting** the synthesis of cholesterol by the liver.

   These <u>agents</u> **inhibit** the synthesis of cholesterol by the liver. (*slightly different meaning*)

   COMMENT: Not "hepatic synthesis of cholesterol"; too abstract.

13. This <u>net difference in osmolarity</u> **forces** water into the cerebrospinal fluid, thus **increasing** pressure.

   COMMENT: "Thus" is needed to keep the notion of causality.

   This <u>net difference in osmolarity</u> **increases** pressure by **drawing** water into the cerebrospinal fluid.

   Because of the net difference in osmolarity, <u>water</u> **flows** into the cerebrospinal fluid, thus **increasing** pressure.

   <u>Driven</u> by a difference in osmolarity, <u>water</u> **flows** into the cerebrospinal fluid, thus **increasing** pressure.

   COMMENT: "Driven by" is more powerful than "because of" because "driven" is a verb form and also because it is a concrete term that evokes an image.

14. A capsule of amyl nitrite was crushed and held in front of the nose for 20 s *while* the <u>patient</u> **breathed** normally.

   COMMENT: "While normal respiration was maintained" is not as good; too abstract.

15. *As* calcium is translocated across the membrane, a <u>phosphorylated enzyme intermediate</u> **is formed**. Then, *as* calcium is released into the lumen, the <u>phosphorylated enzyme intermediate</u> **is decomposed** into the unphosphorylated enzyme and ADP plus phosphate.

   When calcium is translocated across the membrane, an <u>enzyme</u> **is phosphorylated**. Then, *when* calcium is released into the lumen, the <u>phosphorylated enzyme</u> **is decomposed** into enzyme, ADP, and phosphate.

   When <u>calcium</u> **moves** across the membrane, an enzyme is phosphorylated. Then, when calcium is released into the lumen, the <u>phosphorylated enzyme</u> **breaks down** into enzyme, ADP, and phosphate.

   COMMENT: The source of the problem in both sentences 14 and 15 is the word "with." The solution in both sentences is to add a verb.

Exercise 2.2: Untangling Noun Clusters

1. Blood clotting <u>in</u> the shunt occurred after 5 days.
   COMMENT: The cluster is untangled but the action is in the subject.
   <u>Blood</u> <u>in</u> the shunt **clotted** after 5 days. (*action in the verb*)

2. The precipitate was further purified by centrifugation <u>on</u> sucrose density gradients (OR on density gradients <u>made of</u> sucrose).
   COMMENT: Although "sucrose density gradients" is an accepted technical term, it is clearer to write it the long way ("density gradients made of sucrose") the first time and then to use the cluster.

3. "Regulation <u>of</u> the pH <u>of</u> the Cerebrospinal Fluid <u>by</u> the Blood-Brain Barrier"
   COMMENT: *Not "pH Regulation" because this cluster could mean either regulation <u>of</u> the pH or regulation <u>by</u> the pH.*

4. The antigen was prepared from homogenates <u>of</u> **whole liver** <u>from</u> rats. The antigen was prepared from <u>homogenized</u> **whole liver** <u>from</u> rats.
   COMMENT: *Not "whole rat liver" because then either the rat or the liver could be whole.*

5. T$_4$ stimulated incorporation <u>of</u> choline into **primary cultures** <u>of</u> fetal lung cells.
   COMMENT: *Not "primary cell cultures" because then either the cells or the cultures could be primary. "Fetal lung cells" is OK because if the lungs are fetal, the cells must be fetal, and vice versa.*

6. Serum samples <u>from</u> normal **subjects** and <u>from</u> **patients** who had ulcerative colitis were studied by (OR with) paper electrophoresis.

7. There was no significant difference between lactate **concentrations** in resting **subjects** and in exercising **subjects**.
   COMMENT: *Not "Lactates did not differ significantly when sampled at rest or during exercise" because it is not clear who is resting and who is exercising. In sentences 6 and 7, the subjects must be mentioned.*

Exercise 2.4: Clear Antecedents of Pronouns

1. To decrease blood volume by about 10% in a few minutes, blood was pooled in the subjects' legs by placing wide congesting cuffs around the thighs and inflating <u>the cuffs</u> to diastolic brachial arterial pressure.
   To decrease blood volume by about 10% in a few minutes, blood was pooled in the subjects' legs by <u>inflating wide congesting cuffs</u>, <u>placed around the thighs</u>, to the diastolic pressure of the brachial artery.
   COMMENT: *The second revision avoids repeating "cuffs" and also untangles the adjective cluster "diastolic brachial arterial pressure."*

2. These <u>findings</u> suggest that. . . .
   This <u>difference in recovery</u> suggests that. . . .
   These <u>different degrees of reduction</u> suggest that. . . .
   This <u>selective reduction of apolipoprotein A-I</u> suggests that. . . .
   COMMENT: *These revisions are in order of least to most specific. The last revision is best because two terms from the previous sentence are repeated ("apolipoprotein A-I" and "reduced"). (See Chap. 3, "Repeating Key Terms.")*

3. The <u>size of the bolus</u> is limited. . . .
   The <u>size of the relative error</u> is limited. . . .
   The <u>size of the CT number</u> is limited. . . .
   However, the size of the bolus is limited because large boluses are harder to administer and patients do not tolerate them well.
   COMMENT: *The first revision is the one the author intended, but any of the revisions is reasonable. The last revision is lighter and easier to read than the others because the action is expressed by verbs and an adjective ("are harder," "tolerate").*

Exercise 2.5: Parallelism in Sentences

1. Cardiac output was less in the E. coli group than <u>in</u> the Pseudomonas group.

2. Left ventricular function was impaired in the dogs that received en-dotoxin and <u>in</u> the control dogs.

3. Pulsation of the cells or cell masses <u>can</u> be quick and erratic or <u>slow and regular</u>.

4. The tubes were spun on a Vortex mixer for 10 s, stored at 4°C for 2 h, and then centrifuged at 500 × *g* for 10 min.
   COMMENT: It is OK to omit "then" as well as "they were," but it is not necessary.

5. Tracheal ganglion cells have been classified on the basis of their spontaneous discharge (12), their electrical properties (5), and the presence or absence of vasoactive intestinal peptide (8).
   COMMENT: "or absence" may be omitted.
   Tracheal ganglion cells have been classified on the basis of three properties: spontaneous discharge (12), electrical characteristics (5), and vasoactive intestinal peptide content (8).

6. Phenylephrine increased the rate of mucus secretion <u>and</u> the output of nondialyzable ^{35}S; <u>it also caused</u> a net transepithelial movement of Na towards the mucosa.
   Phenylephrine increased the rate of mucus secretion, increased the output of nondialyzable ^{35}S, <u>and caused</u> a net transepithelial movement of Na towards the mucosa.

7. The fractions were centrifuged, <u>the pellets were</u> resuspended in a small volume of buffer, and a sample of cells was counted in an electronic cell counter.

8. Even the highest dose of atropine had no effect <u>either</u> on baseline pulse rate <u>or</u> on the vagally stimulated pulse rate.
   Even the highest dose of atropine had no effect <u>on pulse rate</u> either during baseline or during vagal stimulation.
   COMMENT: The second revision avoids repetition of "pulse rate."

9. An impulse from the vagus nerve to the muscle has to travel both through ganglia and and <u>through</u> postganglionic pathways.
   COMMENT: "Through both ganglia and postganglionic pathways" is theoretically OK but undesirable here because "through both ganglia" could imply two ganglia.

10. The internal pressure must <u>depend not only</u> on volume but also <u>on</u> the rate of filling.

Exercise 2.6: Parallelism in Comparisons

1. The greater stability in this study <u>than in</u> the previous study resulted from more accurate marker digitization.

2. Total microsphere losses were greater at 34, 64, and 124 min <u>than at</u> 4 min.
   Total microsphere losses at 34, 64, and 124 min <u>were greater than those at</u> 4 min.

3. We frequently observed that mean coronary arterial pressure <u>was lower than</u> mean aortic pressure after carbochromen injection. (*maybe neither decreased*)
   We frequently observed <u>a decrease in</u> mean coronary arterial pressure <u>but not in</u> mean aortic pressure after carbochromen injection. (*one decreased*)
   We frequently observed <u>a greater decrease in</u> mean coronary arterial pressure <u>than in</u> mean aortic pressure after carbochromen injection. (*both decreased*)

4. The loss of apolipoprotein A-I from high-density lipoproteins during ultracentrifugational isolation **was greater than** <u>the</u> losses during other isolation methods.

5. Losses of apolipoprotein A-I during other isolation methods **were smaller than** losses during ultracentrifugation.

6. The protein composition of heavy meromyosin, **like** <u>that of</u> subfragment 1, was homogeneous.

   <u>**Like** the protein composition of</u> subfragment 1, the protein composition of heavy meromyosin was homogeneous.

CHAPTER 3

Exercise 3.1: Paragraph Organization

PART 1

Version 1 is least clear. Versions 2 and 3 are reasonably clear.

Version 1

Strengths   ?

Weaknesses

No clear pattern of organization: Sentence A presents the results for the first two variables. Sentence B contrasts half of the results for the third variable with all of the results for the first two variables. Sentence C presents the other half of the results for the third variable.

Inconsistent point of view: sentence A, cause; sentences B, C, effect.

No statement that changing pH affects lactate and pyruvate concentrations.

Version 2

Strengths

Topic sentences (A, B) that clearly state the contrasting results.

Logical organization: A and B = results; C and D = details supporting the result in B.

Parallel form: The details in C and D are in parallel form.

Weaknesses

The topic sentence is split into two sentences (A, B).

Details overload sentence A.

In C and D, "at" gives no sense of whether pH was increased or decreased.

Too many numbers.

Version 3

Strengths

Easy to understand on first reading.
Simple organization: two parallel sentences: A = all results for decreased pH; B = all results for increased pH.

Weaknesses

No topic sentence, so the point is diffused.
Very long sentences.
Unnecessary repetition in B ("again had no effect on. . .").

Version 4

(An attempt to combine the strengths of Versions 2 and 3)

A, B Topic sentence (results)

C, D Supporting sentences (details—in parallel form)

*A*Changing the pH of the perfusion fluid had no effect on either electrical potential difference or oxygen consumption, *B*but it did affect lactate and pyruvate concentrations. *C*When the pH was lowered from 7.4 to 6.9, lactate and pyruvate concentrations decreased, but their ratio remained the same (Fig. 1). *D*When the pH was raised from 7.4 to 7.9, the lactate concentration increased by one-third and the pyruvate concentration decreased by about the same fraction, thus doubling the lactate-pyruvate ratio.

Strengths

The topic sentence clearly states the contrasting results (as in Version 2).
The organization is logical (as in Versions 2 and 3).
The organization is simple (as in Version 3).
The paragraph is easy to understand (as in Version 3).
Results for each experimental situation are presented separately (as in Versions 2 and 3).
Supporting sentences are parallel (as in Versions 2 and 3).

Weaknesses Avoided

A topic sentence is used.
The topic sentence is not split into two sentences.
Details do not overload the topic sentence.
Supporting sentences clearly indicate whether pH was increased or decreased.
There is no unnecessary repetition of numbers or of results.
Sentences are not too long.

Note that after reading the topic sentence of Version 4, we expect the paragraph to be organized by the independent variable (pH). That is, we expect that we will hear first about the effects of changing pH in one direction and then about the effects of changing pH in the other direction. This organization is exactly what we get, so our expectation is fulfilled.

PART 2

The point of the topic sentence of paragraph 2 is to contrast what happened to lung lymph dynamics during air infusion and during recovery. Organizing the paragraph part by part (that is, variable by variable), as in the original version, does not make the contrast clear. The contrast is clearer when the paragraph is organized whole by whole (that is, first all results during air infusion and then all results during recovery), as in Revision 1 below. In addition, the causal sequence leading to the changes in lymph protein clearance is easier to follow. (Note: For other paragraphs of comparison and contrast, the organization that works best will not necessarily be whole by whole. The best organization can be discovered by trial and error.)

Revision 1

A Topic sentence
B–D During air infusion

E During recovery

*A*Both the alpha adrenergic agonist and the antagonist affected lung lymph dynamics slightly during the air infusion but not during recovery. *B*During the air infusion, the alpha agonist phenylephrine decreased lung lymph flow by 25% whereas the alpha antagonist phentolamine had the opposite effect (Fig. 2). *C*Neither agent altered the lymph-to-plasma protein concentration ratio. *D*Therefore, phenylephrine decreased lymph protein clearance and phentolamine increased it. *E*During recovery, although neither agent altered lung lymph dynamics, the trend for lung lymph flow to be lower after phenylephrine and higher after phentolamine was maintained.

The reason that the whole-by-whole organization works so well in this paragraph is that since there were no important changes during recovery, only one sentence is needed to contrast the absence of changes during recovery with the three sentences about changes during the air infusion. In fact, the only reason a sentence about recovery is needed at all is that the author is adding a detail that was not included in the topic sentence. If the trend for lymph flow to be altered had not been maintained during recovery, sentence E would not have been necessary.

Note that the category term "lung lymph dynamics" is used in sentence E instead of the names of all three variables. The cluster for one of the variables, "lymph-to-plasma protein concentration ratio," should have been defined earlier in the paper; the definition is "ratio of the concentration of protein in lymph to the concentration of protein in plasma."

Note also that each condition needs to be mentioned only at the beginning of the first sentence that discusses the results for that condition: "during the air infusion" at the beginning of B and "during recovery" at the beginning of E. The reason is that the statement of a condition at the beginning of a sentence holds until you change it (see Chap. 3, "The Duration of a Signal" under "Signaling the Subtopics of a Paragraph"). Omitting the two repetitions of "during the air infusion" and "during recovery" makes the revision both shorter and clearer.

Revision 2

*A*Both the alpha adrenergic agonist and the antagonist affected lung lymph dynamics slightly during air infusion but not during recovery. *B*During air infusion, the alpha agonist phenylephrine decreased lung lymph flow by 25%, did not change the lymph-to-plasma protein concentration ratio, and therefore decreased lymph protein clearance. *C*Conversely, the alpha antagonist phentolamine increased lung lymph flow, did not change the lymph-to-plasma protein concentration ratio, and therefore increased lymph protein clearance.

Revision 2 omits the final sentence about recovery and also describes the results for each agent separately, thus making the causal sequence clearer than in Revision 1.

Exercise 3.2: Repeating Key Terms

Revision 1

*A***Blood products** are used frequently in the care of sick preterm infants, but their use may increase the risk of <u>intracranial hemorrhage</u>. *B*Clinicians may be able to decrease the risk of <u>intracranial hemorrhage</u> by optimizing the <u>timing</u> and the <u>method</u> of **blood product** administration. *C*We therefore studied the effects of <u>timing</u> and <u>method</u> of **blood product** administration on two indicators of <u>intracranial hemorrhage</u>, cerebral blood flow and intracranial pressure, in sick preterm infants. *D*The <u>timing</u> chosen was within the first 7 days after birth. *E*The <u>method</u> was rapid infusion.

In Revision 1, the key terms "blood products," "intracranial hemorrhage," "timing," and "method" from sentences A and B are repeated in sentences C–E, and the key terms "cerebral blood flow" and "intracranial pressure" are identified as indicators of intracranial hemorrhage, thus making the relation between all the sentences in this paragraph easy to see. Also, the term "sick preterm infants" from A is repeated in C rather than being changed to "small preterm infants" as done in the original version. In addition, "timing" and "method" are defined, thus explicitly identifying what each term means rather than leaving them implicit and vague, as in the original version.

Revision 2

*A***Blood products** are used frequently in the care of sick preterm infants, but their use may increase the risk of <u>intracranial hemorrhage</u>. *B*We suspected that this risk varies with <u>postnatal age</u> and <u>rate</u> of **blood product** administration. *C*Therefore, we studied the effects of **blood product** administration in sick preterm infants as a function of <u>age</u> (up to 7 days) and <u>rate</u> of **blood product** administration. *D*The specific effects we measured as indicators of <u>intracranial hemorrhage</u> were cerebral blood flow and intracranial pressure.

In Revision 2, the key terms "timing" and "method" are made more precise: "postnatal age" and "rate." Because these terms are precise, they do not need to be defined, as "timing" and "method" were in Revision 1. As in Revision 1, the four key terms in the first two sentences are repeated in the last two sentences, thus making the relationship between the sentences easy to see.

Revision 3

*A***Blood products** are used frequently in the care of sick preterm infants. *B*However, if **blood products** are infused rapidly, causing sudden <u>increases</u> in **blood volume**, the risk of <u>intracranial hemorrhage</u> may be increased. *C*We suspected that this risk varies with the <u>rate</u> at which **blood volume** is <u>increased</u> and with <u>postnatal age</u>. *D*Therefore, we studied the effects of various <u>rates</u> of increasing **blood volume** on two indicators of <u>intracranial hemorrhage</u>, cerebral blood flow and intracranial pressure, in sick preterm infants at <u>ages</u> 0 to 7 days.

Sentence B of Revision 3 makes clear the relation between blood products and blood volume by adding "causing sudden increases in blood volume." This addition allows the switch from "blood products" in the first two sentences to "blood volume" in the last two sentences. This technique of relating key terms is a clear way of moving from one key term to another without confusing the reader. In contrast, the original version switched from "blood products" (A, B) to "volume expansion" (C) without indicating the relation between the two terms and thus broke the continuity between sentences.

Exercise 3.3: Repeating Key Terms and Keeping a Consistent Order

Revision 1

The study protocol consisted of recordings of atrioventricular infranodal and nodal conduction times made during **sinus rhythm**, during **right atrial overdrive pacing** at progressively shorter coupling intervals, and during **attempts to measure antegrade refractory periods** by the extrastimulus technique. Evidence of ventricular pre-excitation during **sinus rhythm** and during **right atrial overdrive pacing** was also sought.

During **sinus rhythm**, atrioventricular infranodal and nodal conduction times were normal. However, during **atrial overdrive pacing** and **measurement of antegrade refractory periods**, although atrioventricular infranodal conduction time was normal, atrioventricular nodal conduction time was suddenly prolonged. There was no evidence of ventricular pre-excitation either during **sinus rhythm** or during **atrial overdrive pacing**.

In Revision 1, key terms are made the same in both paragraphs. Note that the key term "right atrial overdrive pacing" (para. 1) is shortened to "atrial overdrive pacing" in paragraph 2. This shortening, although risky, is probably not confusing because right atrial overdrive pacing is the only kind of atrial overdrive pacing mentioned in this example.

In addition to key terms being repeated in paragraph 2, the topic of ventricular pre-excitation is added to the end of paragraph 1. For consistent order, ventricular pre-excitation is moved to the end of paragraph 2.

Thus, this revision illustrates three ways in which an expectation can be created and fulfilled:

1. *using the same key terms (or key terms that are shortened in a recognizable way) in both paragraphs*
2. *mentioning all the same details in both paragraphs*
3. *mentioning details in the same order in both paragraphs*

Revision 2

The study protocol consisted of recordings of atrioventricular nodal and infranodal conduction times made during sinus rhythm, **during overdrive pacing of the right atrium** at progressively shorter coupling intervals, and during attempts to measure antegrade refractory periods by the extrastimulus technique. **No evidence of pre-excitation was found** either during sinus rhythm or during **overdrive pacing.**

Nodal conduction time was normal during sinus rhythm but was suddenly prolonged during **overdrive pacing** and during attempts to measure antegrade refractory periods. However, **infranodal conduction times** were unchanged.

In Revision 2, nodal and infranodal conduction times are discussed separately in paragraph 2. Thus, the contrast is clearer.

The contrast is reinforced by the shortened key terms "infranodal conduction time" and "nodal conduction time" instead of "atrioventricular infranodal conduction time" and "atrioventricular nodal conduction time." In addition, the cluster "right atrial overdrive pacing" is untangled to become "overdrive pacing of the right atrium" on first use, so shortening this term to "overdrive pacing" in later sentences does not risk confusing the reader.

Finally, the point about no ventricular pre-excitation is made at the end of paragraph 1, so this topic does not need to appear again in paragraph 2. This is the way to handle pre-excitation (or any other minor point) if you want to mention it only once.

Exercise 3.4: Keeping a Consistent Point of View and a Consistent Order

Example 1

Revision 1

*A*Mortality in this series of patients was 90%. *B*Generally, <u>mortality</u> in clinical series has been <u>greater than 80%</u>. *C*The only <u>exception</u> is the mortality of 46% reported by Boley (2).

Point of View: mortality, mortality, exception
Series of Numbers: 90%, 80%, 46%

Revision 2

*A*Mortality in this series of patients was 90%. *B*Mortality in other clinical series has always been greater than 80% except for the mortality of 46% reported by Boley (2).

Point of View: mortality, mortality, mortality

Example 2

Revision 1

A<u>Bradykinin</u> alone usually induced a *contraction* followed by a longer lasting *relaxation*. *B*<u>Adding indomethacin</u> (2 μg/ml for 20–30 min) along with bradykinin increased the magnitude of the bradykinin-induced *contraction*, when one was present, but reduced the magnitude of the *relaxation* to 7% of that induced by bradykinin alone.

Point of View: the cause (that is, the independent variable)
Order: contraction first; relaxation second

Revision 2

A<u>Contraction</u> followed by a longer lasting relaxation was the usual response induced by bradykinin. *B*<u>The contraction</u> was stronger after indomethacin (2 μg/ml for 20–30 min) was added along with bradykinin, but the relaxation was weaker.

Point of View: the effect (that is, the dependent variable)
Order: contraction first; relaxation second

Revision 2 is easier to understand than Revision 1 because some details have been omitted from sentence B, thus making the contrast clearer.

Example 3

Revision 1

In both groups, <u>cardiac output</u> **reached** its lowest values immediately after the injection of endotoxin. Although <u>cardiac output</u> **recovered** in both groups, <u>it</u> **returned** closer to control values in the first group.

Point of View: cardiac output, cardiac output, cardiac output

Revision 2

<u>Cardiac output</u> **decreased** in both groups immediately after the injection of endotoxin and then **returned** toward control values, though the <u>return</u> **was** closer to control in the first group.

Point of View: cardiac output, cardiac output, return

In Revision 2, changing the point of view from "cardiac output" to "return" is legitimate because "return" is a reasonable topic here. In both revisions, note that the <u>verbs</u> now express the action.

Exercise 3.5: Parallel Form and Signaling Subtopics

1. Parallelism in Two Sentences; Signaling Subtopics

Revision 1   (The version you would expect; that is, the second sentence is exactly parallel to the first sentence.)

In rat papillary muscle, 3 mM <u>caffeine converted load-sensitive relaxation</u> (Fig. 1A, B) <u>to load-insensitive relaxation</u> (Fig. 1C, D). However, **in cat papillary muscle**, <u>caffeine did not convert load-sensitive relaxation to load-insensitive relaxation</u> at concentrations of 3 mM (Fig. 2), 5 mM (Fig. 3), or 10 mM (data not shown).

Revision 1 has two parallel sentences. The sentences begin with parallel signals of the subtopics ("in rat papillary muscle," "in cat papillary muscle") and have the same sentence pattern: subject (caffeine), verb (converted, did not convert), completer. Note that the verbs are exact opposites. Other verbs would be less appropriate: "failed to convert" implies an a priori expectation of conversion, which may not be reasonable; "failed to eliminate" (the original version) is not parallel.

Organized by species; therefore, the <u>signal of the subtopics</u> names the species: "in <u>rat</u> papillary muscle," "in <u>cat</u> papillary muscle."
Point of view: independent variable (caffeine).
The last sentence no longer describes adding 3 mM caffeine at 5 or 10 mM.

Revision 2   (A version organized like Revision 1 but more concise)

In rat papillary muscle, 3 mM caffeine eliminated the load sensitivity of relaxation (Fig. 1A-D). In contrast, in cat papillary muscle, not even 10 mM caffeine eliminated the load sensitivity of relaxation (Figs. 2, 3).

Revision 3 (A version that omits the notion of "conversion" and organizes by the independent variable)

Under control conditions, the <u>relaxation</u> of rat and cat papillary muscles <u>was load sensitive</u> (Figs. 1, 2). **After 3 mM caffeine,** the <u>relaxation</u> of ***rat*** papillary muscle <u>became load insensitive</u> (Fig. 1) but the <u>relaxation</u> of ***cat*** papillary muscle <u>was still load sensitive</u> (Fig. 2) and remained so even after 5 (Fig. 3) or 10 mM caffeine.

> *Organized by the independent variable; therefore, the <u>signal of the subtopics</u> names the independent variable: "under control conditions," "after 3 mM caffeine."*
> *<u>Point of view</u>: dependent variable (relaxation).*

Revision 4 (A version that has a topic sentence that implies the point of view of the independent variable and organization by the species)

<u>Caffeine</u> had different effects on the load sensitivity of relaxation in rat and cat papillary muscle. **In rat papillary muscle**, 3 mM <u>caffeine</u> converted the load sensitivity of relaxation (Fig. 1A, B) to load insensitivity (Fig. 1C, D). However, **in cat papillary muscle**, <u>caffeine</u> did not convert load sensitivity to load insensitivity at concentrations of 3 mM (Fig. 2), 5 mM (Fig. 3), or 10 mM (data not shown).

> *Organized by species.*
> *<u>Point of view</u>: independent variable (caffeine).*

Revision 5 (A version that has a topic sentence that implies the point of view of the dependent variable and organization by the species)

Although papillary muscle <u>relaxation</u> was load-sensitive under control conditions (no caffeine) in both rats (Fig. 1) and cats (Fig. 2), <u>relaxation</u> in these muscles responded differently to caffeine. **In rat papillary muscle**, <u>relaxation became load-insensitive when 3 mM caffeine was added to the bath</u> (Fig. 1). In contrast, **in cat papillary muscle**, <u>relaxation remained load-sensitive after 3 mM (Fig. 2), 5 mM (Fig. 3), or 10 mM caffeine was added to the bath</u>.

> *Organized by species.*
> *<u>Point of view</u>: dependent variable (relaxation).*

2. Parallelism in More Than Two Sentences

Revision 1

*E*Araldite-embedded tissues were sectioned at 1 μm with an ultramicrotome (Porter-Blum MT-1).

Revision 2

*B, C*Tracheal segments fixed in Bouin's fixative were dehydrated in graded ethanol solutions, cleared in alpha-terpineol, embedded in paraffin, and sectioned at 7 μm with a rotary microtome (American Optical). *D, E*Tracheal segments fixed in 0.2% glutaraldehyde were dehydrated in graded acetone solutions, embedded in araldite (Polysciences), and sectioned at 1 μm with an ultramicrotome (Porter-Blum MT-1).

3. Preserving Parallel Form

To avoid destroying the parallel form in this paragraph, use a topic sentence to state the contrast between the fetuses and the mothers and then, after a second topic sentence, describe the details for the fetuses.

Revision

Injection of naloxone altered the arterial blood gas and pH responses of the fetuses but not those of the mothers. The fetal responses depended on the site of injection. After fetal injection of naloxone, fetal arterial blood pH and Po_2 both decreased (from 7.39 ± 0.01 (SD) to 7.35 ± 0.02 and from 23.0 ± 0.5 to 20.8 ± 0.8 mmHg, respectively). There was no change in arterial blood Pco_2. After maternal injection of naloxone, only fetal arterial blood Po_2 decreased (from 24.4 ± 0.8 to 22.2 ± 1.0 mmHg). There were no significant changes in fetal arterial blood pH or Pco_2.

Exercise 3.6: The Value of Transitions

1. **Relationship:**   The second sentence gives the next step.
   How you know: "Then" implies the next step.

2. **Relationship:**   The second sentence explains how the microspheres were prepared.
   How you know: "In brief" implies an explanation.

Note that frequently people use "briefly" for "in brief." Also note that if "in brief" meant "for a short time," the sentence would be written "They were suspended briefly in 1 ml of dextran solution. . . ." However, it is better to specify the duration of the suspension: "They were suspended for 5 s in 1 ml of dextran solution. . . ."

3. **Relationship:**   Hard to tell.
   How you know: No transition word.

Even though most readers might guess right ("in brief" is the true relationship), the point is that the reader should not be guessing. Using the appropriate transition word makes the logical relationship incapable of being misunderstood.

Exercise 3.7: The Meaning of Some Transition Words

1. Change "and" to "so," or begin the sentence with "Because" and omit "and."
2. Change "while" to "but," "whereas," or ";" or change "while" to "and" and replace the first "and" with a comma.
3. Change "while" to "whereas" or "but," or begin the sentence with "Although."
4. Change "As" to "Because" or "Since." Only "because" is completely unambiguous, because "since" also has a time meaning.

Exercise 3.8: Stating the Message

Revision 1

Our findings differ from those of Malik and Kidd (12), who found that carbon dioxide supplemented the effect of hypoxia on pulmonary vascular resistance in spontaneously breathing dogs. <u>The different findings can probably be accounted for by differences in experimental design</u>: not only were the species and age of the animals studied different, but so was the duration of the periods of study.

Revision 2

Our findings differ from those of Malik and Kidd (12), who found that carbon dioxide supplemented the effect of hypoxia on pulmonary vascular resistance in spontaneously breathing dogs. <u>However, the comparison with our findings may not be valid</u> because we studied animals of a different age and species, and the duration of our study period was different.

Exercise 3.9: Displaying Thinking

Structure of the Argument; Message

A_1 Topic

A_2 Message
B Evidence for one side

C Support for B

D, E Evidence for the other side

F Support for E

^{A_1}**Hypothermia** is presently used to prevent **myocardial damage** during surgery requiring circulatory arrest, ^{A_2}but the effect of **hypothermia** per se on the **myocardium** is not clear. ^{B}Some **studies** in dogs have found that **hypothermia** causes **myocardial damage**. ^{C}In those **studies**, subendocardial hemorrhages, calcified necrosis, and fatty degeneration were seen in the heart after 1–4 hours at body temperatures between 21 and 30°C (9, 10). ^{D}However, other **studies** in dogs and rabbits have not found **myocardial damage** under similar conditions of **hypothermia** (6, 8). ^{E}Similarly, **studies** of **patients** who were **hypothermic** as a consequence of various medical disorders have found no evidence of permanent **myocardial damage**. ^{F}In those **patients**, although serum activity of total creatine kinase MB isoenzyme was increased, there was no clinical or postmortem evidence of acute **myocardial** infarction (2, 7).

Techniques of Continuity

A_2 Transition word; Key terms; Consistent order
B Topic signaled; Key terms; Consistent order
C Transition phrase; Key term
D Transition word; Topic signaled; Key terms
E Transition word; Topic signaled; Key terms; Consistent order
F Transition phrase; Key terms

This paragraph has two topic sentences: A_1, which states the topic, and A_2, which states the message. The topic sentence stating the message ("the effect ... is not clear") could imply a pro-con organization, and that is the organization used in this paragraph. The techniques of continuity emphasize the pro-con structure. Sentence B begins with a signal of the "pro" side ("some studies in dogs have found that"). Sentence D must be the "con" side because of the transition word ("however") and because of the parallel signal of the topic ("other studies in dogs and rabbits have not found"). E is also the "con" side because of the transition word "similarly," which implies an equal idea, and also because of the parallel form of the signals of the topics in sentences B, D, *and E and the repetition of the key term "studies" in sentences B, D, and E. In addition, consistent order is used in sentences A, B, and E (hypothermia first, myocardial or myocardium second).*

In keeping with this pro-con structure, sentences B (pro) and D and E (con), along with sentence A (topic and message), are the sentences that move the story forward. Sentences C and F are supporting sentences. Sentence C is linked to sentence B by a transition phrase ("in those studies") and by repetition of a key term ("studies"). Similarly, sentence F is linked to sentence E by a transition phrase ("in those patients") and by repetition of a key term ("patients"). The transition phrase ("in those patients") implies that the sentence will give details about the patients mentioned in sentence E. Nevertheless, some readers think that sentence F is the conclusion, or message, of the paragraph. But a conclusion would have to be about all patients in the category, not about only those in the two referenced studies.

Thus, the pro-con structure is indicated by the techniques of continuity and the sentences that move the story forward (A, B, D, E). The techniques of continuity used are parallel signals of the topics, transition words showing contrast (D) and similarity (E), transition phrases, repetition of key terms ("hypothermia," "myocardial damage," and "studies"), and, to a lesser extent, consistent order.

Exercise 3.10: Condensing

Revision 1   *(31 words versus 44 words in the original version)*

Both pulmonary artery constriction and microvascular injury increased input resistance (to 170% and 215% of control, respectively; the difference between these values was not significant, $P = 0.7$) (Fig. 7).

Revision 2   *(16 words)*

Mean input resistance was increased similarly by both pulmonary artery constriction and microvascular injury (Fig. 7).

CHAPTER 4

Exercise 4.1: Clearly Written Introductions

Structure

A *Known (method)*
  (Topic sentence)

B *Known (finding)*

C *Known (finding)*
D *Problem*

E *Questions*
  (species not stated)

Introduction 1

A<u>**Measuring clearance**</u> from the <u>**lungs**</u> of micronic aerosols of technetium-99m-labeled diethylenetriaminepentaacetic acid (<u>^{99m}**Tc-DTPA**</u>) delivered into the lower <u>**respiratory**</u> tract is used to give an index of <u>**respiratory**</u> epithelial permeability. **B**When <u>**measured**</u> in <u>**upright**</u> normal subjects, the <u>**clearance**</u> of <u>^{99m}**Tc-DTPA**</u> was reported to be <u>**faster**</u> in the <u>**upper regions**</u> of the <u>**lungs**</u> than in the lower regions (22). **C**<u>**Faster clearance**</u> in the <u>**upper regions**</u> of the <u>**lungs**</u> was also reported in <u>**upright smokers**</u> (17). **D**However, the authors did not <u>**correct**</u> their data for the <u>**radioactivity**</u> that <u>**recirculates**</u> after transfer from the <u>**lungs**</u> into the blood. **E**Therefore, we designed this study to determine whether the <u>**respiratory clearance**</u> of <u>^{99m}**Tc-DTPA**</u> is different within <u>**lung regions**</u> after <u>**correction**</u> for <u>**recirculation**</u> of <u>**radioactivity**</u> and also to determine the influence of posture and <u>**smoking**</u> on the <u>**regional respiratory clearance**</u> of <u>^{99m}**Tc-DTPA.**</u>

Structure

1 Known
ᴬ*Known (method)*
ᴮ*Importance of the topic*

2 Problem
ᶜ*Problem*
ᴰ*Support for C*

ᴱ*Importance of the problem*
ᶠ*Support for E*

3 Question
ᴳ*Question and species*
ᴴ*Details of G, Organization of the paper*

Introduction 2

1 ᴬ<u>Preparative **ultracentrifugational** flotation (1) has long been the standard method for **isolating lipoproteins**</u>. ᴮCompositional analyses of the lipoprotein classes are predicated upon this form of isolation (2, 3), and most current metabolic and structural studies use lipoproteins that have been isolated by ultracentrifugation.

2 ᶜ<u>**Ultracentrifugational isolation**, however, has been reported to cause structural changes in **lipoproteins**, specifically, the **loss of apolipoproteins**</u>. ᴰFor example, in studies of both rat and human lipoproteins, a portion of the complement of apolipoproteins A-I and E (apo A-I and apo E) in serum was lost, as evidenced by its appearing at a density greater than 1.21 g/ml after ultracentrifugation (4–6). ᴱFurthermore, the loss of apolipoprotein during ultracentrifugational isolation is greater than the loss caused by other isolation methods. ᶠThe loss of apo A-I from high-density lipoproteins during ultracentrifugational isolation, for example, can reach as much as 50% (7, 8).

3 ᴳ<u>This study was undertaken to identify the **ultracentrifugational** factors that are responsible for the **loss of apolipoprotein** from *human* high-density lipoproteins</u>. ᴴThe effects of four factors were studied: ionic strength, temperature, rotor configuration, and centrifuge tube material.

Comments

Introduction 1

In Introduction 1, all sentences move the story forward. Continuity comes primarily from repetition of key terms (see boldface words above) and from transition words: "also" (C), "However" (D), "Therefore" (E).

The questions follow inevitably from the statements of the known and the problem and are equally specific, as shown by repetition of key terms picked up from those statements (see boldface words above). The questions are signaled by "Therefore, we designed this study to determine whether... and also to determine...." In question 1, the independent variable is the correction for recirculation of radioactivity. In question 2, the independent variables are posture and smoking. In both questions, the dependent variable is regional respiratory clearance of ^{99m}Tc-DTPA. Question 1 is in present tense ("<u>is</u> different"); question 2 does not use a verb. The species (humans) is not stated in the question but is clear from "upright normal subjects" (B) and "upright smokers" (C).

The experimental approach is not stated separately at the end of the Introduction but is evident because the experiments done were the same as those described in sentences B and C, the technique used was the same as the one described in A, and the problem mentioned in D was solved by correcting for recirculation of radioactivity.

What is new and important about the question is evident: true regional respiratory clearance of ^{99m}Tc-DTPA and therefore true respiratory epithelial permeability. The importance of the topic is implied by its use as an index of respiratory epithelial permeability (sentence A).

Introduction 2

In Introduction 2, the first sentence of every paragraph moves the story forward. The other sentences indicate the importance of the work or the topic, or support other statements. Continuity comes partly from repetition of key terms both in the sentences that move the story forward (see boldface words above) and in the entire Introduction. Transition words also provide continuity: "however" (C), "For example" (D), "Furthermore" (E), "for example" (F).

The question follows inevitably from the statements of the known and the problem and is equally specific, as shown by the repetition of key terms picked up from the story ("ultracentrifugational" in A; "loss" and "apolipoproteins" in C) and from one supporting sentence ("high-density lipoproteins" in F). The question is signaled by "This study was undertaken to identify. . . ." The independent variables are the four ultracentrifugational factors; the dependent variable is loss of apolipoprotein. The question is in present tense ("are responsible"). The species (humans) and the material (high-density lipoproteins) are stated appropriately in the question.

The experimental approach is evident from the question.

What is new about the work is evident: identification of factors that cause loss of apolipoproteins. The importance of the work is stated: sentence B states the importance of the method; E states the importance of the loss of apolipoproteins.

Exercise 4.2: Introductions

Introduction 1

Strengths

The outstanding strength of this Introduction is its Lawrence of Arabia opening. This opening awakens interest by using concrete words that evoke powerful mental images: camels, gazelles, hot deserts, burrow, desert sun.

The Introduction is very readable, mainly because the sentences are short (8 of the 10 sentences have fewer than 20 words).

The *newness* of the work is evident.

The Introduction is *short*.

The "if so" idea, though not that exact term, is used to link the related questions.

Weaknesses

The *funnel* leading to the questions is *not rigorous*.

A. The first sentence (A) does not identify the topic of the questions and thus may be too general. But if the Introduction starts closer to the specific topic (see Revision 2 below), it should try to keep at least some of the wonderful image-evoking words.

C. A step is missing before sentence C. The missing step is "So the question arises, how do ungulates regulate their body temperature?"

F. Sentence F interrupts the story. F does not support E. G supports E. F should be omitted, or F can be incorporated into sentence G (see Revision 1, sentence D).

H. Sentence H is circular: "bursts" = "short duration." The subject of the sentence should be "these high speeds," which was a concept in the previous sentence (70–80 km/h). In sentence H, the new information being given about the high speeds is that they occur in short bursts. The new information belongs in the verb and completer, not in the subject (see Revision 1, sentence E).

I. The logical relation between sentences H and I is not stated. A display of thinking is needed here. At minimum, H and I should be in one sentence beginning with "Because." For fuller displays of thinking, see sentence E of Revision 1 and sentence D of Revision 2.

A–G. Key terms for animals are changed. We hear about antelopes (title, E, I), oryxes (A), gazelles (A, F, G), and eland (F). Actually, oryxes, gazelles, and eland are all types of antelope, but some readers may not know that. Only the types of antelope used in this study need to be named in the Introduction, and they should be identified as types of antelope (see Revision 1, sentence D).

The *questions* are *not complete* (question 1) or *clearly derived* (question 2). Information missing from question 1 is the independent variable (running), what heat storage plays a role in (heat balance or temperature regulation), and the species.

The display of thinking leading to question 2 is missing. This display of thinking needs to make clear how the subtitle ("Independence of Brain and Body Temperatures") relates to question 2 (see sentence F of Revision 1 and sentence E of Revision 2).

The questions should not be called "simple."

Sentence C has *a lot of references*. If a review article is available, it should be cited instead of all the individual references. Otherwise, only the most seminal references should be cited. Keep in mind that the reference lists in the papers cited can lead readers to the other papers.

The *experimental approach is not stated*. It should probably be added.

Revision 1

INDEPENDENCE OF BRAIN AND BODY TEMPERATURES PERMITS HEAT STORAGE IN RUNNING ANTELOPE

*A*The existence of antelope and other ungulates in hot deserts has long puzzled physiologists, because, unlike rodents, ungulates are too large to escape the sun by burrowing or by finding shade. *B*Thus, external heat loads pose major problems of temperature regulation for them (for a review, see ref. 1).

*C*However, internal heat loads may pose even greater problems of temperature regulation. *D*For example, a typical desert antelope, the gazelle, running at 70 km/h produces heat at 40 times its basic metabolic rate (2). *E*Because these high speeds are usually of short duration, it is possible that antelope might store heat while running and then dissipate it during periods of relative inactivity. *F*Heat storage, though, would require physiologic mechanisms for coping with high body temperature, such as preferential protection of normal brain temperature.

*G*To determine whether heat is stored in running antelope, we measured their core body temperature during treadmill exercise. *H*Additionally, we measured brain temperature during exercise to determine whether normal brain temperature is maintained.

Comments on Revision 1

The missing step is added (B).
A review article is substituted for individual references (B).
The gazelle is identified as a type of antelope (D).

The point about speed is subordinated to avoid breaking the continuity (D).
A fuller display of thinking leading to question 1 is added (E).
The word "bursts" is omitted to avoid circular statement (E).
The thinking leading to question 2 is added (F).
Question 1 is made more specific, thus eliminating the need to define what heat storage plays a role in (G).
The independent variable (running) and the animals studied (antelope) are included in question 1.
Question 2 is made more specific, thus following clearly from F and relating clearly to the title (H).
The questions are not called "simple" (G).
The experimental approach for each question is stated (G, H).

Revision 2

EFFECT OF RUNNING ON BRAIN AND BODY TEMPERATURE IN ANTELOPES

AIn order for camels, antelopes, and other ungulates to survive in hot deserts, they must be able to regulate their body temperatures. **B**Although most work on the regulation of body temperature in desert ungulates has been concerned with external heat loads (see ref. 1 for a review), internal heat loads may also pose problems for temperature regulation. **C**For example, a typical desert antelope, the gazelle, running at high speed (70 km/h) produces heat at 40 times its basic metabolic rate (2). **D**Because high-speed running usually occurs in short bursts, and because dissipation of this internally produced heat is limited by the high ambient temperature, it seems possible that the antelope might allow its body temperature to rise rather than dissipate this heat. **E**If body temperature does rise, maintenance of the brain at a lower temperature than the rest of the body would be important since the brain is known to be more sensitive to high temperatures than are the other organs. **F**To determine whether body temperature rises in running antelopes and, if so, whether brain temperature rises equally, we measured both brain and body temperatures in antelopes running at high ambient temperatures.

Comments on Revision 2

In addition to the changes noted for Revision 1, Revision 2 states the topic of the paper (temperature regulation) in the first sentence rather than waiting until the third sentence, as in the original version, and thus avoids the problem of the missing step. Revision 2 also presents a detailed display of thinking leading to both questions (sentences D and E). Finally, Revision 2 states both questions before stating the experimental approach.

Note: Because these revisions were written by researchers unfamiliar with this work, the scientific details that they invented may be inaccurate.

Although both of the revisions funnel to the questions clearly and state the questions and the experimental approach clearly, neither is as lively as the original version, so there is still room for improvement. Revision 1 has short sentences and keeps some of the concrete images of the original version (hot deserts, burrowing, sun), but omits others (camels, oryxes, gazelles, bursts) and adds some heavy abstract words (periods of relative inactivity, physiologic mechanisms, preferential protection). Revision 2 clearly displays the thinking leading to the questions but is dull because of abstract words (ungulates, high ambient temperature, maintenance) and long sentences (4 of the 6 sentences have more than 30 words). Thus, although the revisions are more rigorous than the original version, they do not reflect the excitement of scientists fascinated by their work that is so appealing in the original version.

Introduction 2

Strengths

The funnel to the questions is clear (funnel, para. 1; questions, para. 3).

The general question at the beginning of sentence J follows clearly from paragraph 1 (and specifically from sentence E).

The general question includes both the independent variable (alkalosis) and the dependent variable (constriction of the pulmonary circulation).

The newness of the work is evident from the statement of the unknown (C–E).

The importance is stated (para. 2).

The experimental approach is stated (K, L).

The species (newborn rabbits) and the material (isolated, perfused lungs) are stated in the experimental approach (K).

Weaknesses

This Introduction is too long. The details (trees) overshadow the message (forest).

> In paragraph 2, G and H say about the same thing, so G or H can be omitted.
>
> Sentence I can be omitted because it restates H.
>
> In paragraph 3, the first three specific questions (J) are unnecessary, and they are confusing because they are not in parallel form. The experimental approach (L) is clearer.
>
> The fourth specific question is not parallel to the first three specific questions, so it should be presented separately.
>
> The results (M) are unnecessary. Moreover, the results are confusing, partly because they provide more detail than the reader can cope with at this point in the paper and partly because of a change of key terms: the dependent variable mentioned in the first result is not pulmonary vasoconstriction, which is what we expect, but pulmonary vascular resistance; how pulmonary vascular resistance relates to pulmonary vasoconstriction is not indicated. Finally, including results makes the Introduction read like an abstract rather than an Introduction.

The answer (N) does not answer the question asked. In the answer, the *sequence of exposures* to the stimuli (alkalosis and hypoxia) is the independent variable, but in the question only *alkalosis* is the independent variable. Also, the question does not match the title, though the answer does. Since it is not clear what the question is, the Introduction does not prepare the reader adequately to understand the rest of the paper.

The reason for using three sequences of stimuli (L) is not stated. It should be.

The statement of the importance (para. 2) interrupts the flow of thought between the funnel (para. 1) and the questions (para. 3).

The writing is heavy because of fancy, abstract words, a low ratio of verbs to nouns, and some long sentences.

Revision 1

ALKALOSIS REDUCES HYPOXIA-INDUCED PULMONARY VASOCONSTRICTION IN LUNGS FROM NEWBORN RABBITS BUT NOT IF ALKALOSIS IS INDUCED BEFORE HYPOXIA

1   *A*Alveolar hypoxia causes pulmonary vasoconstriction. *B*Numerous studies have been done to determine whether alkalosis or acidosis can increase or reduce hypoxia-induced pulmonary vasoconstriction (1–14). *C*Only a few of these studies have been done in newborn animals (10, 13, 14). *D*The results of these studies have been variable. *E*Alkalosis has been shown both to reduce and to have no effect on constriction of the neonatal pulmonary circulation in response to alveolar hypoxia.

2   *F*Understanding the effect of alkalosis on the neonatal pulmonary circulation and on the response of the pulmonary circulation to hypoxia is important because alkalosis, produced primarily by mechanical hyperventilation, is widely used in the treatment of newborns who have the syndrome of persistent pulmonary hypertension (15, 16). *G*If alkalosis is responsible for the clinical improvement in these infants, it is possible that some of the deleterious effects of mechanical hyperventilation could be avoided by using alternative means of inducing alkalosis.

3   *H*The purpose of this study was to determine whether or not alkalosis reduces constriction of the neonatal pulmonary circulation in response to hypoxia. *I*In addition, we determined whether both respiratory and metabolic alkalosis have the same effect on the pulmonary circulation and its response to hypoxia. *J*Because the variable results of previous studies may have resulted from the different sequences in which the lungs were exposed to hypoxia and alkalosis, we tested the vasoconstrictive responses to these stimuli in three different sequences in isolated, perfused lungs from newborn rabbits: respiratory or metabolic alkalosis before, during, and after alveolar hypoxia. *K*We found that both respiratory and metabolic alkalosis reduce hypoxia-induced pulmonary vasoconstriction in isolated, perfused lungs from newborn rabbits, but not if alkalosis is induced before hypoxia.

Structure of Revision 1

Paragraph 1:   *Known (A–C), Problem (D, E).*
Paragraph 2:   *Importance.*
Paragraph 3:   *Questions (H, I), Experimental Approach (J), Answer (K).*

Comments on Revision 1

Revision 1 condenses the Introduction by omitting the following details:

> *unnecessary words (B, C),*
> *two unnecessary sentences (original sentences G and I),*
> *the first three specific questions (original sentence J),*
> *the experimental approach (original sentences K, L),*
> *the answer (original sentence N).*

In addition, Revision 1 condenses the results into an answer (K) that answers the questions (H, I) and adds the reason for using three sequences of exposures to the stimuli (J).

However, the reason for using the three sequences of stimuli should be stated as a question, not as experimental approach; the importance (para. 2) still interrupts the flow of thought from the funnel (para. 1) to the questions (para. 3); and the writing is still heavy.

Revision 2

EFFECT OF ALKALOSIS ON HYPOXIA-INDUCED PULMONARY VASOCONSTRICTION IN LUNGS FROM NEWBORN RABBITS

1 *A*Understanding the effect of alkalosis on the neonatal pulmonary circulation and on the response of the pulmonary circulation to hypoxia is important because alkalosis, produced primarily by mechanical hyperventilation, is widely used in the treatment of newborns who have the syndrome of persistent pulmonary hypertension (15, 16). *B*Although mechanical hyperventilation is often clinically effective in the treatment of these infants, it is not clear whether the clinical improvements during mechanical hyperventilation are due to the alkalosis resulting from the therapy. *C*The results of the few studies of the effect of alkalosis on hypoxia-induced pulmonary vasoconstriction in lungs of newborn animals have been variable. *D*Alkalosis has been shown either to reduce (10) or to have no effect (13, 14) on constriction of the neonatal pulmonary circulation in response to alveolar hypoxia. *E*These variable results may have been caused by the different sequences in which the lungs were exposed to hypoxia and alkalosis.

2 *F*Thus, the purposes of this study were to determine whether or not alkalosis reduces constriction of the neonatal pulmonary circulation in response to hypoxia and whether the sequence of exposure to alkalosis and hypoxia determines the effect of alkalosis. *G*To answer these questions, we tested the vasoconstrictive responses of isolated, perfused lungs from newborn rabbits to alkalosis and hypoxia in three sequences: respiratory or metabolic alkalosis before, during, and after alveolar hypoxia.

Structure of Revision 2

Paragraph 1: *Importance (A), Unknown leading to question 1 (B–D), Clue leading to question 2 (E).*

Paragraph 2: *Questions (F), Experimental approach (G).*

Comments on Revision 2

Revision 2 has been reorganized to begin with the importance. Thus, the questions come directly after the funnel.

Revision 2 adds a question about the three sequences of stimuli (F) and displays thinking leading to this question (E).

Revision 2 mentions the effects of metabolic and respiratory alkalosis only in the experimental approach, not as a question.

Revision 2 is shorter than Revision 1 because the studies of adults (original sentence B) and the answer have been omitted.

Thus, Revision 2 resolves most of the weaknesses of the original version. However, the writing is still heavy.

Revision 3

1 *A*Respiratory alkalosis produced by mechanical hyperventilation is widely used to treat infants with pulmonary vasoconstriction that has been either caused or aggravated by hypoxia (15, 16). **B** Although this respiratory alkalosis is thought to be responsible for the frequent success of mechanical hyperventilation in treating these infants, experimental studies in newborn animals have provided conflicting evidence of the ability of alkalosis to reduce hypoxia-induced pulmonary vasoconstriction (10, 13, 14). **C** We do not know what determines the ability of alkalosis to reduce hypoxia-induced vasoconstriction in some situations but not to affect it in others. **D** Nor do we know whether the respiratory aspect of the alkalosis is important or if similar beneficial effects might be obtained with metabolic alkalosis. **E** If metabolic alkalosis could be shown to reduce hypoxia-induced pulmonary vasoconstriction, many of the deleterious side effects of mechanical hyperventilation could be avoided.

2   **F** Because the sequences of lung exposure to alkalosis and hypoxia varied in the previous studies (10, 13, 14), we hypothesized that the sequence of lung exposure to alkalosis and hypoxia determines the ultimate effect of alkalosis on hypoxia-induced pulmonary vasoconstriction in newborn animals. **G** We also hypothesized that metabolic alkalosis is as effective as respiratory alkalosis in reducing pulmonary vasoconstriction. **H** To test these hypotheses, we measured the ability of both respiratory and metabolic alkalosis to reduce hypoxia-induced pulmonary vasoconstriction in isolated, perfused lungs of newborn rabbits when hypoxia and alkalosis were introduced in three different sequences: hypoxia before alkalosis, hypoxia after alkalosis, and simultaneous hypoxia and alkalosis.

Structure of Revision 3

Paragraph 1:   *Importance of the topic (A), Problem (B), Unknown leading to question 1 (C), Unknown leading to question 2 (D), Importance of question 2 (E).*

Paragraph 2:   *Clue and Question 1 (F), Question 2 (G), Experimental approach (H).*

Comments on Revision 3

Revision 3 adds a question about metabolic and respiratory alkalosis (G), displays the thinking leading to this question (D, E), and omits the general question about whether alkalosis reduces hypoxia-induced pulmonary vasoconstriction.

Revision 3 also includes "newborn animals" in the first question (F), thus avoiding the implication that the question is about humans.

The writing is still heavy.

CHAPTER 5

Exercise 5.1: A Clearly Written Methods Section

TOPIC +
Signal of
the Topic

Techniques of
Continuity

Methods

Preparation
Organized chronologically.
No topic sentences.
Minimal use of techniques of continuity.

1 ANESTHESIA
  A *Verb*

1 A Nine **dogs** (14–25 kg) were **anesthetized** with thiopental sodium (25 mg/kg i.v.) followed by **chloralose** (80 mg/kg i.v.). B Supplemental doses of **chloralose** (10 mg/kg i.v.) were given hourly to maintain **anesthesia**. C The **dogs** were paralyzed with decamethonium bromide (0.1 mg/kg) 10 min before measurements of tracheal secretion.

A–C *Key terms repeated*

A, C *Consistent point of view*

2 VENTILATION
  D *Verb*

2 D The trachea was cannulated low in the neck, and the lungs were ventilated with 50% oxygen in air by a Harvard respirator (model 613), whose expiratory outlet was placed under 3–5 cm of water. E Percent CO_2 in the respired gas was monitored by a Beckman LB-1 gas analyzer, and end-expiratory CO_2 concentration was kept at about 5% by adjusting the ventilatory rate. F Arterial blood samples were withdrawn periodically and their P_{O_2}, P_{CO_2}, and pH were determined by a blood gas/pH analyzer (Corning 175). G Sodium bicarbonate (0.33 meq/ml) was infused i.v. (1–3 ml/min) when necessary to minimize a base deficit in the blood.

D–G *Key term signaling topic of sentence*

3 INSERTION OF
  CATHETERS
  H *Key term*

3 H The chest was opened in the midsternal line and a **catheter** was inserted into the left atrium via the left atrial appendage. I **Catheters** were *also* inserted into the right atrium via the right jugular vein and into the abdominal aorta via a femoral artery.

H, I *Parallel form; Key term repeated*
I *Transition word*

4 PREPARATION
  OF TRACHEAL
  SEGMENT
  J *Key term*

4 J A **segment** of the trachea (4–5 cm) immediately caudal to the larynx was incised ventrally in the **midline** and transversely across both ends of the **midline** incision. K The dorsal wall was left intact. L Each **midline** cut edge was retracted laterally by nylon **threads** to expose the mucosal surface. M The **threads** were attached to a stationary bar on one side and to a force-displacement transducer (Grass FT03) on the other. N The **segment** was stretched to a baseline tension of 100–125 g.

J, L, M, N *Key terms repeated*

TOPIC +
Signal of
the Topic

Techniques of
Continuity

Methods

Protocol
Organized from most to least important (paras. 5–8) and chronologically (paras. 5–7).
One topic sentence (para. 7).
Continuity primarily from repetition of key terms and transition words and phrases.

---

5 MAIN PROTOCOL
O Transition phrase; Independent variable

Q Baseline ("before"); Dependent variable

S Sham control

5 *O* To stimulate pulmonary C-fiber endings, in each of the 9 **dogs** we **injected capsaicin** (10–20 μg/kg) into the right atrium. *P* **Capsaicin** was taken from stock solutions prepared as described elsewhere (4). *Q* At 10-s intervals for 60 s before and 60 s after each **injection**, we measured **secretions** from tracheal submucosal glands. *R* **Injections** were separated by resting periods of about 30 min. *S* As a control, in the same 9 **dogs** we measured **secretion** in response to **injection** of vehicle (0.5–1.0 ml) into the right atrium.

O–S Key terms repeated

S Transition phrase signaling a subtopic

---

6 VERIFICATION PROTOCOL
U Transition phase
T Background
U Purpose and procedure

6 *T* Although **capsaicin** selectively stimulates pulmonary C-fibers from within the pulmonary circulation, it is likely to stimulate other afferent pathways, including bronchial C-fibers, once it passes into the **systemic** circulation (2, 5). *U* To verify that secretion in our experiments was not caused by **systemic** effects of **capsaicin**, we *next* measured secretion after injecting **capsaicin** (10–20 μg/kg) into the left atrium and again, 30 min later, into the right atrium of all 9 dogs.

T, U Key terms repeated; Transition words

---

7 VERIFICATION PROTOCOL
V Topic sentence
V Purpose
V, W Procedure

X Outcome

7 *V* Finally, to verify that stimulation of pulmonary **C-fibers** was responsible for the secretions, we measured secretion in response to capsaicin (10–20 μg/kg into the right atrium) in the 9 **dogs** before and after **blocking** conduction in both of the cervical **vagus nerves**, which carry the pulmonary C-fibers, either by **cooling** the nerves to 0°C as described elsewhere (8) (4 **dogs**) or by **cutting** the nerves (5 **dogs**). *W* Before the first **blocking experiment** on each **dog**, we cut the recurrent and pararecurrent nerves so that the tracheal segment received its motor supply solely from the superior laryngeal nerves (14). *X* Consequently, when we **cooled** or **cut** the midcervical **vagus nerves** during an **experiment**, we could be certain that the changes in the tracheal responses were caused by interruption of the afferent vagal **C-fibers**.

V–X Key terms repeated; Transition words; Consistent point of view ("we")

V, X Consistent order ("cooled," "cut")

TOPIC +
Signal of
the Topic

Techniques of
Continuity

Methods

8 *VERIFICATION*
PROTOCOL
ᵞ*Transition phrase*

8 ᵞAs a further check on the effects of stimulating (and blocking) pulmonary C-fibers, in each of these protocols, we *also* measured heart rate, mean arterial pressure, and isometric smooth muscle tension of the tracheal segment, which are known to be altered reflexively by stimulation of pulmonary C-fibers (3).

ᵞ*Transition word*

Methods of Measurement

Organized from most to least important.
Strong continuity:
Paragraph 9: From repetition of key terms.
Paragraph 10: From a combination of four
techniques of continuity. This is a model
paragraph.

9 *METHOD OF*
MEASUREMENT
OF MAIN
DEPENDENT
VARIABLE
ᶻ*Topic sentence*

9 ᶻThe rate of **secretion** from sub**mucosal gland ducts** was assessed by **counting hillocks** of **mucus** per unit time as described elsewhere (8). ᴬᴬ*Briefly*, immediately before each experiment, the **mucosal** surface was gently dried and sprayed with **tantalum**. ᴮᴮThe **tantalum** layer prevented the normal ciliary dispersion of **secretions** from the openings of the **gland ducts**, so the accumulated **secretions** elevated the **tantalum** layer to form **hillocks**. ᶜᶜ**Hillocks** with a diameter of at least 0.2 mm were **counted** in a 1.2 cm² field of **mucosa**. ᴰᴰTo facilitate **counting**, the **mucosa** of the retracted segment was viewed through a dissecting microscope, and its **image** was projected by a television camera (Sony AVC 1400) onto a television screen together with the output from a **time-signal** generator (3M Datavision DT-1). ᴱᴱThe **image** and the **time signal** were recorded by a videotape recorder (Sony VO-2600) for subsequent playback and measurement of the rate of **hillock** formation.

ᴬᴬ*Transition word*
ᶻ⁻ᴱᴱ*Key terms repeated*

ᴰᴰ*Transition phrase*
signaling the subtopic
of DD and EE
ᴰᴰ, ᴱᴱ*Consistent order*
("image," "time
signal")

10 *METHODS OF*
MEASUREMENT
OF SECONDARY
VARIABLES
ᶠᶠ*Topic sentence*

10 ᶠᶠ**Heart rate**, mean **arterial pressure**, and **isometric smooth muscle tension** of the tracheal segment were recorded continuously throughout each experiment by a Grass polygraph. ᴳᴳ**Heart rate** was measured by a cardiotachometer triggered by an electrocardiogram (lead II). ᴴᴴ**Arterial pressure** was measured by a Statham P25Db strain gauge connected to the catheter placed in a femoral artery. ᴵᴵ**Isometric smooth muscle tension** in the segment was measured by a Grass FT03

ᶠᶠ⁻ᴵᴵ*Consistent order;*
Key terms repeated

ᴳᴳ⁻ᴵᴵ*Parallel form;*
Key term signaling
topic of sentence

Methods

force displacement transducer attached to the lateral edge of the retracted segment, as described elsewhere (1, 14).

Statistical Analysis

11   *STATISTICAL*
ANALYSIS
KK*Transition*
phrase

11   *JJ*Data are reported as means ± SD. *KK*To determine if there were **significant differences** in secretion before and after stimulation within each protocol, or significant differences in secretion between the experimental protocols, we performed two-way repeated-measures analysis of variance. *LL*When we found a **significant difference** between protocols, we performed the Student-Neuman-Keuls test to identify pairwise differences. *MM*We considered **differences significant at** $P < 0.05$.

KK–MM
Key terms repeated;
Consistent point of view
("we")

Organization and Continuity
Within and Between Paragraphs

This Methods section is divided into four subsections, each signaled by a subtitle (Preparation, Protocol, Methods of Measurement, and Statistical Analysis). Within each subsection, topics are signaled both visually (by new paragraphs) and verbally, and continuity is strong. Topic sentences are used in only three paragraphs: 7, 9, and 10. Sentence A in paragraph 1, for example, is not a topic sentence. It is the first step of anesthesia. A topic sentence would have to say something like "Dogs were anesthetized according to our usual procedure."

The protocol that answers the question (para. 5) is complete and clear. It is easy to see how the protocol will yield the answer to the question. The protocol includes two controls: baseline (sentence Q) and sham (sentence S), and three verification protocols: verification that secretion was not caused by systemic effects of capsaicin (para. 6), verification that stimulation of pulmonary C-fibers was responsible for secretions (para. 7), and verification that stimulation of pulmonary C-fibers affected other variables as expected (para. 8). Some readers might not notice the baseline control because it is not identified. To make the baseline control more noticeable, "(baseline)" could be added after "for 60 s before" in sentence Q.

Note that the number of dogs is stated for each protocol (sentences O, S, U, V).

Throughout the Methods section, repetition of key terms also provides continuity from paragraph to paragraph. The repeated key terms are "dog(s)," "trachea" or "tracheal," "segment," "capsaicin," "C-fiber(s)," "secretion(s)," and "submucosal gland(s)."

Point of view is well handled. "We" is used only in the protocol and statistical analysis, the storytelling subsections of Methods. Note that "we" appears only in the sentences that move the story forward: O, Q, S, U, V, W, X, Y in the protocol and KK, LL, MM in the statistical analysis. In addition, "we" appears at the beginning of only one sentence (MM), so it is not obnoxious.

Thus, we can see that to keep the story line of the paper going, this Methods section focuses in two ways on the methods that answer the question. One way is by the organization of topics from most to least important: the protocol comes early in the Methods section, the protocol that answers the question comes before the other protocols, and the methods for dependent variables that answer the question are described before methods for other dependent variables. The other way that this Methods section keeps the story line going is by signaling the organization so that it is apparent. The visual signals used are subtitles and new paragraphs. The verbal signals used are words (paras. 1–4 in Preparation), transition phrases (paras. 5, 6, and 8 of Protocol and para. 11 of Statistical Analysis), and topic sentences (para. 7 of Protocol and paras. 9 and 10 of Methods of Measurement).

Exercise 5.2: Content and Organization in Methods

1. The topics of each paragraph are 1, preparation; 2, protocol; 3, methods of measurement; 4, sham control (protocol); 5, materials; 6, analysis of data.

2. It is easier to see how the protocol will yield the answer to the question when the repetition in the protocol is omitted.

3. Topic sentence: <u>paragraph 3, sentence M</u>: "Recovery of prostaglandin E_2 from the buffer solution was calculated and prostaglandin E_2 content was measured as follows."

   Transition phrases signaling the topic of the paragraph: <u>paragraph 2, sentence E</u>: "To determine whether exogenous arachidonic acid increases prostaglandin E_2 production"; <u>paragraph 4, sentence U</u>: "In a control series of experiments."

4. It is easy to find the protocol that answers the question (para. 2) because the question is restated at the beginning of the protocol (sentence E).

6. The description of the baseline would be clearer if it were presented all in one place and at the first opportunity. In the original version, the baseline incubation is mentioned in sentence E and is identified as the baseline in sentence F, but the baseline incubation solution, which presumably is the same as the control incubation solution, is not defined until sentence U. In the revisions of paragraph 2, all baseline details are given together (sentence F of Revision 1, sentences E and F of Revision 2).

7. Paragraph 4 should come at the end of paragraph 2 because paragraph 4 describes a control series of experiments, which is part of the protocol.

8. The purpose of incubating ductus tissue with indomethacin is not clear. The purpose is made clear in Revision 1 of paragraph 2 by identifying indomethacin as a prostaglandin synthesis inhibitor (sentence F), thus implying that the incubation is a blocking control, and in Revision 2 by stating the purpose (sentence F). In addition, the purpose of assessing recovery of prostaglandin E_2 is not clear. The purpose is added in the revision of paragraph 3 (sentence N).

9. The sample size is not clear. Sentence E says that eight rings of ductus arteriosus were incubated. Sentence L mentions a mean "per experiment." It is not clear if one experiment equals one ring or if more than

one experiment using eight rings was done. The revisions of paragraph 2 make the sample size clear: eight experiments, each done on eight rings of ductus arteriosus taken from one fetal lamb.

10. Three pieces of information at first seem inappropriate to the Methods section—sentences L, S, and W. Sentence L tells the mean weight, which seems like a result. However, it is not a result that answers the question and therefore is not desirable in the Results section. Rather, the mean wet weight is a value used to express prostaglandin E_2 production. Therefore, it is more useful in Methods than in Results. Similarly, sentence S, which tells the percent recovery of prostaglandin E_2, is not a result that answers the question. Rather, it tells something about the material the author is working with and thus is appropriate in the Methods section. Finally, sentence W, which states that the maximum concentration of ethanol had no effect on prostaglandin E_2 production, is also not a result that answers the question. Knowing that ethanol had no effect is important because it indicates a valid experimental design. Therefore, this information is also more appropriate in Methods than in Results. Conclusion: Information that looks like results but does not help answer the question is less disruptive in Methods than in Results, so present such information in the Methods section.

REVISIONS

The main revision needed in this Methods section is in the protocol. First, the repetition of details needs to be avoided so that the overview of what was done to answer the question is clear. In addition, the description of the baseline, the purpose of adding indomethacin, and the number of experiments should be clarified. Finally, the control series of experiments (para. 4) needs to be included in the protocol (at the end of para. 2). These changes are illustrated in the two revisions of paragraph 2.

Revisions of other paragraphs are also included to illustrate alternative ways of writing these paragraphs. All revisions use "we."

Paragraph 1: Preparation

Revision 1

We prepared rings of ductus arteriosus from 16 breed-dated fetal lambs of 122 to 145 days of gestation (term is 150 days) that were delivered by cesarean section from spinally anesthetized ewes. After exsanguinating a lamb, we removed the entire ductus arteriosus, dissected it free of adventitial tissue, and divided it into eight 1-mm-thick rings, whose average wet weight was 22.1 ± 8.2 (SD) mg. Then we placed the rings in glass vials containing 4 ml of buffer (50 mM Tris HCl, pH 7.39, containing 127 mM NaCl, 5 mM KCl, 2.5 mM $CaCl_2$, 1.3 mM $mgCl_2 \cdot 6 H_2O$, and 6 mM glucose) at 37°C. We allowed the preparation to stabilize for 45 min before we began the experiments.

In this revision of paragraph 1, the first sentence is a topic sentence that states the topic of the paragraph (preparation of rings of ductus arteriosus). Note also that the number of fetal lambs and the number of rings are stated. In addition, the weight of the rings of ductus arteriosus is included here rather than in the protocol (para. 2), where it is less relevant.

Revision 2

From 16 exsanguinated 122- to 145-day fetal lambs (term is 150 days), we excised the ductus arteriosus, dissected it free of adventitial tissue, and sliced it <u>circumferentially</u> into eight 1-mm-thick rings. We incubated these rings in glass vials containing 4 ml of buffer A (50 mM Tris HCl, pH 7.39, containing 127 mM NaCl, 5 mM KCl, 2.5 mM $CaCl_2$, 1.3 mM $mgCl_2 \cdot 6\ H_2O$, and 6 mM glucose) at 37°C for 45 min before all experiments.

Each day we prepared stock solutions of arachidonic acid (0.33 mg/ml; Sigma) and indomethacin (16 mg/ml; Sigma) in ethanol. Ethanol alone had no effect on prostaglandin E_2 production.

This revision of the preparation condenses the preparation from 106 to 81 words by making "exsanguinated" an adjective instead of a verb and by omitting some details (pregnant ewes, spinal anesthetics, breed-dated, cesarean section, stabilized). In addition, this revision includes materials (original para. 5) in the preparation (30 more words), which is a reasonable organization.

Paragraph 2: Protocol

Revision 1   (Repetition is avoided (E), details are added (underlined), and the topic sentence gives an overview.)

^{E}Topic Sentence: Question; Independent variable; Dependent variable

^{F}Details of independent variable

^{G}Detail

^{H}n
$^{I, J}$Weight

^{K}Control

^{E}To determine whether exogenous arachidonic acid increases production of prostaglandin E_2 <u>in the ductus arteriosus</u>, we incubated eight rings of ductus tissue <u>from a fetal lamb</u> at 37°C for 90 min in each of three <u>consecutive</u> buffers and then collected the buffers for measurement of prostaglandin E_2. ^{F}The buffers we used were, first, fresh buffer <u>bubbled with oxygen (baseline)</u>, then fresh buffer containing 0.2 μg/ml arachidonic acid (Sigma) (0.67 μM), and finally fresh buffer containing 0.2 μg/ml arachidonic acid and 2 μg/ml of the <u>prostaglandin synthesis inhibitor</u>, indomethacin (Sigma) (5.6 μM). ^{G}<u>Between incubations in the last two buffers, we washed the rings in fresh buffer for 30 min.</u> ^{H}<u>We did this experiment eight times, each time with tissue from a different fetus.</u> ^{I}At the end of each experiment, we blotted the rings dry and weighed them. ^{J}The mean wet weight was 22.1 ± 8.3 (SD) mg of tissue per experiment. ^{K}<u>In eight control experiments, we measured prostaglandin E_2 production in other rings submitted to the same sequence of incubations and washes but in oxygenated buffer alone.</u>

Revision 1 of paragraph 2 avoids repetition by stating the incubation step once (sentence E), stating the measurement of the dependent variable once (sentence E), and naming the three incubation solutions (independent variable) in one sentence (F). Avoiding repetition makes the overview clear. Revision 1 also adds the tissue to the question (E), adds the species (E), describes the baseline clearly (F), states the purpose of using indomethacin (F), clarifies the number of experiments (H), and includes the control series (K). Note that if the second revision of paragraph 1 (Preparation) is used, "(Sigma)" can be omitted from the Protocol.

Revision 2   (Two-sentence overview)

^{E}Question; Independent variable

^{E}To determine whether exogenous arachidonic acid increases production of prostaglandin E_2 in the ductus arteriosus, we incubated eight ductus arteriosus rings from a fetal lamb sequentially in buffer A bubbled with oxygen, buffer A containing 0.2 μg/ml arachidonic acid (0.67 μM), and buffer A containing

F Dependent variable

G n
H Control

I Detail

0.2 μg/ml arachidonic acid and 2 μg/ml indomethacin (5.6 μM) at 37°C for 90 min each. ^{F}After the incubations, we collected the buffer solutions for measurement of baseline production of prostaglandin E_2, arachidonic acid-stimulated production, and net production resulting from simultaneous arachidonic acid stimulation and indomethacin inhibition, respectively. ^{G}We did this experiment eight times, each time with tissue from a different fetal lamb. ^{H}In eight control experiments, we measured prostaglandin E_2 production in ductus arteriosus rings after three 90-min incubations in buffer A bubbled with oxygen. ^{I}We washed all rings in fresh buffer A for 30 min between the last two incubations.

Revision 2 gives the overview in two sentences rather than in one, as in Revision 1, and describes the purpose of each incubation explicitly. Revision 2 also organizes the remaining details differently than in Revision 1 (though both revisions are organized from most to least important) and omits the weight, including it instead in Methods of Measurement. Buffer A would have to be defined in Preparation (as in Revision 2 of para. 1 above).

Paragraph 3: Methods of Measurement

^{M}We measured production of prostaglandin E_2 by the rings of ductus arteriosus as follows. ^{N}First, because not all prostaglandin E_2 is recovered from the buffer solution during extraction, we calculated percent recovery. ^{O}For this calculation, we added a known amount of ^{3}H-prostaglandin E_2 (6000 dpm, 130 Ci/mmol; New England Nuclear) to each buffer solution and acidified the solutions to pH 3.5 with 1 N citric acid. ^{P}We then extracted the prostaglandins in a 1:1 mixture of cyclohexane and ethyl acetate and purified them in silicic acid microcolumns (4). ^{Q}To calculate percent recovery, we compared the radioactivity measured before and after extraction. ^{R}Next, we measured prostaglandin E_2 content by radioimmunoassay using a specific rabbit antiserum against an albumin-conjugated prostaglandin E_2 preparation. ^{S}We determined prostaglandin E_2 production from the prostaglandin E_2 content corrected for percent recovery, which ranged from 50 to 70%. ^{T}We report prostaglandin E_2 production as pg/mg wet weight per 90-min incubation.

In this revision of paragraph 3, the purpose of calculating recovery of prostaglandin E_2 is added (N) for the benefit of readers who do not work in this field, the relation between production and content of prostaglandin E_2 is added (S), correction of prostaglandin E_2 content for recovery is added (S), and the percent recovery is mentioned in the sentence stating the correction (S).

Paragraph 4

See sentence K in Revision 1 of paragraph 2 (Protocol) and sentence H of Revision 2.

Paragraph 5: Materials

We prepared stock solutions of indomethacin (16 mg/ml) and arachidonic acid (0.33 mg/ml) in ethanol on the day of each experiment. To rule out any effect of ethanol on prostaglandin E_2 production, we incubated additional rings of ductus arteriosus in fresh buffer containing the maximum concentration of ethanol. After the 90-min incubation at 37°C, we collected the buffer and measured prostaglandin E_2. Ethanol had no effect on prostaglandin E_2 production (data not shown).

We purchased all chemicals and a prostaglandin E$_2$ radioimmunoassay kit from Sigma (St. Louis, MO). We purchased ^{3}H-prostaglandin E$_2$ (specific activity, 130 Ci/mmol) from New England Nuclear (Boston, MA).

This revision of paragraph 5 presents the ethanol information as a quality control experiment (para. 1). In addition, all materials are included, so "(Sigma)" can be omitted from paragraph 2 and "(130 Ci/mmol; New England Nuclear)" can be omitted from paragraph 3. The "Materials" subsection can be paragraph 1 instead of paragraph 5 (but then "additional" in the second sentence should be changed to "eight").

Paragraph 6: Analysis of Data

We summarized all data as mean $\pm$ SD. To determine whether prostaglandin E$_2$ production differed among the three treatments, we analyzed the data by single-factor repeated-measures analysis of variance. When we found a significant difference, we used the Student-Newman-Keuls test to determine which group was different from the others. We considered differences significant at $P < 0.05$.

This revision of paragraph 6 shows another way to write the statistical methods (third sentence).

CHAPTER 6

Exercise 6.1: An Unclear Results Section

COMMENTS

Paragraphs 3 and 4 are probably the best paragraphs in this Results section. However, most readers think paragraphs 4 and 5 are the best, probably because these are the only two paragraphs that do not begin with a figure legend.

Paragraph 4 has many strengths. It is short, it begins with a result (not a figure legend), data and statistical details are subordinated (though the data should be separated from the results by parentheses, not by commas), and an idea of the magnitude of a difference is given ("20% greater"). In addition, key terms naming the diets are consistent, the point of view in the three sentences is consistent, the three sentences are appropriately in parallel form, the topic of each sentence is signaled by the key term at the beginning, and transition words are used to indicate the logical relationships between the sentences. However, the logic is not rigorous. The "however" at the beginning of the second sentence really applies to the idea in the third sentence. Thus, the last two sentences should read, "However, because the calculated weight loss attributable to fluid losses after the protein diet was also greater than that after the mixed diet, the estimated nonfluid weight loss after the protein diet was no different from that after the mixed diet."

Paragraph 5 is not as clear as paragraph 4. Paragraph 5 has some of the same strengths as paragraph 4. It begins with a result, it subordinates data, and it keeps the names of the diets consistent. However, paragraph 5 has a confusing lack of signals of the topic at the beginning of the first two sentences, which makes the contrast difficult to see. In addition, the point of view in the two sentences is different: sentence U, blood pressure values; sentence V, fall in systolic blood pressure. Finally, "exaggerated postural decline" is unnecessarily fancy and changes the key term. This paragraph can be written more clearly and simply as follows:

When the subjects were supine, <u>blood pressure</u> was not significantly different from prediet values after either the protein diet (119 ± 5 / 72 ± 4 vs. 114 ± 2 / 69 ± 2 mmHg) or the mixed diet (114 ± 3 / 71 ± 3 vs. 114 ± 2 / 69 ± 3 mmHg). However, *when the subjects stood for 2, 5, or 10 min,* <u>blood pressure decreased</u> more after the protein diet than after the mixed diet (by 28 ± 3 vs. 18 ± 3 mmHg, *P* < 0.02). The <u>decrease in blood pressure</u> was accompanied by an increase in adverse symptoms in all seven subjects after the protein diet but in only one of the seven subjects after the mixed diet.

Readers rarely choose paragraph 3 as the best paragraph in this Results section, probably because it begins with a figure legend and contains a lot of data. However, if the first sentence (figure legend) is omitted, paragraph 3 is quite clear. The important result—the mineral balance that changed—is given first (sentence P). Then the mineral balances that did not change are grouped in a single statement (sentence Q). Although the data are numerous, they are listed at the end of the paragraph, so readers can stop reading if they are not interested. A separate table for these data is not advisable because these data do not help answer the question.

Paragraph 2 is not the best paragraph because it contains a fair amount of information that can be omitted or condensed. The first sentence is a figure legend, which is unnecessary. Sentences I–K can be condensed by about one-third. For example, "Neither mean daily nitrogen balance nor the nitrogen balance during the first or last week of the protein diet was significantly different from the corresponding values for the mixed diet (mean, −2.1 ± 0.9 vs. −2.6 ± 0.4 g per day; first week, −4.9 ± 0.5 vs. −4.6 ± 0.3 g per day; and last week, −1.0 ± 0.6 vs. −1.6 ± 0.3 g per day, *P* > 0.1), though nitrogen balance was more negative during the first week than during the last week." Sentence L states a method. The method should be subordinated to the result in the next sentence. For example, "In the subject given each diet for 5½ weeks, daily nitrogen balance was similar after the two diets (Fig. 3)."

Another question that can be raised about this Results section is whether the order of the paragraphs is optimal. The topics in the question are nitrogen and sodium balance and blood pressure and norepinephrine, so these are the topics we would expect to see in the Results section. Why the Results section begins with substrate and hormone levels is not clear. Similarly, why weight loss comes after results for nitrogen and sodium balance and before results for blood pressure and norepinephrine is not clear.

REVISIONS

Paragraph 1

Revision 1 *(79 words)*

Blood and urine ketone acids of the seven subjects were higher after they ate a pure protein diet for 21 days than after they ate a mixed diet, and the decrease in plasma insulin from the baseline values of 0.32 ± 0.06 (SD) IU/liter (protein diet) and 0.29 ± 0.06 IU/liter (mixed diet) was greater (Fig. 1). In addition, plasma glucose was lower (71 ± 5 vs. 76 ± 5 mg/dl, *P* < 0.005), but plasma glucagon was no different (data).

Revision 2   *(84 words)*

Blood and urine ketone acids of the seven subjects were <u>about two times</u> <u>and five times</u> higher, respectively, after 21 days of the protein diet than after the mixed diet, and the decrease in plasma insulin from the baseline values of 0.32 ± 0.06 (SD) IU/liter (protein diet) and 0.29 ± 0.06 IU/liter (mixed diet) was <u>three times</u> greater (Fig. 1). In addition, plasma glucose was <u>slightly</u> lower (71 ± 5 vs. 76 ± 5 mg/dl, $P < 0.005$), but plasma glucagon was no different (data).

Changes in Content

The revisions condense paragraph 1 from 242 words to 79 or 84 words by

- *omitting the figure legend (first sentence) and citing the figure at the end of the new first sentence*
- *omitting data that are shown in the figure*
- *mentioning each diet only once, permitting more than one result per sentence*
- *omitting repetition of "Day 21"*

Baseline data for plasma insulin are included because the data are not given in Figure 1.

The unit of measurement is changed to avoid a multiplier ($\times 10^{-2}$).

Data should also be added for plasma glucagon because they are not shown in a figure or table.

Changes in Continuity

Key terms are consistent:

- *"Protein diet," not "when carbohydrate was eliminated" (sentence E).*
- *"Mixed diet," not "carbohydrate-containing diet" (sentence B).*

The order of comparisons is consistent: all comparisons are from the protein diet to the mixed diet. (In the original version, the comparison in the last sentence is from the mixed diet to the protein diet. Some readers probably misread this comparison as saying that plasma glucose was greater after the protein diet than after the mixed diet.)

A transition word has been added ("in addition").

Topic Sentences

Because these revisions of paragraph 1 are so short, a topic sentence may not be necessary. However, a topic sentence could be added. For example, "Hormone and substrate concentrations in the seven subjects were affected more by the protein diet than by the mixed diet."

Difference Between Revisions 1 and 2

Revision 1: No indication of the magnitude of the differences. Revision 2: General indication of the magnitude of the differences ("two times and five times higher"; "three times greater"; "slightly lower").

Revision 3   *(130 words)*

For those who feel strongly about giving data in the text in addition to showing data in the figures, Revision 3 shows a way to include data without losing the forest for the trees. The tricks are to use a topic sentence (A), omit unnecessary words, state results, and subordinate data in parentheses; thus, three results can be included in one sentence (B). However, because data are included, Revision 3 is not as easy to read as Revisions 1 and 2. Revision 3 also shows a way to display thinking: it states the relation between the results for plasma insulin and plasma glucose (sentence C). Note that the unit of measurement for ketone acids has been changed to mM to agree with the figure; the unit of measurement for plasma glucose has also been changed to mM. P values are included because they are not given in the figure.

A<u>Hormone and substrate concentrations in the seven subjects were affected more by the protein diet than by the mixed diet.</u> **B**Blood ketone acids were twice as high after the protein diet as after the mixed diet (1.94 ± 0.23 (SD) vs. 1.08 ± 0.12 mM, $P < 0.001$), urine ketone acids were five times as high (50.9 ± 12.5 vs. 10.2 ± 2.9 mM, $P < 0.02$), and the decrease in plasma insulin from the baseline values of 0.32 ± 0.06 IU/liter (protein diet) and 0.29 ± 0.06 IU/liter (mixed diet) was three times greater (-0.14 ± 0.05 vs. -0.04 ± 0.05 IU/liter, $P < 0.05$) (Fig. 1). **C**The greater decrease in plasma insulin after the protein diet reflected lower mean plasma glucose concentrations (3.9 ± 0.1 vs. 4.2 ± 0.1 mM, $P < 0.005$). **D**Plasma glucagon concentrations did not change after either diet (data).

Paragraph 6

Revision 1 *(60 words)*

Topic sentence

<u>Plasma norepinephrine concentrations fell below prediet values after the protein diet but not after the mixed diet.</u> However, the lower concentrations occurred only when the subjects lay supine or after the subjects stood for 2 min (Fig. 5). After the subjects stood for 5 or 10 min, the plasma norepinephrine concentrations were no different from those before the diet.

Revision 2 *(57 words)*

Topic sentence

<u>Only the protein diet had an effect on plasma norepinephrine.</u> After the protein diet, plasma norepinephrine concentrations were lower than before the diet both when subjects were supine and after they stood for 2 min (Fig. 5). However, after the subjects stood for 5 or 10 min, the concentrations were equal to those before the protein diet.

Changes in Content

All results are about concentrations, not some about concentrations (sentence AA) and some about increases in the concentrations (sentences Z and BB). Thus, the contrast is clear.

Both revisions use topic sentences. The use of a topic sentence indicating that the mixed diet had no effect on norepinephrine concentrations makes it unnecessary to give details of results for the mixed diet. Thus, both revisions condense the results.

In addition, the revisions condense paragraph 6 (from 104 words to 60 or 57 words) by omitting the figure legend and citing the figure after the first specific result, and by omitting unnecessary words.

(In both revisions, the figure could be cited after the topic sentence, since the topic sentence gives a specific result. But since the second sentence refines the point made in the topic sentence, by limiting the change to two time periods,

citing the figure after the second sentence gives the reader a better idea of what to look for in the figure.)

Change in Continuity

The protein diet is mentioned before the mixed diet, so the order in the comparison is the same as that in paragraphs 1, 3, 4, and 5.

Word Choice

In the original version, "with" in "in response to standing <u>with</u> the hypocaloric mixed diet" (sentence Z) is not clear.

In the original version, "observed" (sentence Z) and "initiation of" and "therapy" (sentences Z and AA) are unnecessary.

Exercise 6.2: Results

Revision 1

1–2   After hypoxia was induced, minute ventilation increased for 5 min and then decreased over the next 50 min in all four subjects (Fig. 1). The decrease was unaltered by injection of 1.2 mg of naloxone (Fig. 2) or 10 mg of naloxone (Fig. 3). The results were the same when no injection was made (Fig. 2) or when placebo was injected instead of 10 mg of naloxone (Fig. 3).

3   The initial increase in minute ventilation during hypoxia was different in magnitude for each subject. Percent change from resting level was 131 ± 61 (mean $\pm$ SD) for nine experiments in subject A, 245 ± 121 for eight experiments in subject B, 57 ± 11 for nine experiments in subject C, and 401 ± 55 for five experiments in subject D. There was no correlation between the initial increase in minute ventilation and resting end-tidal P_{CO_2} (Fig. 4).

4   In two subjects, minute ventilation remained above resting level throughout hypoxia in all experiments (Figs. 2, 3). In the third subject (subject A), minute ventilation remained above resting level in all but one experiment. In this experiment, minute ventilation decreased from 9.8 L/min at rest to 9.6 L/min after 30 min of hypoxia. In the fourth subject (subject C), minute ventilation fell below resting level (from 7.8 ± 0.9 to 7.2 ± 1.1 L/min, $P < 0.05$) after 30 min of hypoxia in all nine experiments. This decrease was accompanied by a negligible increase in end-tidal P_{CO_2} (by 0.3 ± 0.2 mmHg, $P < 0.05$) but no significant change in respiratory rate.

5   There were no significant differences between subjects or between experiments in the same subject for end-tidal P_{O_2}, end-tidal P_{CO_2}, or arterial S_{O_2} during these experiments (Table 1).

The three sentences of paragraph 1–2 are all that is left of the original first two paragraphs. The first sentence is new. It describes the complete response to hypoxia before naloxone was given. The second sentence gives the results that answer the question. The results for both doses of naloxone are given together, thus avoiding repetition. The third sentence states the control results. All methods and figure legends have been omitted.

Paragraph 3 gives results that occurred chronologically before the results in paragraph 1–2, but because the results in paragraph 1–2 are more important to the question, they are presented first. The following details have been changed in paragraph 3: "Mean change (% $\pm$ SD)" is now "Percent change (mean $\pm$

SD)"; "n = 8," "n = 9," and "n = 5" are replaced by "for eight experiments," "for nine experiments," and "for five experiments"; the subjects' initials are replaced by single letters.

In paragraph 4, the sentences have been reorganized to move from least change to most change. Also, the number of subjects whose minute ventilation remained above resting level has been corrected to two (not three), and the results for subject SK (= subject A) have been clarified by adding "minute ventilation remained above resting level in all but one experiment." Finally, the excess digits in the standard deviations have been omitted (for example, "7.8 ± 0.91" is now "7.8 ± 0.9").

In paragraph 5, a statement is made about the variables and the table citation is subordinated in parentheses.

Revision 2

1–2   Naloxone did not prevent the return of minute ventilation to baseline during prolonged hypoxia. During hypoxia alone, minute ventilation increased within 1–5 min and then gradually decreased over the next 50 min in each of the four subjects (Fig. 1). Naloxone did not alter this response whether given at a dose of 1.2 mg (Fig. 2) or at a dose of 10 mg (Fig. 3) 15–35 min after hypoxia began. The results were the same when no injection was made (Fig. 2) and when placebo was injected instead of 10 mg of naloxone (Fig. 3).

3   The initial increase in minute ventilation due to hypoxia varied between subjects and did not correlate with resting end-tidal P_{CO_2} (Fig. 4).

4   In only one subject (subject C) did minute ventilation during hypoxia fall significantly below resting level. This fall was seen after 30 min of hypoxia in all nine experiments and was accompanied by a small but significant increase in end-tidal P_{CO_2}.

5   Neither dose of naloxone affected the changes in end-tidal P_{O_2}, end-tidal P_{CO_2}, or arterial oxygen saturation during the course of hypoxia in any of the subjects (Table 1).

In Revision 2, results are emphasized, the section is brief, and the beginning is strong.

In contrast to Revision 1, Revision 2 starts with the result that answers the question. Thus, the beginning of Revision 2 is stronger than the beginning of Revision 1. In addition, Revision 2 omits all unnecessary detail, so the trees do not overshadow the forest. In Revision 1 some detail is retained, so the forest is not quite so clear.

In paragraph 1–2 of Revision 2, the first sentence is a topic sentence stating the results that answer the question. The second, third, and fourth sentences are supporting sentences. The second sentence describes the results for hypoxia alone, thus clarifying the complete response to hypoxia. The third sentence describes the results for naloxone at both doses, thus avoiding repetition. The fourth sentence describes control results.

In paragraph 3, the data (which appear in Figs. 2 and 3) have been omitted.

In paragraph 4, only the important exception is described. The slight decrease in minute ventilation in subject SK (= subject A) was considered "noise" and was therefore omitted.

In paragraph 5 a clearly relevant statement is made about the variables and the table citation is subordinated in parentheses.

CHAPTER 7

Exercise 7.1: Overall Story in a Complex Discussion

Outline of the Overall Story		**Topic Sentence**
I. Surviving finding (paras. 1–4)	¶1 A	Section TS (paras. 1–4)
A. Reasons the second peak had not been seen before	B	Section TS (paras. 1–3) (Key term TS)
1. Disadvantages of techniques (para. 1)	C	Paragraph TS (para. 1) (Transition word TS; topic only)
	J	Paragraph TS (para. 1) (Transition word + key term TS; message)
2. Experimental conditions (para. 2)	¶2 K	Paragraph TS (Transition word + key term TS)
3. Anesthetics (para. 3)	¶3 M	Paragraph TS (Transition word TS)
	Q	Sub TS (Key term TS)
B. Reasons the second peak was seen now (para. 4)	¶4 T	Paragraph TS (Transition phrase + category term TS: "problems" = the topic of paras. 1–3)
	W	Sub-TS (Category term TS: "technique" = "power spectral analysis" in sentence V)
II. Hypotheses to explain the second peak (paras. 5–9)	¶5 Z	Section TS (paras. 5–9) and Section TS (paras. 5–6) and Paragraph TS (para. 5) (Transition clause + key term TS)
A. Hypothesis 1 to explain the second peak (based on dependent oscillations)		
1. Statement of hypothesis (para. 5)		
2. Evidence against hypothesis 1 (para. 6)	¶6 EE	Paragraph TS (Key term TS)
B. Hypothesis 2 to explain the second peak (based on independent oscillations)	¶7 JJ	Section TS (paras. 7–9) (Transition clause + key term TS)
1. Argument for independence (para. 7)	KK	Paragraph TS (Key term TS)
	LL	Sub TS (message) (Transition phrase TS)
2. Explanation of independence (para. 8)	¶8 QQ	Paragraph TS (Transition clause + key term TS)
3. Statement of hypothesis 2 (para. 9)	¶9 TT	Paragraph TS (Transition phrase + key term TS)

The overall story in paragraphs 1–9 of this Discussion has only two steps and thus two main sections: I, why the authors saw the previously unnoticed second peak in the power spectral densities of the whole nerve signal, and II, what the second peak is. These two steps are the forest. The individual stories within subsections of the Discussion (capital letters in the outline) and within paragraphs (arabic numbers in the outline) are the trees.

Within section I of the Discussion, the story proceeds by the overview technique. Within section II, even though there is a section topic sentence (sentence Z), the story proceeds by the step-by-step technique. If section II proceeded by the overview technique, we would expect to read about hypothesis 2 immediately after reading about hypothesis 1 (para. 5). But this is not what happens. Although we do eventually get to hypothesis 2 (para. 9), we arrive by a circuitous route. That route is indicated step by step by the paragraph topic sentences.

Thus, in both sections, the topic sentences guide us through the overall story. In paragraphs 1–4 (step 1 of the overall story), the first sentence in paragraph 1 is a section topic sentence. Along with the second sentence of paragraph 1 and the first sentence of paragraph 4, it tells the overall story (forest) of the section. In addition, the first sentence in paragraph 2 reminds us of the overall story (forest) by repeating "reason for not noticing the second peak." The other sentences in paragraphs 1–4 (except sentence M) are the trees. Note that the second topic sentence in section I (sentence B) is developed by enumeration: paragraphs 1, 2, and 3 each explain one of the three reasons mentioned in the topic sentence. This pattern of development is an expansion of the pattern we first saw within a single paragraph (see Example 3.1 in Chap. 3).

Similarly, the topic sentences guide us through the overall story in paragraphs 5–9 (step 2 of the overall story). The topic sentence of paragraph 5 (sentence Z) is a transition clause topic sentence that summarizes the point of paragraphs 1–4 (the surprising finding of a second peak) and introduces the topic of paragraphs 5–9 (hypotheses to explain the second peak). Note that "one of the first hypotheses" implies that at least two hypotheses will be presented. Thus, sentence Z is the section topic sentence for paragraphs 5–9, as well as the topic sentence for paragraphs 5 and 6, which are about the first hypothesis, and for paragraph 5, which states the first hypothesis. The topic sentence of paragraph 6 is a key term topic sentence rejecting the first hypothesis. Thus, paragraphs 5 and 6 are organized according to a pro-con structure (see Example 3.3 in Chap. 3).

The topic sentence of paragraph 7 (sentence JJ) is a section topic sentence that introduces the topic of paragraphs 7–9. This is the most difficult topic sentence to understand in this Discussion, because it summarizes an idea that was not in the topic sentence of paragraph 6 (the sources of the oscillations are in the brain stem) and because it does not state the second hypothesis, which is what we expect, but instead states a notion that the second hypothesis is based on (independence of the oscillations). The topic sentence of paragraph 8 (sentence QQ) further delays the expected statement of the second hypothesis by explaining the independence. Finally, the topic sentence of paragraph 9 (sentence TT) introduces the second hypothesis.

The Discussion goes on to describe evidence that supports the second hypothesis but first answers the question originally posed in the Introduction. The beginning of the next paragraph is as follows.

10 Before considering the evidence from the single fiber recordings that supports this hypothesis, we will examine the results of these recordings. The original goal in recording single fibers in the phrenic and recurrent laryngeal nerves was to answer the question of how single fibers and their individual power spectra contribute to the whole nerve power spectrum. We first had to know whether the peaks in the power spectra of single fibers are due to the shape of the action potential or to the firing rate. We determined this information by. . . .

Exercise 7.2: Content and Organization in a Discussion

COMMENTS ON THE ORIGINAL VERSION

Topics of Paragraphs

Paragraphs 1–3:	Introduction
Paragraph 4:	Explanation of a discrepancy
Paragraph 5:	Results for question 2
Paragraph 6:	Speculation on steal as the reason for the answer to question 2
Paragraph 7:	Speculation on other sites of steal
Paragraphs 8–9:	Conclusion

Answers to the Questions

The answer to question 1 is not stated. The results for question 1 are mentioned in sentence N of paragraph 4, which explains how the author's study differs from a previous study. The results for question 1 are stated more noticeably at the beginning of paragraph 8. These comments are too little and too late.

The answer to question 2 is not stated. The results for question 2 are presented in paragraph 5. Note that "absent" should be added after "decreased" in sentence W (compare sentence N in para. 4 with sentence II in para. 8). The answer is hinted at in sentence Y, the last sentence of paragraph 5. However, saying that your results support a previous conclusion makes your work sound unoriginal. In fact, the results go beyond the previous findings and thus are new, not confirmatory. Sentence Y can be omitted. The relation to a previous conclusion can be dealt with either as a discrepancy (see para. 2 of Revisions 1 and 2) or as an extension of previous work (see sentences A and B of Revision 3). The first sentence of paragraph 5 should be revised to state the answer to question 2. The verb must be in present tense, and the population must be expanded to all preterm infants who have a large shunt through a patent ductus arteriosus.

To emphasize the answers to the question more, they should be stated at the beginning of the Discussion (para. 1).

Beginning of the Discussion

The beginning of the Discussion (paras. 1–3) is introductory information. This information should be omitted. It is simply a review of the evidence for retrograde blood flow in the descending aorta and for decreased blood flow in the cerebral arteries. The condensed version of this evidence in the Introduction is sufficient.

Middle of the Discussion

In paragraph 6, the first sentence should be a topic sentence indicating that the author is going to present a possible explanation for the parallel relation between cerebral and aortic blood flows. Two possible topic sentences are given in the revisions below (see the first sentence of para. 3 in Revisions 1 and 2).

In paragraph 7, the first sentence should be a topic sentence indicating that this paragraph is speculation about a tangential topic—other sites of steal. In the original version, it is nearly impossible to see how paragraph 7 fits into the overall story. Paragraph 7 should also be revised to clarify what the other sites of steal are (see para. 4 of Revisions 1 and 2).

End of the Discussion

The conclusion (paras. 8–9) is too long and irrelevant. In paragraph 8, the first sentence should be revised to state the <u>answer</u> to question 1 (not the <u>results</u> for question 1), and the answer to question 2 should be added. The other sentences in paragraph 8 should be made relevant or omitted. In paragraph 9, the first sentence is irrelevant to the purposes of this paper, so it should be made relevant or omitted. The second sentence in paragraph 9 is similar to sentence JJ in paragraph 8 except that now steal is inaccurately said to be <u>shown</u> rather than <u>suggested</u> by the findings. Both sentences about steal are unnecessary in the conclusion. The final sentence, which states possible complications of abnormal cerebral blood flow, may be kept as is. Two good endings for this Discussion are illustrated in the last paragraph of Revisions 1 and 2.

REVISIONS

Revision 1

Questions

1. "To determine if retrograde diastolic blood flow **can occur** in the cerebral arteries of preterm infants who have a large shunt through a patent ductus arteriosus"
2. "To relate alterations in cerebral blood flow to alterations in aortic blood flow"

Discussion

1 **Answers and supporting results**
A Answer to question 1
B Answer to question 2
C, D Supporting results
A–C Good signals of the answers and results

1 **A**<u>In this study we have shown that</u> diastolic blood flow in the cerebral arteries of preterm infants who have a large shunt through a patent ductus arteriosus **can be** not only decreased but also absent or even retrograde. **B**<u>We also have evidence that</u> these changes in cerebral blood flow closely **parallel** changes in aortic blood flow. **C**<u>We found that</u> in all infants with a large ductal shunt, who had retrograde diastolic blood flow in the descending aorta, the cerebral blood flow was greatly decreased, absent, or retrograde. **D**Moreover, after closure of the patent ductus arteriosus in these infants, so that they no longer had retrograde blood flow in the descending aorta, the diastolic blood flow was also forward in the cerebral arteries.

2 **Explanation of a discrepancy**
E Key term topic sentence
F Subtopic sentence
H Subtopic sentence

J Good condensing

2 **E**<u>Our observations extend beyond</u> those of Perlman et al. (6), who were able to find only a decrease in cerebral blood flow during diastole and did not report any retrograde or absent blood flow. **F**Two factors may be responsible for the differences between these findings. **G**First, the infants in our series may have had larger left-to-right ductal shunts and therefore greater changes in cerebral blood flow. **H**Second, the different methods of detection may have led to different findings. **I**Whereas Perlman et al. (6) used a continuous-wave Doppler velocitometer, we measured cerebral blood flow with a range-gated pulsed-Doppler system. **J**Compared to the pulsed-Doppler system, continuous-wave analysis is limited by <u>lower resolution</u> and <u>a potential for signal loss</u> (15, 16), either of which could result in undermeasured cerebral blood flow.

3 **Speculation on cerebral steal**
K Key term topic sentence

3 **K**<u>The changes in aortic and cerebral blood flows during diastole in preterm infants who have a large shunt through a patent ductus arteriosus may be explained by the difference in resistance between the pulmonary and the systemic vasculature.</u> **L**In these infants the pulmonary vascular bed, which has low resistance to blood flow, freely communicates with the systemic vascular bed, which has higher resistance. ^{M}Therefore, the presence of a large shunt through a patent ductus arteriosus results in a steal of blood from the aorta during diastole and in a concomitant decrease in diastolic blood flow in the cerebral arteries. ^{N}Eventually, the cerebral blood flow reverses and may lead to diastolic steal of blood from the cerebral circulation.

<table>
<tr><td>

4   *Speculation on coronary steal*
^{O}*Transition phrase topic sentence*

</td><td>

4 ^{O}<u>As opposed to diastolic steal in the cerebral and systemic circulations, we found no evidence of diastolic steal from the coronary arteries in preterm infants who have a large shunt through a patent ductus arteriosus.</u> ^{P}In Doppler tracings taken from the ascending aorta just above the aortic valve, no differences in diastolic blood flow were apparent between control infants and infants who had a large ductal shunt. ^{Q}However, retrograde blood flow from the coronary arteries may have been too small to be detected by our technique.

</td></tr>
<tr><td>

5   *Conclusion*
^{R}*Key term topic sentence*
$^{R-T}$*Clinical implications*

^{U}*Application of the method*

</td><td>

5 ^{R}<u>Some of the clinical complications of a patent ductus arteriosus, such as cerebral ischemia, may be explained by our findings that cerebral blood flow during diastole can be decreased, absent, or retrograde.</u> ^{S}The extent of these changes in blood flow appears to be related to the size of the ductal shunt, and thus a large shunt may predispose infants to serious complications. ^{T}It is therefore important to recognize these changes in blood flow within a vessel. ^{U}Because range-gated pulsed-Doppler echocardiography is a safe, noninvasive means of assessing not only the patency of the ductus arteriosus but also alterations in blood flow within a vessel, this echocardiographic technique can be used to improve the diagnosis and management of complications of a patent ductus arteriosus.

</td></tr>
</table>

Comments on Revision 1

Beginning

Paragraph 1 of Revision 1 states the answers to both questions at the beginning and then states the results that support the answers. The same results happen to support both answers, so this presentation is very efficient. In addition, results for aortic blood flow are subordinated at the beginning of each sentence (C, D), thus focusing the sentences on the important results—those for cerebral blood flow. Note that results for the control infants, which are not necessary in the Discussion, have been omitted.

The answer to question 1 uses the same key terms as in the question but changes the point of view slightly: from "retrograde diastolic blood flow" to "diastolic blood flow," and therefore changes the verb from "can occur" to "can be." The question should be changed accordingly. The answer to question 2 uses the same key terms as in the question but instead of using the verb "is related to," specifies the relationship: "parallels." Note that this specific term ("parallels") creates a picture in the reader's mind, whereas "is directly related to," though also a valid answer, does not.

Middle

Paragraphs 2 and 3 present two important topics: the explanation of the discrepancy and the speculation on steal. The order of these two topics could also be reversed. Note that in paragraph 2, the introduction to the comparison clearly specifies the difference between the two studies ("Our observations extend beyond") (sentence E). In addition, the explanation of the limitations of the previous method is nicely condensed by stating only the essential feature of each limitation (sentence J). Also note that the authors of the previous paper are always referred to as "Perlman et al.," never "Perlman," as in the original version.

Paragraph 4 uses a very clear transition phrase topic sentence to introduce a secondary point (whether steal also occurs in the coronary arteries) and explains the point clearly. This topic was not clearly signaled or explained in the original version (para. 7, sentences GG and HH).

Thus, the middle of this Discussion uses two key term topic sentences and one transition phrase topic sentence to create the overall story. (In the topic sentence in para. 2, a category term, "observations," rather than a key term is used to refer to the changes in blood flow mentioned in para. 1. In the topic sentence of para. 3, a category term, "changes," is used and several key terms are repeated: "aortic," "cerebral," "blood flows," "diastole," "preterm infants," "large shunt," "patent ductus arteriosus.") Note that you can see the overall story of the Discussion by reading the first sentence of each paragraph.

End

Paragraph 5 (conclusion) presents clinical implications and an application of the method. The first answer is incorporated into the first sentence describing clinical implications (R). This presentation of the answer is less obvious than a straightforward restatement of the answers. Also note the smooth connection between the clinical implications and the application of the method (T). Thus the method, which seemed irrelevant in the original version (para. 9, sentence PP), is now made relevant.

Revision 2

1 Answers
A *Context*
  A₁ *Aorta subordinated*
  A₂ *Cerebral arteries emphasized*
B *Answers*
  B₁ *Answer to question 1*
  B₂ *Answer to question 2*
C *Subtopic sentence*
D–F *Supporting sentences (note condensing)*

1 ^{A_1}Although retrograde blood flow in the descending aorta during diastole is a common finding in preterm infants who have a patent ductus arteriosus (4, 5, 9–14), ^{A_2}it has only recently been suggested that blood flow in the cerebral arteries may be similarly altered (6). ^{B}<u>The results of our study indicate ^{1}that retrograde blood flow during diastole can occur in the cerebral arteries of preterm infants who have a large shunt through a patent ductus arteriosus and ^{2}that alterations in cerebral blood flow closely parallel alterations in aortic blood flow.</u> ^{C}<u>The parallel relationship between cerebral and aortic blood flows, and the importance of shunt size, are apparent from our findings.</u> ^{D}Thus, in control infants and infants who had a small ductal shunt, there was no evidence of abnormal diastolic blood flow in the cerebral arteries or in the descending aorta. ^{E}However, in infants who had a large ductal shunt, diastolic blood flow was reduced, absent, or retrograde in the cerebral arteries, and retrograde in the descending aorta. ^{F}Moreover, after closure of the ductus, normal diastolic blood flow was re-established at both sites.

2 Explanation of a discrepancy
G *Transition phrase + key term topic sentence*
H *Subtopic sentence*

2 ^{G}In contrast to our results, Perlman et al. (6) reported only reduced diastolic blood flow in the cerebral arteries of preterm infants who have a large ductal shunt. ^{H}Two factors might explain the more severe alterations in cerebral blood flow that we observed (<u>absent and retrograde flow</u>): <u>the size of the shunt</u> and <u>the technique used</u>. ^{I}First, the infants in our study may have had a larger ductal shunt, and consequently greater changes in cerebral blood flow, than the infants in Perlman et al.'s study. ^{J}Second, whereas Perlman et al. used a continuous-wave Doppler velocimeter, we measured cerebral blood flow with a range-gated pulsed-Doppler system. ^{K}Compared to the pulsed-Doppler system, continuous-wave analysis is limited by lower resolution and a potential for signal loss (15, 16), either of which could result in undermeasured cerebral blood flow.

3 *Speculation on cerebral steal*
^{L}*Key term topic sentence*

3 ^{L}<u>A likely explanation for our results is that</u>, in the presence of a large shunt through a patent ductus arteriosus, the high resistance systemic circulation communicates with the lower resistance pulmonary circulation, thereby <u>diverting</u> blood away from the aorta and reducing diastolic blood pressure. ^{M}As the diastolic blood pressure falls, diastolic blood flow in the cerebral arteries decreases and eventually reverses, thereby diverting blood away from the cerebral arteries as well. ^{N}The failure of the cerebral arteries to decrease resistance and maintain forward diastolic flow is probably due to maximum vasodilation or impaired autoregulation, both of which are believed to occur in preterm infants who have a large ductal shunt (6, 17, 28).

4 *Retrograde blood flow in other arteries*
^{O}*Transition word + key term topic sentence*

4 ^{O}<u>Our results suggest that blood flow may also be diverted from other arteries during diastole.</u> ^{P}We found forward blood flow in the transverse aorta proximal to the ductus arteriosus during diastole, <u>when there is normally no blood flow.</u> ^{Q}We believe that this blood flow reflects blood diverted from the carotid and subclavian arteries toward the ductus <u>via the transverse aorta.</u> ^{R}Similar findings have been reported previously (5, 10, 11). ^{S}However, in measurements taken from the ascending aorta just above the aortic valves, we found no differences between control infants and infants who had a large ductal shunt. ^{T}Thus, if blood is also diverted from the coronary arteries during diastole, it was too little to be detected by our technique.

5 *Conclusion*
$^{U,\,V}$*Sumary of conclusions*

^{W}*Clinical implication*

5 ^{U}<u>In summary, this study shows that</u> retrograde blood flow can occur in the cerebral arteries, as well as in the descending aorta, of preterm infants who have a large shunt through a patent ductus arteriosus. ^{V}In addition, the retrograde blood flow in the cerebral arteries closely parallels the changes in aortic blood flow. ^{W}This altered cerebral blood flow may lead to complications such as ischemia or hemorrhagic brain injury.

Differences Between Revisions 1 and 2

Beginning
Paragraph 1 of Revision 2 begins with context (A) and then states the answers (B) and the supporting results (C–F). A subtopic sentence (C) is used to introduce the supporting results. The statement of the results has been nicely condensed.

Middle
Paragraph 2 explains the discrepancy essentially as in Revision 1 but adds the topic of each explanation to the subtopic sentence (H), thus providing a clear overview.

Paragraph 3 presents the speculation on steal but changes the term "steal" to "diverting." This revision includes the sentence on maximum vasodilation and impaired autoregulation, which is omitted in Revision 1.

Paragraph 4 uses a transition word + key term topic sentence to introduce a secondary point—whether blood flow is also diverted from other arteries. This topic sentence clearly identifies the topic of the paragraph because the topic sentence makes a point, rather than stating a result, as in the original version (para. 7). The paragraph includes all of the arteries mentioned in the original version, not just the coronary arteries, as in Revision 2. Details have been added (underlined) to make the explanation clearer.

Whereas Revision 1 uses two key term topic sentences and one transition phrase topic sentence, Revision 2 uses two transition topic sentences and only one key term topic sentence to tell the overall story.

End

Paragraph 5 (conclusion) presents a straightforward summary of conclusions followed by a clinical implication. Since clinical implications are also mentioned at the end of the first paragraph of the Introduction, the story comes full circle.

The Overall Story

In both revisions, you can see the overall story by reading the first sentence or two of each paragraph. Both revisions proceed by the step-by-step technique.

Revision 3

^AContext

^BAnswers

^AIn this study, we have extended previous work showing decreased blood flow in the cerebral arteries of preterm infants who have a large shunt through a patent ductus arteriosus (6). ^BOur results demonstrate that, in these infants, cerebral blood flow can be not only decreased but also absent or even retrograde and that these changes in cerebral blood flow closely parallel changes in aortic blood flow.

Revision 3 shows another way to begin this Discussion: by presenting the answers to the questions as an extension of previously published work on the topic of abnormal cerebral blood flow in preterm infants. This is a very straightforward presentation.

CHAPTER 8

Exercise 8.1: Design of Figures and Tables and Their Relation to the Text

COMMENTS

In this Results section, the figure and table are not clearly designed and do not relate well to the text.

Figure 2

Type of Graph. *A bar graph would show the increases in airflow resistance and the before and after values more clearly than a line graph does.*

Axis. *At first glance, the axis looks logarithmic, but it is actually linear. To make it* look *linear, tick marks and scale numbers should be placed at equal intervals.*

More tick marks could be added to make the 2-fold and 8-fold increases easier to see.

Relation to the Text. *Once tick marks are added, it is easy to see that "8-fold" is a bit of an exaggeration. The real value is between 7 and 8 fold. It is better to underestimate than to overestimate, so that readers will not think you are trying to inflate the data.*

Using the same key terms in the text, figure legend, and axis label would make the relation between the figure and the text clearer. The indicator ("airflow resistance") should be used in the figure legend, not the variable ("bronchoconstriction"), because airflow resistance is what was measured. The key term "airflow resistance" should also be used in the axis label. If the abbreviation

(Rrs) is used, it should be defined in the figure legend. Similarly "dose of smoke inhaled" in the text does not correlate well with "number of smoke inhalations" in the figure.

    Figure Legend. *The point ("increases") could be added to the figure legend. The figure legend could be revised to give most experimental details before the statistical details. In addition, the times of measurement could be added.*

    To show the variability of the data, rather than how close the measured mean is to the true mean, SD could be shown (as in Table 1) instead of SE.

Table I

    Type of Illustration. *A line graph shows time course more clearly than a table does.*

    Relation to the Text. *The text says that the maximum was reached within 1 min, but the means show that the maximum was reached within ½ min. If instead you look at individual data, you would have to say that the mean was reached within 2 min (dogs 2–4, ½ min; dog 1, 1 min; dog 5, 2 min). Similarly, airflow resistance decreased to one-half the maximal value within 2 min (the mean of 188% at 2 min is not different from 190% at 4 min).*

    In the title, "bronchoconstriction" should be changed to "airflow resistance."

Revision

Results

    Inhalation of cigarette smoke into the lungs of anesthetized dogs caused 2- to 7-fold increases in airflow resistance of the total respiratory system depending on the number of tidal volumes of smoke inhaled (Fig. 2). Airflow

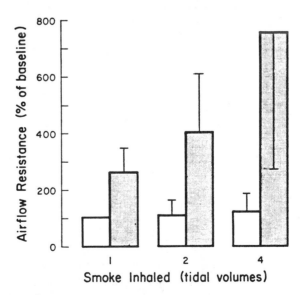

Figure 2. ^{A}Increases in airflow resistance of the total respiratory system after inhalation of cigarette smoke in 5 anesthetized dogs. ^{B}The dogs were given 1, 2, or 4 tidal-volume inhalations of cigarette smoke. ^{C}Inhalations were separated by 20 min. ^{D}Values are means ± SD ½ min before (□) and ½ min after (▨) each series of inhalations.

resistance increased rapidly after the start of smoke inhalation; <u>on average,</u> the maximum was reached within ½ min (<u>Fig. 3</u>). Airflow resistance remained increased transiently, decreased to one-half the maximal value within <u>2</u> min (<u>Fig. 3</u>), and returned to baseline before the next dose 20 min later [*figure citation omitted*].

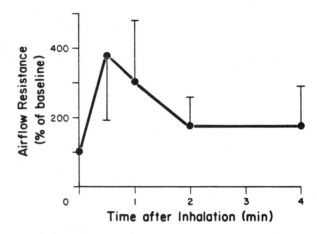

Figure 3. Time course of <u>airflow resistance of the total respiratory system</u> after inhalation of 2 tidal volumes of cigarette smoke in 5 <u>anesthetized</u> dogs. Data are means ± SD.

Exercise 8.2: Table Design and Relation to the Text

Revision

Table II. Effects of Peritoneal Dialysis and Hemodialysis on Plasma Apoproteins in Patients Who Have Renal Disease

Treatment	Plasma Apoprotein (mg/dl)					Apo A-I/ Apo B
	Apo A-I	Apo A-II	Apo B	Apo D	Apo E	
Control	163 ± 23	36.4 ± 2.0	98 ± 32	5.6 ± 1.2	7.3 ± 1.6	1.7 ± 0.6
Peritoneal Dialysis	123 ± 20	36.0 ± 4.0	94 ± 8	9.5 ± 1.0*	7.5 ± 0.9	1.3 ± 0.2
Hemodialysis	102 ± 17*	34.8 ± 6.5	89 ± 14	6.7 ± 1.3	6.8 ± 0.8	1.2 ± 0.2†

Values are means ± SD from 10 control subjects, 6 peritoneal dialysis patients, and 15 hemodialysis patients.
*$P < 0.0005$, †$P < 0.01$ vs. control.

Comments

The original table is generally clear, but it can be made clearer.

Title and Column Headings. *In the revision, to make the title complete, the independent variables (peritoneal dialysis and hemodialysis) have been added and the control subjects have been omitted. As a result, the key terms in the title correlate with the terms in the first column on the left (peritoneal dialysis, hemodialysis).*

In addition, the column heading "Plasma Apoprotein" has been added, correlating with that term in the title, and the unit of measurement (mg/dl) is included after this general heading rather than being stated after each individual apoprotein.

Instead of a title in the form "Effects of X on Y in Z," the title could be in the form "Y after X in Z," and the point ("Greater Changes") could be included:

> *Plasma Apoproteins After Peritoneal Dialysis or Hemodialysis in Patients Who Have Renal Disease*
>
> <u>*Changes in*</u> *Plasma Apoproteins After Peritoneal Dialysis or Hemodialysis in Patients Who Have Renal Disease*
>
> <u>*Greater Changes*</u> *in Plasma Apoproteins After Hemodialysis than After Peritoneal Dialysis in Patients Who Have Renal Disease.*

Relation to the Text. *To make the table show the decreases in apo A-I and in apo A-I/apo B described in the text, the control values have been moved to the first row (as is conventional), peritoneal dialysis values are in the middle ("intermediate"), and the hemodialysis values are last ("much lower").*

Showing Significant Differences. *To show statistically significant differences, symbols (*,†) have been placed after the values that are different, and footnotes have been added to state the P values and what numbers are being compared.*

Presentation of Numbers. *To make the numbers align neatly on the decimal point and on the ±, the columns and rows of the table have been switched: independent variable in the first column on the left, dependent variables across the columns on the right.*

Once the data are aligned in columns, it is easier to see that data for apo A-II and for apo A-I/apo B have different numbers of decimal places. In the revised table, all values have the same number of decimal places.

CHAPTER 10

Exercise 10.1: The Content of Abstracts

Abstract 1

Grade: C

+ *States the name (A), the purpose (A), the species (A), and the advantages (B) of the device.*
− *Gives no visual image of the device; that is, does not describe its key features or tell how it works.*
− *Does not tell how it was tested or how well it works.*
− *Does not state the advantages clearly:*
> *Is incorporation of an injection unit an advantage or part of the description of the device (a key feature)?*
> *What is the difference between nontraumatic immobilization and lack of physiological disturbance? (Note the heavy words.)*
> *What does "feasibility of repeated attempts at insertion with only one venipuncture" mean?*
− *Does not make the emphasis clear: the title emphasizes injection; the abstract emphasizes immobilization.*

Revision 1   (Not based on the text of the paper)

A "STRAITJACKET" THAT IMMOBILIZES RATS FOR INTRAVENOUS INJECTION

A_1*Name*
A_2*Purpose; Species*
B, C Key features
D*Advantages*

E_1*How well it works*
E_2*How it was tested*

A_1 We developed a "straitjacket" A_2 to immobilize rats for intravenous injection. B The jacket, made of leather, fits snugly and is attached to a metal frame for stability. C There is an injection port over the tail for intravenous injection and an attached metered syringe. D The advantages of the jacket are nontraumatic immobilization, <u>easy access</u> for injection, <u>accurate dosing</u> of drugs, and <u>easy handling</u> by a single operator. E_1 The jacket was effective for injection into E_2 all 100 rats tested.

Comments

Revision 1 adds a description of the jacket (B, C) and tells how the jacket was tested (E_2) and how well it works (E_1). Revision 1 also revises the advantages. It omits two advantages: incorporation of an injection unit (included as a key feature in sentence C) and lack of physiological disturbance (considered the same as nontraumatic immobilization). It uses simpler words to describe three of the remaining four advantages: "exactness of dosage quantitation" is changed to "accurate dosing of drugs," "feasibility of repeated attempts at insertion with only one venipuncture" is changed to "easy access for injection," and "requirement of only a single operator" is changed to "easy handling by a single operator." Finally, Revision 1 makes the emphasis clear because the emphasis is the same in the title and in the abstract—immobilization.

Revision 2   (Based on the text of the paper)

A RESTRAINING DEVICE TO IMMOBILIZE RATS FOR INTRAVENOUS INJECTION

A_1*Purpose; Species*
A_2*Name*
B*Key features*
C*How it works*

D*Advantages*

E_1*How well it works*
E_2*How it was tested*

A_1 To immobilize rats for intravenous injection of drugs, A_2 we have designed a restraining device. B This device consists of three rubber belts (to restrain the body) and a rubber ring tourniquet attached to a sliding tailholder projecting from a wooden board mounted on a stand. C To inject a drug, the operator places a finger inside the rubber ring below the tailholder and presses the ring down, thus congesting the tail vein and permitting easy insertion of the needle. D The advantages of this restraining device are that it <u>allows</u> the experimenter <u>to immobilize</u> conscious rats without <u>disturbing</u> their physiological function, it <u>avoids</u> loss of blood or drug by <u>permitting</u> repeated attempts at venipuncture without <u>removing</u> the needle from the tail, and it <u>requires</u> only one operator. E_1 The restraining device was successful for injections into E_2 all 100 rats tested.

Comments

In Revision 2, the key features of the restraining device (B) and how it works (C) are described. The statement of the advantages is clarified by omitting some advantages and rewording the others. "Incorporation of an injection unit" (a key feature), "nontraumatic immobilization" (= lack of physiological disturbance?), and "exactness of dosage quantitation" are omitted. "Feasibility of repeated attempts at insertion" is reworded and its advantage is stated (D). This advantage ("avoids loss of blood or drug") replaces "exactness of dosage quantitation." Verbs (underlined) are used to list all advantages. How the restraining device was tested and how well it works are stated (E). Because the term "strait-jacket," though vivid, is slightly misleading (since the rat's legs are not re-strained), this term is replaced by the (less vivid) term "restraining device."

Abstract 2

Grade: C

+*Easy to read.*

+*States what was found briefly and completely.*

+*Has clear organization indicated by new sentences for what was done, what was found, and what was concluded.*

−*The question is stated vaguely: the independent variable is missing.*

−*Species?*

−*The overview of what was done (A) is not clear:*

    How was one lung exposed—surgically?

    What was it exposed to?

−*The overview of what was done is incomplete: What happened to the other lung is not described until sentence C; it should be in sentence A.*

−*Some details of what was done are missing:*

    What was the concentration of ozone?

    How long was the exposure?

    What was the state of the animals during the study?

    What cells were studied?

−*The answer is not stated or not clearly signaled or both:*

    The last sentence (E) signals an answer, but it states an implication, as indicated by the verb "could be" and by the facts that in this study bacteria were not given and mortality was not assessed. The answer should probably be about the effect of ozone on the defense mechanism of the lungs (see the title), though it is questionable whether the results of bronchoalveolar lavage should be extended to the lungs as a whole. The intended answer seems to be that ozone impairs the defense mechanism of the lungs, though an increased number of polymorphonuclear leukocytes may be a good thing for lung defense.

    Sentence D has an unclear signal ("were found to be"): it could be either results or the answer.

    It is also possible that there are two questions and two answers, one about the effect of ozone on the defense mechanism and the other about direct toxicity (sentence D) (see Revision 2).

±*The writing is generally clear but contains some <u>jargon</u> ("unilateral lung exposure technique," "bacterial challenge") and <u>unclear word choice</u> (what does "depress various intracellular hydrolytic enzymes" mean: decrease the numbers of enzymes? decrease enzyme activity?). Also the <u>signal</u> of what was found would be clearer if it were at the beginning of the sentence. In the title, "defensive mechanism" should be "defense mechanism."*

Revision 1

OZONE SUPPRESSES THE DEFENSE
MECHANISM IN RABBITS' LUNGS

A₁ *Question; Species*

A₂ *What was done; Condition*

B, C *What was found; Details of methods*

A₁ We studied <u>the effects of low concentrations of ozone</u> on the endogenous defense mechanism of <u>rabbits'</u> lungs **A₂** by <u>ventilating one lung with ozone and the other lung with air during light anesthesia.</u> **B** We found that ozone <u>(0.5–3.0 ppm for 3 h)</u> decreased the viability <u>of alveolar macrophages,</u>

decreased <u>the activity</u> of intracellular hydrolytic enzymes (lysozyme, beta-glucuronidase, and acid phosphatase), and increased the absolute number and percentage of polymorphonuclear leukocytes in pulmonary lavage fluid. ^{C}All these effects were dose related, appeared only in the lung ventilated with ozone, and resulted from direct toxicity of ozone and not from a generalized systemic response. ^{D}We conclude that <u>ozone suppresses the defense mechanism of rabbits' lungs</u>. ^{E}We <u>suggest</u> that this suppression may be responsible for the <u>high death rate</u> of rabbits <u>infected with bacteria</u> after their lungs are ventilated with ozone.

^{D}*Answer*
^{E}*Implication*

Comments

In Revision 1, the independent variable is added to the question (A_1), and the species (A_1), methods details (A_2, B), and the answer (D) are also added. In A_2 the overview of what was done is now complete, and precise word choice makes clear how the lungs were exposed and what each lung was exposed to. In A_2 and B, the following details of methods are now included: the condition of the rabbits (lightly anesthetized), the concentration of ozone (0.5–3.0 ppm), the duration of exposure to ozone (3 h), and the type of cells studied (alveolar macrophages). The answer (D) answers the question asked: the key terms for the independent and dependent variables are the same in the question and the answer, and the point of view is the same. Also, the signal of what was found ("We found that") is moved to the beginning of the sentence (B), and the result for hydrolytic enzymes is described more precisely ("<u>decreased</u> the <u>activity</u> of intracellular hydrolytic enzymes"). Finally, in the implication (E), word choice is simplified ("high death rate" instead of "increased mortality"), jargon is avoided ("infected with bacteria" instead of "given a bacterial challenge"), and an appropriate signal is used ("We suggest that").

Revision 2

OZONE DIRECTLY IMPAIRS ENDOGENOUS DEFENSES IN RABBIT LUNGS

^{A}In rabbits exposed to ozone and then given an injection of bacteria, mortality is increased. ^{B}The increased mortality may result from ozone-induced impairment of the lungs' defense mechanisms. ^{C_1}We therefore asked <u>whether ozone exposure impairs endogenous defense mechanisms in rabbits' lungs</u> and, ^{C_2}<u>if so, whether the impairment is caused by direct toxicity of ozone or by a generalized systemic response</u>. ^{D_1}For this study, we assessed components of the lungs' defense mechanisms in lavage fluid from both lungs of lightly anesthetized rabbits ^{D_2}after ventilating one lung with ozone (0.5–3.0 ppm for 3 h) and the other lung with air. ^{E}We found that low concentrations of ozone decreased the viability of alveolar macrophages, decreased the activity of various intracellular hydrolytic enzymes (lysozyme, beta-glucuronidase, and acid phosphatase), and increased the absolute number and percent of polymorphonuclear leukocytes within pulmonary lavage fluid. ^{F}All these effects were dose related and were found only in the lung exposed to ozone. ^{G}These results indicate that <u>ozone exposure impairs endogenous defense mechanisms in rabbits' lungs and that this impairment is caused by direct toxicity</u>. ^{H}We speculate that these impaired lung defenses may be responsible for the increased mortality of rabbits infected with bacteria after exposure to ozone.

A, B Background
A Known
B Unknown
C_1 Question 1; Species
C_2 Question 2
D What was done
D_1 Dependent variable; Condition
D_2 Independent variable
E, F What was found

G Answers

H Speculation

Comments

Revision 2 asks two questions (C_1, C_2) and gives two answers (G). In Revision 2, question 1 is stated more specifically than the same question in Revision 1 and thus anticipates the answer more clearly. The reason the question in Revision 2 is more specific is that it uses the same verb ("impairs") as the answer.

Also in Revision 2, background information is added (A, B) to prepare for the speculation at the end of the abstract (H). Note that sentence B states the ultimate question the author is interested in and sentence H speculates on a possible answer to the ultimate question.

Other details added in Revision 2 are the same as those in Revision 1.

Abstract 3

Grade: F

– *Too much detail. You cannot see the forest for the trees.*

> *In what was done (A), give the general approach, not every variable, and indicate the relationship between variables.*

> *In what was found (B–F), give data for only the most important findings, give percentages instead of means and SE, or omit data altogether. Omit* P *values. Omit all "significantly's." State "mean ± SE" (if used) only once.*

– *Too many abbreviations. $\dot{Q}s/\dot{Q}t$ can be replaced by "shunt fraction." $\dot{V}A/\dot{Q}$ and C_{air} are never mentioned again, and $Pst(L)$ and TLC are used only once each, so they are unnecessary. S_{air} and SO_2 are bizarre.*

– *The question is not stated.*

– *The last sentence is unclear: is it the implication of this study or of other studies? If other studies, it does not belong in the abstract.*

Revision

A *Background*
B₁ *Question*

B₂, C *What was done*

D *What was found*

E *Answer*

NO RELATION BETWEEN INCREASED LUNG ELASTIC RECOIL PRESSURE AND SHUNT FRACTION IN HEALTHY MEN WITH STRAPPED CHESTS

A Elastic recoil pressure of the lungs increases when total lung capacity decreases. **B₁** To determine whether this increased pressure is due to atelectasis, **B₂** we measured elastic recoil pressure and the right-to-left intrapulmonary shunt fraction (an index of atelectasis) before and during chest strapping (a condition that decreases lung capacity) in healthy men. **C** Experiments were done while the men breathed room air (baseline) or 100% oxygen (to induce atelectasis). **D** We found that despite a 50% increase in elastic recoil pressure during chest strapping, there was no increase in shunt fraction while the men breathed room air and a minimal increase in shunt fraction while they breathed 100% oxygen. **E** We conclude that increased elastic recoil pressure in the lungs is not due to atelectasis during conditions of decreased total lung capacity.

Comments

The revision is much easier to read because the question is stated (B_1), the experimental approach gives an overview (B_2, C), indicators are identified (B_2, C), and unnecessary details (less important variables, data, statistical information, the implication at the end) and all abbreviations are omitted.

Exercise 10.2: Length of Abstracts

Abstract

-1
-2
-3
-2
-6
-14

The disposition of morphine was investigated by means of radioimmu-noassay after an ~~single~~ intravenous dose (10 mg/70 kg) was administered to 10 ~~adult~~ normal <u>men</u> ~~male subjects~~ who had not received other drugs for 2 weeks ~~preceding the study~~. A multiphasic decline in serum concentrations of morphine occurred. Detectable blood concentrations of morphine, ~~or of~~ a metabolite, or ~~of~~ both persisted for 48 hours ~~after a single intravenous dose~~.

Number of Words in the Original Version: 69
Number of Words Omitted: 14
Number of Words Remaining: 55

Critique of the Original Version

Even if the word limit for this abstract were 150 words, this abstract, at 69 words, would be too long, because the message can be expressed clearly and completely in 55 words; 14 words in the original version are unnecessary.

In addition, some of the words are imprecise. For example "disposition" means distribution and elimination. Did the author mean disappearance? pharmacokinetics? clearance? Similarly, what does "normal" mean: healthy? drug-free? Also, the men may not have <u>received</u> drugs (from someone else) but they may have <u>taken</u> (ingested, injected) drugs. Finally, the men probably had not taken <u>any</u> drugs for 2 weeks, so omit "other."

The word "multiphasic" is a precise technical term used to describe a curve that has two or more slopes along its course. However, some authors might prefer a simpler, less technical term such as "gradual" or "stepwise."

Other problems are as follows: Action is expressed in a noun ("decline") and an adjective ("detectable") rather than forcefully, in verbs. A key term is changed (serum, blood). The dose should be in mg/kg, not in mg/70 kg.

Revision 1   *(52 words)*

The <u>disappearance</u> of morphine was investigated by means of radioim-munoassay after an intravenous dose <u>(0.14 mg/kg)</u> was administered to <u>each of</u> 10 <u>healthy men</u> who had <u>taken no</u> drugs for 2 weeks. The concentration of morphine in the serum <u>decreased gradually</u>. Morphine, a metabolite, or both <u>were detectable</u> for 48 hours.

Revision 2   *(42 words)*

To study the <u>pharmacokinetics</u> of morphine, <u>we</u> measured its concentration by radioimmunoassay after an i.v. dose (0.14 mg/kg) to 10 drug-free men. <u>We found</u> a <u>stepwise</u> decrease in serum morphine. Either morphine or a metabolite was detectable for 48 hours.

Comments

Revision 2 uses "we" and adds a signal for what was found.

CHAPTER 11

Exercise 11.1: Titles

Abstract 1

Question: B_2 the effect of CPAP on renal function in newborns.
Answer: FCPAP can impair renal function in newborns.

Title:

1. Continuous Positive Airway Pressure Impairs Renal Function in Anesthetized Newborn Goats (88)
2. Impaired Renal Function From Continuous Positive Airway Pressure in Anesthetized Newborn Goats (94)

Comments

The title for Abstract 1 should be fairly easy to write because the abstract is clearly written.

Functions

Both titles identify the main point of the paper.
Both titles aim to attract appropriate readers by putting an important word first.
> *Putting "continuous positive airway pressure" first should attract neonatologists.*
> *Putting "impaired renal function" first should attract nephrologists.*

Content

Both titles include the necessary information:
> *The independent variable (continuous positive airway pressure).*
> *The dependent variable (renal function).*
> *The species (newborn goats).*
> *The condition of the animals (anesthetized).*
> *The point (impairs, impaired).*
The first title is a sentence and expresses the point in a verb in the present tense ("impairs").
The second title is a phrase and expresses the point in an adjective ("impaired").

Hallmarks

Both titles accurately, completely, and specifically identify the main point of the paper.
> *The same terms are used in the title as in the question and the answer.*
> *The species and the condition are taken from what was done (sentence C). The condition is included in the title because anesthesia can affect the variables measured. However, some authors might prefer to omit "anesthetized."*
Both titles are unambiguous.
> *No noun clusters, misplaced adjectives, or abbreviations are used. Even though "CPAP" is a standard abbreviation in neonatology and is used in the abstract, the abbreviation is not used in the title because it is unlikely to be familiar to readers in other fields and therefore could be meaningless to readers of sources such as Index Medicus.*

In contrast to the titles given above, the title "Impairment of Renal Function Induced by Continuous Positive Airway Pressure" is ambiguous. In this title, it is not clear what was induced by continuous positive airway pressure—the impairment or the renal function.
Both titles are concise.
  They compact the necessary words by using a category term ("renal function") instead of naming all the dependent variables (urine flow, sodium excretion, glomerular filtration rate).
  In addition, the second title uses the shortest possible terms: "impaired" rather than "impairment of" (8 vs. 13 characters and spaces) and "from" rather than "induced by" (4 vs. 10).
Both titles begin with an important word.

Abstract 2

Question: A_1 To determine whether sulfur dioxide and cold dry air interact in causing bronchoconstriction in people who have asthma.

Answer: F Thus, cold dry air increases the bronchoconstriction induced by inhaled SO_2 in people who have asthma.

Title:

1. Sulfur Dioxide and Cold Dry Air Exaggerate Bronchoconstriction in Asthmatics (84)
2. Cold Dry Air Increases Sulfur-Dioxide-Induced Bronchoconstriction in Asthmatics (79)
3. Increased Bronchoconstriction in Asthmatics Breathing Sulfur Dioxide in Cold Dry Air (84)
4. Synergistic Effects of SO_2 and Cold Dry Air on Bronchoconstriction in Asthmatics (80)

Running Title:

1. SO_2 and Cold Dry Air Exaggerate Bronchoconstriction (51)
2. Cold Dry Air Increases SO_2-Induced Bronchoconstriction (54)
3. Bronchoconstriction From Breathing SO_2 in Cold Dry Air (54)
4. Synergistic Effects of SO_2 and Cold Dry Air (43)

Comments

The title for Abstract 2 is more difficult to write than the title for Abstract 1 because the answer in Abstract 2 does not answer the question exactly as it was asked. Thus, the title based on the question (first title) makes a slightly different point than the titles based on the answer (second and third titles).

Titles that state the point in other ways are also possible (fourth title). The statement of the answer in the abstract (and in the paper) should then be changed to agree with the point in the title.

Functions

All titles identify the main point of the paper and put an important word first.

Content

All titles include the necessary information:
  The independent variables (sulfur dioxide, cold dry air).

The dependent variable (bronchoconstriction).
The population (asthmatics).
The point (exaggerate, increases, increased, or synergistic effects).
The third title also includes the experimental approach (breathing).
The first and second titles are sentences and express the point in a verb in present tense ("exaggerate" or "increases").
The third and fourth titles are phrases and express the point in an adjective ("increased") before the dependent variable (bronchoconstriction) or in an adjective and a noun ("synergistic effects").

Hallmarks

All titles accurately, completely, and specifically identify the main point of the paper. (The titles are as accurate as possible considering the discrepancy between the question and the answer.)
All titles are unambiguous.
> *No noun clusters or misplaced adjectives are used.*
> *One title uses a standard abbreviation (SO_2).*
All titles are concise.
All titles begin with an important term.

Running Title

The running titles are all shortened versions of the titles.
The first, second, and fourth running titles are the same as the beginning of the corresponding titles.
The third running title uses the same key terms as in the corresponding title but joins them with "from."

Abstract 3

Abstract 3, which is from Science, *does not follow the usual format (question, what was done, what was found, answer). Instead it states only the results (A) and an implication (B).*

Title: Glue Sniffing Causes Heart Block in Mice (40)

Comments

This revised title illustrates three points:
> *It is unnecessary for the title to fill the space allowed. Short titles have more impact than long ones.*
> *A title for a paper published in a general journal can be catchy.*
> *A title must be based on solid results, not on an implication or a speculation. Although some people try to include humans and sudden death in the title by using a question in a subtitle ("A cause of sudden death in humans?"), even tentative implications do not belong in the title, so the subtitle should be omitted.*

Note that it is impossible to fit all three results from the abstract into the title. The solution is either to choose one of the results, as done in the title above (causes heart block), or to use a category term, for example, "impaired cardiac conduction," "cardiac conduction abnormalities," or "cardiac rhythm disturbance." However, because these terms are all more abstract than "heart block," they are not as catchy. Similarly, it is difficult to include both of the independent variables in the title. But since toluene is the solvent in airplane glue, either "toluene" or "airplane glue" can be omitted from the title. "Airplane glue" is catchier than the less familiar "toluene."

Note also the careful compacting of words in this title. "Glue sniffing" is not only catchy but also condenses the longer term "inhalation of airplane glue." "Causes" is a condensed way of saying "sensitizes the heart to." For some readers "causes" may seem like overstatement, especially since "asphyxia-induced" is omitted. These readers may prefer "leads to," which is less direct than "causes." Finally, "heart block" is a condensed way of saying "atrioventricular block" without using an abbreviation ("A-V block").

Even though this title is catchy and thus should attract readers, it also follows the guidelines for the content and hallmarks of a good title. All the necessary information is included: "glue" is the independent variable, "sniffing" is the experimental approach, "causes" is the point, "heart block" is the dependent variable, and "mice" is the species. In addition, although some readers will dispute the accuracy of the title and perhaps also the completeness, the title specifically identifies the main point of the paper, is unambiguous, is concise, and begins with an important term.

CHAPTER 12

Exercise 12.1: Seeing the Big Picture

Strengths

Overall

The paper is fairly short, meaty, and clear.
There are no loose ends.
Most key terms are kept consistent or are shortened recognizably (for example, "umbilical cord occlusion," "cord occlusion").
Only three abbreviations are used: pO_2, pCO_2, SD (partial pressure of oxygen, partial pressure of carbon dioxide, standard deviation).

Introduction

What is known (A–D) and the importance (E) are clearly stated.
The Introduction starts close to the specific topic.
The funnel in the first half of paragraph 2 (F–J) is clear.
The signal of the question (O) is clear.
The statement of the experimental approach (P) clearly addresses the problem mentioned in paragraph 2 (J).

Materials and Methods

Subtitles clearly identify the subsections of Materials and Methods.
Verbal signals are used in some subsections:
  Animals: Key term ("Sixteen fetal sheep").
  Surgical Preparation: Topic sentence ("The surgical protocol has been described previously. Briefly, . . .").
  Experimental Protocol: A topic sentence that gives a brief overview ("Four experiments were performed in the sequence presented below.").
For each protocol, we know what was done and what the independent and dependent variables and the controls are.

Each protocol is organized according to the independent variables listed in the question (ventilation, oxygenation, umbilical cord occlusion).

Purposes (para. 4, 5, 7) and reasons (para. 6, 7, 9, 10, 12) are included for specific procedures.

Thinking is clearly displayed in "Calculations" and "Analysis of Data."

Results

The order of independent variables within paragraphs 1, 2, and 3 is consistent (ventilation, oxygenation, umbilical cord occlusion).

Thinking is clearly displayed in "Major vs. Minor Responders During Ventilation Alone" to explain why the author is reporting some results that do not help answer the question. Because the question for these results could not have been designed into the study, stating the question and describing the methods in the Results section is appropriate.

Discussion

The Discussion has the three standard parts: the answer to the question at the beginning, explanation and expansion of the answer in the middle, and a restatement of the answer followed by speculation at the end.

Topics are organized from most to least important to the question and answer.

Reading the topic sentence at the beginning of each paragraph gives an overview of the story.

Paragraph 1:
Clear statement of the context (A).
Clear statement of the answer (B).

Paragraph 2:
Clear topic sentence (D).

Paragraph 3:
Clear.
A limitation of the study design is included (X).
Although the topic of paragraph 3 is tangential, the author considered it at least as important as the question and answer, so it is included in the Discussion.

Paragraph 4:
Clear.

Paragraph 5:
The last sentence brings the story full circle by mentioning the syndrome of persistent pulmonary hypertension of the newborn, which was first mentioned in the Introduction (E).

References

All references in the list are in the text, and vice versa.

Figures and Tables

The figures are parallel.

The tables are clear and clearly support the statements in the text, and their form is parallel.

The variables and the values in the figures and tables are the same as those in the text. The key terms and the units of measurement are also the same.

The species is stated in all figures and tables.

In all figures and tables data are identified as mean ± SD, and *n* (the sample size) is given.

Figure legends and footnotes of tables give enough information to make the figures and tables understandable without reference to the text.

Data in figures do not repeat data in tables.

Abstract

The signals of what was found (E) and of the answer (K) are clear.

The background statement (A) is clear.

The statement of what was found (E–J) is clear.

Results and data in the abstract are the same as those in the Results section.

The species is stated in what was done (C).

Data are presented as percent change rather than as mean and standard deviation.

Weaknesses

Overall

The statements of the question are not all the same.
>   Abstract: "to determine whether ventilation and oxygenation of the fetal lungs could cause this decrease in resistance" (C).
>   Introduction: "to determine whether the sequential exposure of the fetus to gaseous ventilation, oxygenation, and umbilical cord occlusion could decrease pulmonary vascular resistance to levels seen at birth" (O).

The statements of the answer are not all the same.
>   Abstract: "The changes in pulmonary vascular resistance and blood flow that occur at birth can be achieved by *in utero* ventilation and oxygenation" (K).
>   Discussion: "Ventilation and oxygenation together can account for the decrease in pulmonary vascular resistance, and thus for the large increase in pulmonary blood flow, that normally occur at birth" (B).
>   Discussion: "The changes in pulmonary vascular resistance and blood flow that are critical to the adaptation of the fetus to the postnatal environment can be achieved by *in utero* ventilation and oxygenation (EE). Moreover, much of the vasodilatory response can be achieved without an increase in fetal pO₂" (FF).

The answers do not answer the questions asked. The verbs in all the answers are different from the verbs in the questions. In addition, the end of the Discussion (FF) includes an answer for which there is no question. This is a major discrepancy in the overview.

The overview in the text is not as clear as the overview in the abstract. Organization from most to least important should be used more in the text. Also, more techniques of continuity need to be used in the text to make the overview clear: topic sentences, verbal and visual signals of topics, exact repetition of key terms. Finally, long explanations should be condensed.

The writing could be livelier.

Introduction

The review of the literature (evidence that the pulmonary vascular response to ventilation, oxygenation, and umbilical cord occlusion may be altered by the metabolic effects of acute surgery and anesthesia (K–N)) is unnecessary. This topic is dealt with more relevantly in the Discussion (para. 2).

The references in the review of the literature (11–25) are unnecessary.

The question (O) relates to the first answer only. To relate to both answers (Discussion, para. 5, EE and FF), the question needs to be quantitative, not all or nothing (not <u>whether</u> but <u>the extent to which</u> ventilation, oxygenation, and umbilical cord occlusion can account for the decrease in pulmonary vascular resistance that occurs at birth). Alternatively, there could be two questions: <u>whether</u> and, if so, <u>which event is most important</u>.

The question should be in present tense.

Materials and Methods

Surgical Preparation: The brief description does not seem brief.

Experimental Protocol:

More overview is needed at the beginning.

Verbal signals would be helpful for each protocol, in addition to the subtitles.

Details of the overview and details of methods should be moved to other subsections (see Revision 2).

Calculations:

Organizing from most to least important would emphasize the dependent variable (pulmonary vascular resistance) more.

More overview would be useful, specifically, a topic sentence in paragraph 9 saying that pulmonary blood flow was measured in two ways, a companion topic sentence in paragraph 10 announcing the second way of measuring pulmonary blood flow, and a transition phrase in the third sentence of paragraph 9 stating the purpose of injecting microspheres into the left atrium.

Results

Putting the results for pulmonary vascular resistance in the middle of the Results section and also burying them at the end of the paragraph on pressures (para. 3) makes the important results hard to find. Organizing from most to least important would emphasize the results that answer the question both in the Results section and in the figures (pulmonary vascular resistance, the most important dependent variable, would be in Fig. 1). The variables on which the calculation of pulmonary vascular resistance was based (pulmonary blood flow and mean pulmonary arterial and left atrial pressures) can come next, and blood gases and pH can come last. For this organization, a topic sentence linking pulmonary blood flow to pulmonary vascular resistance should be added (see Revision 1). In addition, within paragraphs 2 and 3, subtopics (ventilation, oxygenation, umbilical cord occlusion) should be signaled at the beginning. Also, a new paragraph is needed for left atrial pressure (para. 3).

Even better than reorganizing from most to least important would be to reorganize according to the independent variable, as in Methods, rather than according to the dependent variable (see Revision 2). This reorganization would make the Results correspond more clearly with the question, the abstract, Methods, and the calculation of pulmonary vascular resistance.

A subtitle is needed for the beginning of the Results section to parallel the subtitle for the major and minor responders.

The species should be mentioned at the beginning of Results.

The data for pulmonary blood flow and for pulmonary vascular resistance do not need to be mentioned; citing the figures is sufficient.

In paragraph 2, Figure 1 should be cited after an experimental result (the effect of ventilation), not after a control result. In paragraph 3, Figure 2 should be cited after the result for ventilation alone (the dramatic decrease), not at the end of the sentence.

In paragraph 5, the first sentence (methods) should be subordinated to the second sentence (results), and Table 4 should be cited after the result, not after the method. The remaining sentences can be omitted because the details are included in the Discussion (para. 3).

Discussion

Paragraph 1:

A stronger signal of the answer in B and a stronger link between B and A would be helpful (see Revision 1).

The species should be mentioned in the signal of the answer.

Instead of stating a result, sentence C should state an answer. The variable should be pulmonary vascular resistance and the verb should be in present tense.

Paragraphs 2–4:

Condensing would make these paragraphs clearer.

Paragraph 3:

Identifying the great variability in the response of fetal pulmonary blood flow as an unexpected finding (sentence M) would make the overview clearer.

Paragraph 4:

To make the topic sentence sound less negative and to focus the story on the topic of paragraph 4, the first point in sentence Y can be subordinated to the second point.

Paragraph 5:

"In utero" belongs in the experimental approach, not in the answer (EE).

The answer should be signaled and the species should be named in the signal.

Changing the key term (from "ventilation" to "without an increase in fetal pO_2") makes the second answer (FF) difficult to understand.

Pulmonary vascular resistance should be added to the last sentence (II) to relate the speculation to the dependent variable in the answer before relating it to a clinical problem based on the dependent variable.

Figures and Tables

In the tables, <u>all</u> sample sizes less than 16 should be accounted for. (The sample size of 12 during umbilical cord occlusion in Table 1 is accounted for in para. 7 of Methods. The sample size of 10 for left atrial pressure during ventilation and oxygenation is accounted for in para. 3 of Results.)

Tables 1–3 could be redesigned so that the independent variable runs down the first column on the left (see Revision 1).

Figures 1 and 2 should be bar graphs (see Revision 1).

The data for the answer to the question should not be split into two figures and a table (Figs. 1, 2 and Table 3). To make the calculation of pulmonary vascular resistance from pulmonary blood flow and the difference between left atrial pressure and systemic arterial pressure clear, all the data can be presented in a table (see Revision 2).

In Figure 3, the point that individual changes in pulmonary blood flow were extremely variable is difficult to see because the overlap of curves makes following and comparing individual curves difficult. One way to make the point in Figure 3 clear is to redraw the graph as two separate graphs, one for major responders and the other for minor responders (see Revision 1). Another way to make the point in Figure 3 clear is to draw a column of eight bar graphs for the eight major responders and another column of eight bar graphs for the eight minor responders.

Abstract

The question in the abstract (C) does not reflect the paper accurately because the question omits one of the independent variables (umbilical cord occlusion), thus creating only a partial expectation of the topics in the paper.

What was done should mention pulmonary vascular resistance (D).

Changing the key term "ventilation" to "ventilation . . . with a gas mixture that produced no changes in arterial blood gases" (E) and to "without an increase in fetal pO_2" (L) is confusing.

"Unexpectedly" should be added at the beginning of the results in sentence I.

In the answer (K), the point of view should be the same as that in the question; the verb should also be the same. In addition, "*in utero*" belongs only in what was done, not in the answer.

The abstract is longer than necessary. Sentences B (background) and M (speculation) can be omitted. Sentences E–H (results) can be condensed.

Title

The title indicates the topic of the paper only vaguely.

"Changes" should be changed to "decreases."

"Pulmonary Circulation" should be changed to "Pulmonary Vascular Resistance" (the dependent variable).

It is OK to keep "Birth-Related Events," but for a more specific title, the specific independent variables that decreased pulmonary vascular resistance should be named.

For the most specific title, the point can be made in a verb ("decrease").

The species must be included in the title.

Revision 1

In Revision 1, most of the weaknesses in the original version have been avoided.

Text

All statements of the question are now the same.

All statements of the answers are the same.

The answers answer the question asked.

The overview in the text is clearer because organization from most to least important is used more (Calculations, Results), more topic sentences (Calculations, Results) and verbal signals (Methods, Results, Discussion) and visual signals (Results) of topics (including the unexpected finding) are used, an overview of the protocol is added (Methods, para. 3), and key terms are repeated exactly (Abstract, Discussion).

In addition, the paper has been shortened:

> *In the Introduction, the review of the literature is omitted, and a review article is cited instead of many references.*
>
> *In Methods, the surgical preparation is condensed to about one-third of its original length.*
>
> *In Results, most of the second paragraph about the major and minor responders is omitted.*
>
> *In the Discussion, the explanation of the discrepancy (para. 2) has been substantially condensed.*

Figures and Tables

Because Results is reorganized to put the most important result (pulmonary vascular resistance) first, Figure 1 rather than Figure 2 now shows the data for pulmonary vascular resistance, and Table 2 is now Table 3, and vice versa.

All three figures have been redrawn and Tables 1–3 have been redesigned.

Abstract

The abstract is clearer and briefer.

Title

The new title is more precise than the original title.

Writing

The writing could still be livelier.

In Revision 1 below, additions and revisions are in boldface type; the overview is underlined in Methods, Results, and Discussion.

VENTILATION AND OXYGENATION DECREASE PULMONARY VASCULAR RESISTANCE IN NEAR-TERM FETAL SHEEP

Abstract

^{A}Background

^{B_1}Question

$^{B_2}, {}^C$What was done

$^{D–I}$What was found

^{A}At birth, **pulmonary vascular resistance decreases dramatically,** allowing pulmonary blood flow to increase and oxygen exchange to occur in the lungs. ^{B_1}To determine the **extent to which sequential ventilation of the fetus's lungs, oxygenation of the lungs, and umbilical cord occlusion can account for** this decrease in resistance, ^{B_2}we studied **16** chronically instrumented, near-term sheep fetuses *in utero*. ^{C}**We calculated pulmonary vascular resistance from measurements of vascular pressures and measurements of pulmonary blood flow obtained by injecting radionuclide-labeled microspheres.** ^{D}We found that ventilation **alone** caused a large but variable increase in pulmonary blood flow, to 401% of control, no change in pulmonary arterial pressure, and a doubling of left atrial pressure. ^{E}Thus, pulmonary vascular resistance fell dramatically, to 34% of control. ^{F}Oxygenation caused a modest further increase in pulmonary blood flow and a decrease in mean pulmonary arterial pressure, so resistance fell to 10% of control. ^{G}Umbilical cord occlusion caused no **further changes in pressure, flow, or resistance.** ^{H}Unexpectedly, the fetuses' **pulmonary blood flow responses to ventilation** fell into 2 groups: **during ventilation the mean increase was maximal in 8 of the 16 fetuses but was only 20% of the**

J, K *Answers*

maximal increase in the other 8. [I]We **found** no differences between the 2 groups of fetuses to explain their different responses. [J]We conclude that **ventilation and oxygenation together can account for the decrease in pulmonary vascular resistance to levels that occur at birth.** [K]Moreover, **ventilation alone accounts for most of this decrease on average, though not necessarily in every fetus, for unknown reasons.**

Introduction

(All of the introduction is overview.)

1   **Known**
[A]*General topic*
B, C*Fetus: high resistance*

[D]*Newborn: decreased resistance*

[E]*Importance*

1   [A]In the circulation of both fetuses and newborns, the main role of the right ventricle is to deliver blood to the gas exchange circulation for uptake of oxygen and removal of carbon dioxide. [B]In the fetus, this delivery is achieved by virtue of the pulmonary vascular resistance being very high. [C]Right ventricular output is thus diverted away from the lungs and toward the placenta, through the ductus arteriosus (1–4). [D]Immediately at birth, as the lungs become the organ of gas exchange, pulmonary vascular resistance must fall dramatically, allowing pulmonary blood flow to increase and oxygen exchange to occur in the lungs. [E]If pulmonary vascular resistance does not fall, the syndrome of persistent pulmonary hypertension of the newborn occurs, often leading to death.

2   **Unknown**
[F]*Unknown*
[G]*Possible answers*

H, I*Known (previous work)*

[J]*Problem with previous work*

[K]*Question*

[L]*Experimental approach*

2   [F]Which of the many events that occur at birth are responsible for the normal decrease in pulmonary vascular resistance is not fully understood. [G]Three major events of the birth process that could be responsible are ventilation, or rhythmic gaseous distension, of fetal lungs, oxygenation of the lungs, and occlusion of the umbilical cord. [H]Two of these events—ventilation and oxygenation—have been studied in acutely exteriorized fetal sheep. [I]The studies suggested that oxygenation rather than ventilation of the fetal lungs is the major event responsible for the decrease in pulmonary vascular resistance (5–10). [J]However, the metabolic effects of acute anesthesia and surgery may have altered the pulmonary vascular response in these studies, because this response is considered to be at least partly mediated by vasoactive metabolites (11).

3   [K]**The purpose of this study was to determine the extent to which sequential ventilation of fetal lungs, oxygenation of fetal lungs, umbilical cord occlusion, or a combination of these events can account for the decrease in pulmonary vascular resistance, and thus for the large increase in pulmonary blood flow, that normally occur at birth.** [L]To remove the superimposed effects of acute anesthetic and surgical stresses and of other components of the birth process, such as prenatal hormonal surges, labor, delivery, and cold exposure, we studied near-term fetal sheep *in utero* 2–3 days after surgery.

Methods

Animals

1   Sixteen fetal sheep were studied at 134.9 ± 1.2 (SD) days of gestation (term is about 145 days). The fetuses were of normal weight (3.6 ± 0.6 kg) and had normal blood gases (see Results) and hemoglobin concentrations (10.9 ± 1.6 g/dl) at the onset of the study.

Surgical Preparation

2 The surgical protocol has been described previously (4, 12). Briefly, **under anesthesia, catheters were inserted as follows. For measurement of pulmonary blood flow and vascular pressures, catheters were inserted into the ascending aorta, the descending aorta, the inferior vena cava, the left atrium, the pulmonary artery, and the amniotic cavity (for zero pressure reference). The ascending aortic catheter was also used to obtain blood samples for determination of pH, pCO_2, pO_2, hemoglobin concentration, and hemoglobin oxygen saturation. A catheter was also inserted into the pleural cavity for drainage. An endotracheal tube attached to 2 polyvinyl tubes was inserted for drainage of tracheal fluid postoperatively. An occluder was placed around the umbilical cord.**

Experimental Protocol

3 48–72 h after surgery, we performed four sequential experiments in each fetus: control, ventilation alone **(that is, ventilation with the same gas concentrations as in the fetus),** oxygenation **(ventilation with 100% oxygen),** and umbilical cord occlusion. **During each experiment, for the calculation of pulmonary vascular resistance, we measured pulmonary blood flow by injection of radionuclide-labeled microspheres and measured mean pressures in the pulmonary artery and the left atrium. We also assessed indicators of oxygenation and acid-base status.** Before beginning experimental measurements, we waited for at least 15 min after the intervention for pressures and blood gases to stabilize.

Control

4 The ewe was placed in a study cage and allowed free access to alfalfa pellets and water. During all 4 experiments, after vascular catheters were connected to Statham P23Db strain-gauge transducers (Statham Instruments, Oxnard, CA), pressures were recorded continuously on a direct-writing polygraph (Beckman Instruments, San Jose, CA). For control experiments, fetal blood samples were obtained from the ascending aorta for determination of pH, pCO_2, and pO_2 (Corning 158 pH/blood gas analyzer, Medfield, MA), and of hemoglobin concentration and hemoglobin oxygen saturation (Radiometer OSM2 hemoximeter, Copenhagen, Denmark). Radionuclide-labeled microspheres (selected from [57]Co, ^{51}Cr, [153]Gd, [114]In, [54]Mn, [95]Nb, [113]Sn, [85]Sr, and [65]Zn), 15 μm in diameter, were then injected into the inferior vena cava while reference blood samples were withdrawn from the ascending aorta, descending aorta, and pulmonary artery at a rate of 4 ml/min. Fetal or maternal blood was then given to replace the blood loss.

Ventilation

5 **To assess the effects of ventilation on pulmonary vascular resistance**, the 2 polyvinyl tubes connected to the tracheal tube were opened and the tracheal fluid was allowed to drain by gravity. A mixture of nitrogen, oxygen, and carbon dioxide was balanced to match the fetal blood gases obtained during the control experiment. The gas mixture was approximately 92% nitrogen, 3% oxygen, and 5% carbon dioxide. Before ventilation was begun, this gas mixture was briefly allowed to flow through the polyvinyl tubing at a rate of about 10 L/min so that the fetus would not be exposed to high concentrations of oxygen at the onset of ventilation. The tubing was then connected to a specially designed respirator, and ventilation was adjusted as described previously (12). Ventilatory settings are presented in Table 1. After variables

TABLE 1. *Ventilatory settings for variables in the fetal sheep during ventilation, oxygenation, and umbilical cord occlusion*

Experiment	Respiratory Rate (breaths/min)	Peak Inspiratory Pressure[a] (mmHg)	End Expiratory Pressure[a] (mmHg)
Ventilation[b]	50 ± 8 (15)[c]	27 ± 10 (15)	3 ± 6 (15)
Oxygenation	57 ± 12 (13)	26 ± 9 (14)	4 ± 6 (14)
Cord Occlusion	57 ± 13 (11)	25 ± 9 (12)	4 ± 6 (12)

[a] Pressures are referenced to amniotic cavity pressure.

[b] During ventilation, fetuses received a mixture of nitrogen, oxygen, and carbon dioxide balanced to match their blood gases during the baseline experiment.

[c] Data are mean ± 1 SD for the number of fetuses given in parentheses. There were no statistically significant differences between experiments for any of the variables.

stabilized, blood samples were obtained as for the control and two sets of radionuclide-labeled microspheres were injected, one into the inferior vena cava and the other into the left atrium, during withdrawal of reference blood samples as described for the control. Replacement blood was then infused into the fetus.

Oxygenation

6 **To assess the effects of oxygenation on pulmonary vascular resistance**, the gas mixture was then changed to 100% oxygen and ventilation was continued. Carbon dioxide was not added to the oxygen because its addition in the first few studies increased fetal pCO_2. This increase probably occurred because placental blood flow fell during oxygenation (4), impairing carbon dioxide removal. After variables stabilized, blood samples were obtained, microspheres were injected into the inferior vena cava and the left atrium, and replacement blood was infused.

Umbilical Cord Occlusion

7 **To assess the effects of umbilical cord occlusion on pulmonary vascular resistance**, the balloon around the umbilical cord was fully inflated to occlude the umbilical blood vessels and thus abolish placental blood flow (4). After variables stabilized, the experimental protocol was repeated. In 4 of the 16 fetuses, cord occlusion could not be studied, because of a faulty balloon in 2 and the development of pneumothoraces, which led to cardiovascular decompensation, in 2.

8 Upon completion of the last experiment, the ewe was killed by injection of large doses of sodium pentobarbital and the fetus was removed from the uterus and weighed. The lungs were removed from the carcass, and the lungs and carcass were separately weighed and placed in formalin. They were then separately carbonized in an oven, ground into a coarse powder, and placed in plastic vials to a uniform height of 3 cm. Radioactivity of the lungs and the reference blood samples was counted in a 1000-channel multichannel pulse-height analyzer (Norland, Fort Atkinson, WI). Specific activity of each isotope within a sample was calculated by the least-squares method (13).

Calculations

9 Pulmonary vascular resistance was calculated as the difference between mean pulmonary arterial pressure and mean left atrial pressure divided by pulmonary blood flow. For the 6 fetuses in which we were unable to measure left atrial pressure for technical reasons, we used the mean values obtained from the other fetuses during the same experiment.

10 **Pulmonary blood flow was measured in 2 ways.** During the control experiment, because there is no left-to-right shunt through the ductus arteriosus (14), pulmonary blood flow was measured by injecting microspheres into the inferior vena cava and withdrawing blood samples from the pulmonary artery. This injection and withdrawal technique excludes bronchial flow. **To measure bronchial flow**, in 6 fetuses we also injected microspheres into the left atrium during the control experiment. We found that bronchial flow was relatively constant and quite small, always less than 3% of combined ventricular output. We then subtracted this value from the pulmonary blood flow measurements in the remaining experiments.

11 **During ventilation, oxygenation, and umbilical cord occlusion, a different technique for measuring pulmonary blood flow was used. The reason is that** upon ventilation, pulmonary vascular resistance falls and blood flow increases dramatically. Thus, a left-to-right shunt through the ductus arteriosus cannot be excluded. To measure pulmonary blood flow in the presence of a left-to-right shunt requires a technique that determines the contribution of left ventricular output to pulmonary blood flow. Therefore, during ventilation, oxygenation, and umbilical cord occlusion, we injected microspheres labeled with different radionuclides simultaneously into both the inferior vena cava and the left atrium and calculated pulmonary blood flow as the difference between combined ventricular output and the sum of blood flows to the fetal body and placenta (4). Combined ventricular output was calculated as the sum of left and right ventricular outputs. Blood flows to the fetal body and placenta were calculated from the left atrial injections and reference blood withdrawals from the ascending and descending aorta (4).

Analysis of Data

12 In this study, we assessed the sequential effects of ventilation, oxygenation, and umbilical cord occlusion. Determination of their independent effects was not possible because the order of the experiments could not be randomized. One reason is that we were concerned that oxygenation of the fetal lungs might induce multiple and perhaps irreversible metabolic and hemodynamic consequences, so that subsequent ventilation without oxygenation could not be studied. Another reason is that the umbilical cord cannot be occluded before oxygenation. Thus, the protocol is composed of 4 sequential experiments, each serving as the control for the next. Data from each of these experiments were analyzed by the Mann-Whitney U test, comparing only the data obtained during one experiment with data obtained during the experiment immediately preceding it. Statistical significance was considered present when the P value was ≤ 0.01. All data are presented as mean ± 1 SD.

Results

Effects of Ventilation, Oxygenation, and Umbilical Cord Occlusion

1 In the 16 sheep fetuses studied, pulmonary vascular resistance decreased dramatically (to 34% of control values) during ventilation alone (**Figure 1**), decreased further during oxygenation (to 10% of control), and did not change further after cord occlusion (11%).

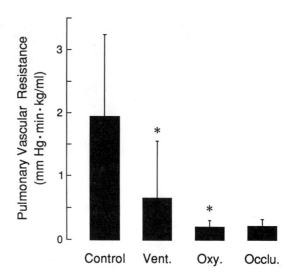

Figure 1. Pulmonary vascular resistance during sequential ventilation, oxygenation, and umbilical cord occlusion in the 16 fetal sheep. Data are mean ± 1 SD. * $P \leq 0.001$ vs. the experiment immediately preceding it.

2 **These changes in pulmonary vascular resistance were calculated from and reflect changes in pulmonary blood flow and vascular pressures.** Pulmonary blood flow in the control experiment (33 ± 17 ml/min/kg fetal body weight) was similar to that previously measured in chronically instrumented fetuses of similar gestational ages (2, 3), constituting 9% of combined ventricular output. **Ventilation alone** increased pulmonary blood flow dramatically, to 401% of control values (**Figure 2**). The variability of this increase in pulmonary blood flow was marked, however, which led us to separate the fetuses into 2 groups, as described below. Oxygenation increased pulmonary blood flow further, to a mean of 623% of control. Umbilical cord occlusion did not cause any further change in pulmonary blood flow.

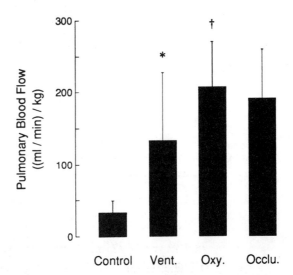

Figure 2. Pulmonary blood flow during sequential ventilation, oxygenation, and umbilical cord occlusion in the 16 fetal sheep. Data are mean ± 1 SD. *$P \leq 0.001$, † $P \leq 0.005$ vs. the experiment immediately preceding it.

3 Mean <u>pulmonary arterial pressure</u> was normal in the control experiment and did not change during ventilation (Table 2). **<u>During oxygenation</u>** there was a small but significant decrease in pressure. Because this decrease was similar to that seen in mean systemic arterial pressure, it cannot be explained by partial closure of the ductus arteriosus. **<u>After umbilical cord occlusion</u>**, there was no further change in mean pulmonary or mean systemic arterial pressure.

TABLE 2. *Mean vascular pressures during the experiments*

Experiment	Pressure[a] (mmHg)		
	Pulmonary Arterial	Systemic Arterial	Left Atrial
Control	53 ± 8 (15)[b]	52 ± 6 (15)	4 ± 5 (12)
Ventilation	55 ± 9 (15)	53 ± 6 (15)	$9 \pm 4^*$ (10)
Oxygenation	$47 \pm 6^*$ (15)	$48 \pm 6^*$ (15)	10 ± 5 (10)
Cord Occlusion	48 ± 16 (12)	58 ± 16 (12)	9 ± 5 (7)

[a] Pressures are referenced to amniotic cavity pressure.

[b] Data are mean $\pm$ 1 SD for the number of fetal sheep given in parentheses.

* Significantly different from the value during the immediately preceding experiment, $P \leq 0.01$.

4 <u>Left atrial pressure</u> could be measured in only 10 fetuses for technical reasons. In association with the large increase in pulmonary blood flow during ventilation alone, mean left atrial pressure doubled (Table 2). It did not change further during oxygenation or cord occlusion.

5 <u>Systemic arterial blood gases and hemoglobin oxygen saturation</u> were normal in the control experiment and did not change during ventilation alone (Table 3). <u>Oxygenation</u> caused a large increase in pO_2 and hemoglobin oxygen saturation but did not change pCO_2 or pH. <u>Cord occlusion</u> did not change these variables significantly, but there was much greater variability in pCO_2 and pH, probably because of the inability of some fetuses to maintain adequate CO_2 exchange in the lungs, because of pulmonary immaturity.

TABLE 3. *Ascending aortic pH, blood gases, and hemoglobin oxygen saturations during the experiments*

Experiment	pH	pO_2 (mmHg)	pCO_2 (mmHg)	Hgb O_2 sat.[a] (%)
Control	7.37 ± 0.06[b] (15)	18 ± 3 (16)	55 ± 26 (15)	47 ± 13 (16)
Ventilation	7.35 ± 0.07 (16)	19 ± 4 (16)	54 ± 6 (16)	46 ± 12 (16)
Oxygenation	7.34 ± 0.09 (16)	$215 \pm 154^*$ (16)	51 ± 10 (16)	$97 \pm 6^*$ (16)
Cord Occlusion	7.29 ± 0.15 (13)	263 ± 168 (13)	58 ± 21 (12)	95 ± 10 (16)

[a]Hgb O_2 sat., hemoglobin oxygen saturation.

[b]Data are mean $\pm$ 1 SD for four sequential experiments on the number of fetal sheep given in parentheses.

*Significantly different from the value during the immediately preceding experiment, $P \leq 0.01$.

Major vs. Minor Responders During Ventilation Alone

6 The individual changes in pulmonary blood flow were extremely variable. In some fetuses the majority of the increase occurred during ventilation alone, whereas in others there was almost no increase until oxygenation. This finding led us to separate the fetuses according to their response to ventilation and examine the reasons for this variability. We arbitrarily divided the fetuses into 2 groups: major responders, which showed an increase in pulmonary blood flow during ventilation alone that was at least 50% of the cumulative increase (the difference between pulmonary blood flow during control measurements and after cord occlusion), and minor responders, which showed an increase of less than 50%. Interestingly, 8 fetuses were major responders and 8 were minor responders (**Figure 3**). The major responders had an increase in flow during ventilation that was equal to the cumulative increase (103 ± 52%), whereas the minor responders had a much smaller increase (20 ± 17%). **When** we examined the measured variables that could have caused this disparity between the major and minor responders, **we found that** none of those variables showed statistically significant differences between the 2 groups (Table 4).

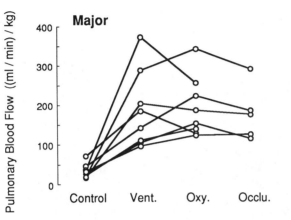
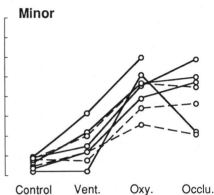

Figure 3. Individual changes in pulmonary blood flow in each of the **8 major responders and the 8 minor responders** during sequential ventilation, oxygenation, and umbilical cord occlusion.

Discussion

A Context

B, C Answers

1 *A*Three major events of the birth process are ventilation, or rhythmic gaseous distension of the lungs, oxygenation, and loss of the umbilical-placental circulation. *B*In this study in fetal sheep, we found that 2 of these events, ventilation and oxygenation, together can account for the decrease in pulmonary vascular resistance, and thus for the large increase in pulmonary blood flow, that normally occur at birth. *C*Moreover, **most of the decrease in pulmonary vascular resistance**, on average nearly two-thirds, **is accounted for by** ventilation alone.

2 **Explanation of a discrepancy**

2 *D*Our finding that about two-thirds of the decrease in pulmonary vascular resistance occurs during ventilation alone is much larger than the previously accepted value of about one-third (6). *E*The reason we found a larger decrease than previously accepted may be that previous studies were performed on acutely exteriorized fetuses (5, 6, 8–10). *F*An acute stress such as that caused by the anesthesia and surgery used to exteriorize a fetus can greatly alter production and inhibition of various metabolic agents, including prostaglandins, leukotrienes, and bradykinin. *G*All of these agents may affect pulmonary vascular resistance (11, 15–18). *H*Thus, it is possible that anesthesia or surgical stress or both indirectly inhibited the ventilation-induced decrease in pulmonary vascular resistance in the previous studies. *I*Because our study was done in awake, unstressed fetuses *in utero*, our finding of a large decrease in pulmonary vascular resistance during ventilation may be more accurate.

3 *Explanation of the unexpected finding*

3 [J]An unexpected finding of this study is the great variability in the response of fetal pulmonary blood flow to the effects of ventilation alone. [K]In one-half of the fetuses, the mean increase in pulmonary blood flow during ventilation alone was maximal, whereas in the other half it was only about 20% of the cumulative response. [L]Interestingly, Cook et al. (19) found similar variability in their study of nitrogen and air ventilation: of the 6 fetuses studied, 2 showed no effect of nitrogen ventilation but a large effect upon changing to air, 2 showed a small effect of nitrogen and a larger response to air, and 2 showed a large increase in pulmonary blood flow during nitrogen ventilation with no further change upon exposure to air. [M]To explain these findings, Cook et al. noted that nitrogen had the greatest effect on the smallest fetuses. [N]However, we were unable to identify the reasons for the variability we found. [O]It was not on a purely arithmetic basis. [P]That is, the major responders did not begin with lower control flows or have lower maximal flows. [Q]In fact, the 2 groups had remarkably similar pulmonary blood flows both during control measurements and during ventilation with 100% oxygen. [R]The groups were also not different in their overall maturity, with respect to either gestational age or weight. [S]In addition, differences in pO_2 were not responsible for the differences between major and minor responders, since both during control measurements and during ventilation alone, the minor responders were neither more hypoxic nor more hypercapnic than the major responders. [T]Lastly, adequacy of alveolar ventilation was probably not responsible for the difference between the groups. [U]Although we were not able to determine the adequacy of alveolar ventilation during ventilation alone, during oxygenation, pO_2 and pCO_2 values were similar in the 2 groups, without the method of ventilation having been changed in either group.

4 *Implications for future studies*

4 [V]Although our data cannot explain the reason for the marked difference between the pulmonary vasodilatory responses of the 2 groups of fetuses, this difference may have important implications for future studies. [W]First, it may be important in uncovering the metabolic processes responsible for the decrease in pulmonary vascular resistance at birth. [X]Second, evaluation of the concentrations and fluxes of the putative metabolic agents involved may demonstrate different fates of these agents in major and minor responders. [Y]However, careful evaluation of lung mechanics is critical in future studies to ensure that the differences between the responses of the pulmonary vascular bed are not caused solely by differences in pulmonary function. [Z]In this regard, it would be of interest to determine whether static gaseous distension of the lungs (that is, distension without ventilation) can induce a similar decrease in pulmonary vascular resistance. [AA]Static distension does increase lung compliance in fetal sheep (20) and has been shown to decrease pulmonary vascular resistance to some degree in acutely exteriorized fetal sheep (21).

5 *Conclusion*
[BB, CC]*Answers*

[DD, EE]*Unexpected finding*
[FF]*Implication*

5 [BB]In summary, this study in fetal sheep shows that 2 major events during the birth process, ventilation and oxygenation of the fetus's lungs, together can account for the decrease in pulmonary vascular resistance, and thus for the large increase in pulmonary blood flow, that normally occur at birth. [CC]Moreover, ventilation alone accounts for most of this change—nearly two-thirds. [DD]The increase in pulmonary blood flow during ventilation is variable. [EE]This variability is probably mediated in part by alterations in a variety of vasoactive metabolites. [FF]By using an *in utero* preparation to investigate the metabolic differences between fetuses that do and do not respond to ventilation alone, the processes responsible for **an incomplete decrease in pulmonary vascular resistance and thus** for the syndrome of persistent pulmonary hypertension of the newborn may be better elucidated.

References

1. Reuss ML, Rudolph AM. Distribution and recirculation of umbilical and systemic venous blood flow in fetal lambs during hypoxia. J Dev Physiol 1980;2:71–84.
2. Anderson DF, Bissonnette JM, Faber JJ, Thornburg KL. Central shunt flows and pressures in the mature fetal lamb. Am J Physiol 1981;241: H60–6.
3. Heymann MA, Creasy RK, Rudolph AM. Quantitation of blood flow patterns in the foetal lamb *in utero*. In: Foetal and neonatal physiology: proceedings of the Sir Joseph Barcroft centenary symposium. Cambridge: Cambridge University Press, 1973:129–35.
4. Teitel DF, Iwamoto HS, Rudolph AM. Effects of birth-related events on central blood flow patterns. Pediatr Res 1987;22:557–66.
5. Lauer RM, Evans JA, Aoki H, Kittle CF. Factors controlling pulmonary vascular resistance in fetal lambs. J Pediatr 1965;67:568–77.
6. Dawes GS, Mott JC, Widdicombe JG, Wyatt DG. Changes in the lungs of the new-born lamb. J Physiol 1953;121:141–62.
7. Dawes GS. The pulmonary circulation in the foetus and newborn. In: Foetal and neonatal physiology: a comparative study of the changes at birth. Chicago: Yearbook Medical Publishers, 1968:79–90.
8. Cassin S, Dawes GS, Mott JC, Ross BB, Strang LB. The vascular resistance of the foetal and newly ventilated lung of the lamb. J Physiol 1964;171: 61–79.
9. Assali NS, Kirschbaum TH, Dilts PV Jr. Effects of hyperbaric oxygen on uteroplacental and fetal circulation. Circ Res 1968;22:573–88.
10. Heymann MA, Rudolph AM, Nies AS, Melmon KL. Bradykinin production associated with oxygenation of the fetal lamb. Circ Res 1969;25:521–34.
11. Heymann MA. Control of the pulmonary circulation in the perinatal period. J Dev Physiol 1984;6:281–90.
12. Iwamoto HS, Teitel DF, Rudolph AM. Effects of birth-related events on blood flow distribution. Pediatr Res 1987;22:634–40.
13. Baer RW, Payne BD, Verrier ED, et al. Increased number of myocardial blood flow measurements with radionuclide-labeled microspheres. Am J Physiol 1984;246:H418–34.
14. Assali NS, Sehgal N, Marable S. Pulmonary and ductus arteriosus circulation in the fetal lamb before and after birth. Am J Physiol 1962;202: 536–40.
15. Leffler CW, Tyler TL, Cassin S. Effect of indomethacin on pulmonary vascular response to ventilation of fetal goats. Am J Physiol 1978;234: H346–51.
16. Leffler CW, Hessler JR. Perinatal pulmonary prostaglandin production. Am J Physiol 1981;241:H756–9.
17. Leffler CW, Hessler JR, Terragno NA. Ventilation-induced release of prostaglandinlike material from fetal lungs. Am J Physiol 1980;238:H282–6.
18. Leffler CW, Hessler JR, Green RS. The onset of breathing at birth stimulates pulmonary vascular prostacyclin synthesis. Pediatr Res 1984;18: 938–42.
19. Cook CD, Drinker PA, Jacobson HN, Levison H, Strang LB. Control of pulmonary blood flow in the foetal and newly born lamb. J Physiol 1963;169:10–29.

20. Ikegami M, Jobe A, Berry D, Elkady T, Pettenazzo A, Seidner S. Effects of distention of the preterm fetal lamb lung on lung function with ventilation. Am Rev Respir Dis 1987;135:600–6.

21. Colebatch HJH, Dawes GS, Goodwin JW, Nadeau RA. The nervous control of the circulation in the foetal and newly expanded lungs of the lamb. J Physiol 1965;178:544–62.

Revision 2

In Revision 2, more of the weaknesses in the original version have been avoided than in Revision 1.

Text

A stronger, more picturesque verb is used in the question and answer.
All three independent variables are included in the answer.
The explanation of the reason for the sequential study design is included in the Introduction rather than in Analysis of Data in Methods.
In the Protocol and throughout the paper, "control" is changed to "baseline."
Methods of measurement are removed from the baseline protocol and put in a separate subsection.
Details of the overview are removed from the baseline protocol and added to the overview of the protocol.
In Results, paragraph 1 is organized according to the independent variable, thus correlating more clearly with the rest of the paper.
The Results section is organized from most to least important (pO_2 etc. last).
The text is condensed more than in Revision 1 (Introduction, Surgical Preparation, Results, Discussion paras. 2–4).

Figures and Tables

Table 3 is redesigned to include all data needed for the calculation of pulmonary vascular resistance; therefore, Figs. 1 and 2 are omitted.

Abstract

The abstract is further condensed by omitting results for pulmonary blood flow and pressures and for the unexpected finding.

Title

This revision gives another precise version of the title.

DECREASES IN PULMONARY VASCULAR RESISTANCE DURING VENTILATION AND OXYGENATION IN NEAR-TERM FETAL SHEEP

Abstract

*A*Pulmonary vascular resistance decreases rapidly at birth to permit the increase in pulmonary blood flow necessary to start oxygen exchange in the lungs. *B*We asked whether ventilation or oxygenation of the fetal lungs, umbilical cord occlusion, or a combination of these three major events that occur at birth triggers this decrease in pulmonary vascular resistance and which event is the main cause. *C*To answer these questions, we studied 16 chronically instrumented, near-term fetal sheep *in utero*. *D*We calculated pulmonary vascular resistance from measurements of pulmonary blood flow, pulmonary arterial pressure, and left atrial pressure made during baseline, ventilation, oxygenation, and umbilical cord occlusion. *E*We found that pulmonary vascular resistance decreased during ventilation alone (to 34% of baseline), decreased further during oxygenation (to 10% of baseline), and did not change further during umbilical cord occlusion. *F*We also found that ventilation alone caused about two-thirds of the decrease in pulmonary vascular resistance. *G*We conclude that ventilation and oxygenation of the fetal lungs, but not umbilical cord occlusion, trigger the decrease in pulmonary vascular resistance that occurs at birth and that ventilation is the main cause.

Introduction

*A*At birth, the elevated pulmonary vascular resistance of the fetus decreases, thus permitting blood from the right ventricle to enter the lungs (1–4). *B*Of the numerous events, including ventilation, oxygenation, and umbilical cord occlusion, that occur at birth, the events responsible for this decrease in pulmonary vascular resistance are not known. *C*Ventilation and oxygenation have been studied in acutely exteriorized sheep by several groups, most of whom found that oxygenation rather than ventilation is the main factor responsible for the decrease in pulmonary vascular resistance (5–10). *D*However, the metabolic effects of anesthesia and surgery in these acutely exteriorized sheep may have affected their pulmonary vascular resistance and thus altered the results (11).

*E*This study was undertaken to determine whether ventilation or oxygenation of the lungs, umbilical cord occlusion, or a combination of these events triggers the decrease in pulmonary vascular resistance that occurs at birth and which of these events is the main cause. *F*To avoid the metabolic effects of anesthesia and surgery, we used near-term fetal sheep *in utero* 2–3 days after surgery. *G*We could not study the independent effects of ventilation, oxygenation, and umbilical cord occlusion because the order of the experiments could not be randomized. *H*One reason is that we were concerned that oxygenation of the fetal lungs might induce multiple and perhaps irreversible metabolic and hemodynamic consequences, so that subsequent ventilation without oxygenation could not be studied. *I*Another reason is that the umbilical cord cannot be occluded before oxygenation. *J*Thus, the study is composed of 4 sequential experiments: baseline, ventilation, oxygenation, and umbilical cord occlusion.

Methods

Animals (as in Revision 1)

Surgical Preparation

*A*All surgical procedures on the fetuses were carried out as described previously (4, 12). *B*Briefly, catheters were placed in the ascending and descending aorta, inferior vena cava, pulmonary artery, left atrium, and amniotic cavity (for zero pressure reference). *C*The trachea was intubated and a silicone rubber balloon occluder was placed around the umbilical cord. *D*After surgery, the fetuses were returned to the ewes' abdominal cavity.

Experimental Protocol

*A*The experiments were done on the fetuses 2–3 days after surgery. *B*Four experiments were performed on each fetus in the following sequence: baseline, ventilation (that is, ventilation with the same gas concentrations as in the fetus), oxygenation (ventilation with 100% oxygen), and umbilical cord occlusion. *C*During each experiment, for the calculation of pulmonary vascular resistance, we measured pulmonary blood flow by injection of radionuclide-labeled microspheres and measured mean pressures in the pulmonary artery and the left atrium. *D*We also assessed indicators of oxygenation and acid-base status. *E*Before the first experiment, the ewe was placed in a study cage and allowed free access to alfalfa pellets and water. *F*Before beginning the experimental measurements, we waited for at least 15 minutes after the intervention for pressures and blood gases to stabilize. *G*After blood samples were taken, fetal or maternal blood was given to replace blood loss.

Baseline

*A*For baseline experiments, blood pressures were recorded in all the vessels catheterized except the inferior vena cava. *B*Fetal blood samples were obtained from the ascending aorta for determination of pH, pCO_2, pO_2, hemoglobin concentration, and hemoglobin oxygen saturation. *C*Pulmonary blood flow was measured.

Ventilation and *Oxygenation*   (the same as paras. 5 and 6 except that "control" is changed to "baseline," "pulmonary blood flow was measured" replaces the microsphere injections, and infusion of replacement blood is omitted)

Umbilical Cord Occlusion   (the same as para. 7 of Revision 1)

Paragraph 8   (the same as in Revision 1)

Methods of Measurement

*A*Blood pressures were measured by connecting the vascular catheters to Statham P23Db strain-gauge transducers (Statham Instruments, Oxnard, CA) and recording the tracings continuously on a direct-writing polygraph (Beckman Instuments, San Jose, CA). *B*Blood gases and pH were analyzed on a Corning 158 pH/blood gas analyzer (Medfield, MA) and hemoglobin oxygen saturations on a Radiometer OSM2 hemoximeter (Copenhagen, Denmark).

Calculations   (the same as in Revision 1 except that "control" is changed to "baseline")

Analysis of Data

*A*Data from each experiment were analyzed by the Mann-Whitney U test, comparing only the data obtained during one experiment with data obtained during the experiment immediately preceding it. *B*Statistical significance was considered present when the *P* value was ≤ 0.01. *C*All data are presented as mean $\pm$ 1 SD.

Results

*A*Ventilation alone decreased pulmonary vascular resistance to 34% of baseline in the 16 fetal sheep studied (Table 2). *B*This decrease resulted from a 4-fold increase in pulmonary blood flow; pulmonary arterial pressure did not change. *C*Oxygenation decreased pulmonary vascular resistance further (to 10% of baseline) because of a further increase in pulmonary blood flow and a small decrease in pulmonary arterial pressure. *D*Umbilical cord occlusion did not cause any further decrease in pulmonary vascular resistance.

TABLE 2. *Changes in Pulmonary Vascular Resistance and Its Components During Ventilation, Oxygenation, and Umbilical Cord Occlusion in Fetal Sheep*

Experiment	Systemic Arterial Pressure[a] (mmHg)	Pulmonary Arterial Pressure[a] (mmHg)	Left Atrial Pressure[a] (mmHg)	Pulmonary Blood Flow ((ml/min)/kg)	Pulmonary Vascular Resistance (mmHg · min · kg/ml)
Baseline	52 ± 6 (15)[b]	53 ± 8 (15)	4 ± 5 (12)	33 ± 17 (16)	1.93 ± 1.31 (16)
Ventilation	53 ± 6 (15)	55 ± 9 (15)	9 ± 4* (10)	133 ± 94† (16)	0.66 ± 0.90† (16)
Oxygenation	48 ± 6† (15)	47 ± 6† (15)	10 ± 5 (10)	206 ± 64‡ (16)	0.20 ± 0.77† (16)
Cord Occlusion	58 ± 16 (12)	48 ± 16 (12)	9 ± 5 (7)	190 ± 69 (16)	0.22 ± 0.11 (16)

[a]Pressures are referenced to amniotic cavity pressure.
[b]Data are mean ± 1 SD for the number of fetal sheep given in parentheses.
*$P \leq 0.05$, †$P \leq 0.001$, ‡$P \leq 0.01$ vs. the experiment immediately preceding it.

[E]The fetuses did not respond uniformly to ventilation. [F]In one group, the major responders, ventilation alone increased pulmonary blood flow maximally (Fig. 1) and thus decreased pulmonary vascular resistance maximally. [G]In the other group, the minor responders, ventilation alone increased pulmonary blood flow to only 20% of the maximal response and decreased pulmonary vascular resistance by only 25%. [H]From the variables measured, we were unable to find any disparity that could explain the different responses to ventilation (Table 3).

[I]As indicated by the arterial blood gases and pH, the baseline condition of all the fetuses that we studied was normal (Table 4). [J]Ventilation did not change these variables. [K]However, oxygenation increased fetal arterial pO_2 and hemoglobin oxygen saturation significantly.

Discussion

1   [A]In this study of fetal sheep, we found that ventilation and oxygenation of the fetal lungs, but not umbilical cord occlusion, trigger the decrease in pulmonary vascular resistance that occurs at birth. [B]Ventilation of the fetal lungs decreased pulmonary vascular resistance to 34% of baseline, and oxygenation further decreased it to 10% of baseline. [C]Thus, ventilation is the main cause of the decrease in pulmonary vascular resistance, accounting for nearly two-thirds of the decrease.

2   [D]Our finding that ventilation alone decreases pulmonary vascular resistance by nearly two-thirds is much higher than the previously accepted value of about one-third (6). [E]One reason for this difference in findings may be the use of acutely exteriorized fetuses in the previous studies (5, 6, 8–10), whereas we studied fetuses *in utero*. [F]In acutely exteriorized fetuses, anesthesia and surgery carried out to exteriorize the fetus can slow the rate of decrease in pulmonary vascular resistance (7), whereas this effect is not seen in fetuses *in utero*. [G]This slower decrease in pulmonary vascular resistance is probably mediated through prostaglandin metabolites and leukotrienes produced during anesthesia and surgery (11, 15–18).

3   [H]An unexpected finding of this study was that ventilation alone dramatically decreases pulmonary vascular resistance in some fetuses, but not in others. [I]In one-half of the fetuses (the major responders) the decrease in pulmonary vascular resistance during ventilation was maximal, whereas in

the other half (the minor responders) it was only 20% of maximal (Fig. 1). ^{J}Cook et al. (19) found similar variability in their studies of ventilation in fetal sheep. ^{K}They concluded that ventilation had a greater effect on smaller fetuses. ^{L}However, we were unable to identify the reason for the difference between the major and minor responders in our study. ^{M}The 2 groups did not differ with respect to their maturity or postoperative stability, their initial pulmonary vascular tone, their ventricular function, or the adequacy of their ventilation (Table 3).

4 ^{N}Thus, the marked difference in effect of ventilation on pulmonary vascular resistance between the 2 groups of fetuses is unexplained. ^{O}Uncovering an explanation for this difference is important for 2 reasons. ^{P}First, the explanation may reveal the cause of persistent pulmonary hypertension of the newborn. ^{Q}Second, the explanation may reveal the specific metabolic agent or agents responsible for decreasing pulmonary vascular resistance at birth.

5 ^{R}In conclusion, in this study in fetal sheep, we found that ventilation and oxygenation of the lungs, but not umbilical cord occlusion, trigger the decrease in pulmonary vascular resistance that occurs at birth. ^{S}We also found that ventilation causes nearly two-thirds of the decrease, though the ventilation-induced decrease in pulmonary vascular resistance varies greatly from fetus to fetus.

LITERATURE CITED

THE GOAL: CLEAR WRITING

Woodford FP. Sounder thinking through clearer writing. Science 12 May 1967;156(3776)743–5.

A lively, clear article that explains the negative effects of poor writing in scientific journal articles and offers suggestions on how to improve scientific writing.

CHAPTER 1: WORD CHOICE

Webster's third new international dictionary of the English language unabridged. Springfield, Massachusetts: Merriam, 1976.

A standard unabridged dictionary of American English. Includes clear definitions of both scientific and general terms, quotations showing how words are used in sentences, and excellent synonym notes.

The American heritage dictionary of the English language. Boston: American Heritage and Houghton Mifflin, 1975.

A standard desk dictionary, particularly useful for words in general use. Includes numerous excellent usage notes and synonym notes. Beautifully illustrated.

Strunk W Jr, White EB. The elements of style. 3rd ed. New York: Macmillan, 1979.

Succinctly states and illustrates rules for clear, graceful writing. Although first published in 1918, this book is still extremely useful.

CHAPTER 2: SENTENCE STRUCTURE

Woodford FP, ed. Scientific writing for graduate students: a manual on the teaching of scientific writing. Bethesda, Maryland: Council of Biology Editors, 1986.

Useful for students as well as for teachers. A procedural approach to writing scientific research papers. Has excellent chapters on "Further Revision: Polishing the Style" (illustrated in excellent annotated "before" and "after" versions of three sample articles in "Editing Assignments") and on "Design of Tables and Figures." Available from the Council of Biology Editors, 9650 Rockville Pike, Bethesda, Maryland 20814.

Strunk and White. *See* Chapter 1.

CHAPTER 4: THE INTRODUCTION

DeBakey L. The scientific journal: editorial policies and practices: guidelines for editors, reviewers, and authors. St. Louis: Mosby, 1976.
A cogent book that deals succinctly and objectively with problems of reviewing manuscripts for publication and of running a journal.

CHAPTER 5: MATERIALS AND METHODS

Glantz SA. Primer of biostatistics. 2nd ed. New York: McGraw-Hill, 1987.
Focuses on problems commonly encountered in analyzing data in biomedical research. Written in a chatty style.

Gardner MJ, Altman DG. Confidence intervals rather that P values: estimation rather than hypothesis testing. Br Med J 15 March 1986;292:746–50.
A clear explanation of why and how to use confidence intervals.

CBE Style Manual Committee. CBE style manual: a guide for authors, editors, and publishers in the biological sciences. 5th ed. Bethesda, Maryland: Council of Biology Editors, 1983.
Includes numerous tables on units of measurement, nomenclature, abbreviations, and proofreaders' symbols.

Young DS. Implementation of SI units for clinical laboratory data: style specifications and conversion tables. Ann Intern Med 1987;106:114–29.
Explains what SI units (Système International d'Unités) are and why and how to use them.

CHAPTER 6: RESULTS

Glantz. *See* Chapter 5.
Gardner and Altman. *See* Chapter 5.

CHAPTER 8: FIGURES AND TABLES

Scientific Illustration Committee of the Council of Biology Editors. Illustrating science: standards for publication. Bethesda, Maryland: Council of Biology Editors, 1988.
Gives standards for publishing effective line art, graphs, maps, halftones, and computer graphics that present scientific data.

Woodford. Scientific writing for graduate students. *See* Chapter 2.

Briscoe MH. A researcher's guide to scientific and medical illustrations. New York: Springer-Verlag, 1990.
Gives clear, specific explanations for effective presentation of all types of illustrations used in biomedical research papers. Includes clear examples of each type of illustration. Also includes a section on tables.

CHAPTER 9: REFERENCES

Lock S. A difficult balance: editorial peer review in medicine. Philadelphia: ISI Press, 1986.
> *Studies peer review in medical journals to determine whether peer review validates published articles and whether validation is worth the price. Concludes that only time validates articles but that peer review is the best means available for selecting articles to publish and for improving the science and writing in journal articles.*

International Committee of Medical Journal Editors. Uniform requirements for manuscripts submitted to biomedical journals. Ann Intern Med 1988;108: 258–65.
> *Presents stylistic requirements, including reference style, for the preparation of manuscripts to be submitted to more than 300 English-language biomedical journals worldwide. Also includes statements on prior and duplicate publication, authorship, and acknowledgments. See also* Bailar JC III, Mosteller F. Guidelines for statistical reporting in articles for medical journals: amplifications and explanations. Ann Intern Med 1988;108:266–73.

CHAPTER 10: THE ABSTRACT

Uniform Requirements. *See* Chapter 9.

REACHING THE GOAL: SUGGESTIONS FOR WRITING

Huth EJ. How to write and publish papers in the medical sciences. 2nd ed. Baltimore: Williams & Wilkins, 1990.
> *Tells how to write research papers, case reports, review articles, editorials, book reviews, and letters to the editor, and describes the steps of preparing and publishing these papers from literature review and preparing to write through proofs and reprints.*

Index

Note: A page number in italics indicates a figure or table.

Words Explained in the Text